Surgical Oncology for the General Surgeon

Editors

NEAL WILKINSON
RANDALL ZUCKERMAN

SURGICAL CLINICS
OF NORTH AMERICA

www.surgical.theclinics.com

Consulting Editor
RONALD F. MARTIN

June 2020 • Volume 100 • Number 3

ELSEVIER

1600 John F. Kennedy Boulevard • Suite 1800 • Philadelphia, Pennsylvania, 19103-2899

http://www.surgical.theclinics.com

SURGICAL CLINICS OF NORTH AMERICA Volume 100, Number 3
June 2020 ISSN 0039–6109, ISBN-13: 978-0-323-71070-1

Editor: John Vassallo, j.vassallo@elsevier.com
Developmental Editor: Nicole Congleton

Surgical Clinics of North America (ISSN 0039–6109) is published bimonthly by Elsevier Inc., 360 Park Avenue South, New York, NY 10010-1710. Months of publication are February, April, June, August, October, and December. Business and Editorial Offices: 1600 John F. Kennedy Blvd., Suite 1800, Philadelphia, PA 19103-2899. Periodicals postage paid at New York, NY and additional mailing offices. Subscription prices are $430.00 per year for US individuals, $891.00 per year for US institutions, $100.00 per year for US & Canadian students and residents, $507.00 per year for Canadian individuals, $1130.00 per year for Canadian institutions, $536.00 for international individuals, $1130.00 per year for international institutions and $250.00 per year for foreign students/residents. To receive student/resident rate, orders must be accompanied by name of affiliated institution, date of term, and the *signature* of program/residency coordinator on institution letterhead. Orders will be billed at individual rate until proof of status is received. Foreign air speed delivery is included in all *Clinics* subscription prices. All prices are subject to change without notice. POSTMASTER: Send address changes to *Surgical Clinics*, Elsevier Health Sciences Division, Subscription Customer Service, 3251 Riverport Lane, Maryland Heights, MO 63043. **Customer Service (orders, claims, online, change of address): Telephone: 1-800-654-2452 (U.S. and Canada); 314-447-8871 (outside U.S. and Canada). Fax: 314-447-8029. E-mail: journalscustomerservice-usa@elsevier.com (for print support); journalsonlinesupport-usa@elsevier.com (for online support)**.

Reprints. For copies of 100 or more, of articles in this publication, please contact the Commercial Reprints Department, Elsevier Inc., 360 Park Avenue South, New York, New York 10010-1710. Tel. 212-633-3874, Fax: 212-633-3820, E-mail: reprints@elsevier.com.

The Surgical Clinics of North America is also published in Spanish by McGraw-Hill Interamericana Editores S.A., P.O. Box 5-237 06500 Mexico D.F. Mexico; and in Portuguese by Interlivros Edicoes Ltda., Rua Comandante Coelho 1085, CEP 21250, Rio de Janeiro, Brazil; and in Greek by Paschalidis Medical Publications, Athens Greece.

The Surgical Clinics of North America is covered in *MEDLINE/PubMed (Index Medicus)*, *EMBASE/Excerpta Medica*, *Current Contents/Clinical Medicine*, *Current Contents/Life Sciences*, *Science Citation Index*, and *ISI/BIOMED*.

Contributors

CONSULTING EDITOR

RONALD F. MARTIN, MD, FACS
Colonel (Retired), United States Army Reserve, Executive Vice President, Kalispell Regional Healthcare, Chief Physician Executive, Kalispell Regional Medical Group, Division of HPB Surgery and Surgical Oncology, Kalispell, Montana, USA

EDITORS

NEAL WILKINSON, MD, FACS
Chair of Surgery, Kalispell Regional Healthcare, Kalispell, Montana, USA

RANDALL ZUCKERMAN, MD, FACS
Chair of Surgery, Kalispell Regional Healthcare, Kalispell, Montana, USA

AUTHORS

ADNAN ALSEIDI, MD, EdM, FACS
Division of Pancreas, Liver and Biliary Surgery, Virginia Mason Medical Center, Virginia Mason HPB Surgery, Seattle, Washington, USA

MORGAN BONDS, MD
Hepatopancreatobiliary Fellow, Section of General, Vascular, and Thoracic Surgery, Virginia Mason Medical Center, Seattle, Washington, USA

KENNETH CARDONA, MD, FACS
Associate Professor, Division of Surgical Oncology, Department of Surgery, Winship Cancer Institute, Emory University, Atlanta, Georgia, USA

ELIZABETH GLEESON, MD, MPH
Surgical Oncology Fellow, Division of Surgical Oncology, Mount Sinai Hospital, New York, New York, USA

HISAKAZU HOSHI, MD
Clinical Professor, Division of Endocrine and Surgical Oncology, Department of Surgery, University of Iowa Hospitals and Clinics, Iowa City, Iowa, USA

MELISSA C. HULVAT, MD, FACS
Medical Director, Bass Breast Center, Kalispell Regional Healthcare, Kalispell, Montana, USA

ELIZABETH JACOB, MD
General Surgery Department, Bassett Medical Center, Cooperstown, New York, USA

DHIRESH ROHAN JEYARAJAH, MD
Department of Surgery, Methodist Richardson Medical Center, Dallas, Texas, USA

BRIAN J. KAPLAN, MD, FACS
Professor, Department of Surgery, Division of Surgical Oncology, Virginia Commonwealth University, Richmond, Virginia, USA

RUSSELL C. KIRKS, MD
Division of Pancreas, Liver and Biliary Surgery, Virginia Mason Medical Center, Virginia Mason HPB Surgery, Seattle, Washington, USA

SABA KURTOM, MD, MS
Resident, Department of Surgery, Virginia Commonwealth University, Richmond, Virginia, USA

DANIEL LABOW, MD
Chair, Eugene W. Friedman Professor of Surgical Oncology, Surgery Department, Mount Sinai Hospital, Mount Sinai West and Morningside, New York, New York, USA

JUAN C. MEJIA, MD, FACS
Providence Sacred Heart Medical Center, Spokane, Washington, USA

RAUL MONZON, MD
General Surgery Department, Bassett Medical Center, Cooperstown, New York, USA

LUIS OCEGUERA, MD
General Surgery Department, Bassett Medical Center, Cooperstown, New York, USA

HOUSSAM OSMAN, MD
Department of Surgery, Methodist Richardson Medical Center, Dallas, Texas, USA; Trinity Surgical Consultants, Richardson, Texas, USA

JENNIFER PASKO, MD
Providence Sacred Heart Medical Center, Spokane, Washington, USA

ERIC PLETCHER, MD, MS
General Surgery Resident, Surgery Department, Mount Sinai West and Morningside, New York, New York, USA

BENJAMIN J. POMERANTZ, MD
Assistant Professor of Radiology, Department of Radiology, Vascular and Interventional Radiology, University of Michigan, University Hospital, Ann Arbor, Michigan, USA

NIKDOKHT RASHIDIAN, MD, FEBS
Department of GI Surgery, Ghent University Hospital, Ghent, Belgium

FLAVIO G. ROCHA, MD
Staff Surgeon, Section of General, Vascular, and Thoracic Surgery, Virginia Mason Medical Center, Clinical Associate Professor of Surgery, University of Washington, Seattle, Washington, USA

CHRISTINA L. ROLAND, MD, MS
The University of Texas MD Anderson Cancer Center, Houston, Texas, USA

LEVI SMUCKER, MD
General Surgery Department, Bassett Medical Center, Cooperstown, New York, USA

MICHAEL K. TURGEON, MD
Katz Foundation Research Fellow, Division of Surgical Oncology, Department of Surgery, Winship Cancer Institute, Emory University, Atlanta, Georgia, USA

CHRISTINE VAN COTT, MD, FACS
Chief of General Surgery, Director, Department of Surgery, St. Vincent's Medical Center, Bridgeport, Connecticut, USA; Professor of Surgery, Director of Surgical Education, Frank H. Netter MD School of Medicine, Quinnipiac University, North Haven, Connecticut, USA

NEAL WILKINSON, MD, FACS
Chair of Surgery, Kalispell Regional Healthcare, Kalispell, Montana, USA

PATRICK WILLAUER, MD
General Surgery Department, Bassett Medical Center, Cooperstown, New York, USA

GEORGE YOUNAN, MD, FACS
Department of Surgery, Inova Fair Oaks Hospital, Division of Hepato-Pancreato-Biliary Surgery, Virginia Surgery Associates, Fairfax, Virginia, USA

ANNE N. YOUNG, MD, MSCR
General Surgery Department, Bassett Medical Center, Cooperstown, New York, USA

Contents

> The incidence of many types of cancer continues to increase, and despite many successes in the realms of screening, prevention, and treatment, cancer remains the second leading cause of death in North America. Cancer types affecting this population have varied over time, with a trend toward more malignancies caused by modifiable risk factors related to a western lifestyle. Despite the increasing incidence of cancer, a combination of population-based screening and improved therapeutics has made the disease more survivable, and created an ever-increasing community of cancer survivors. These cancer survivors face unique challenges and require ongoing care.

> For most individuals, cancer development is multifactorial; however, up to 10% of all cancers are related to an inherited genetic mutation. As health care shifts to having a greater emphasis on prevention, care providers, including general surgeons, will need to play a role in identifying patients at high risk for cancer development. Genetic testing provides a tool to determine those patients with a genetic mutation and to whom appropriate preventive care and treatment may be offered. It is imperative for general surgeons to understand the role genetics plays in the care of individual patients and their relatives.

> The past decade has brought about dramatic changes in the diagnosis and management of cancer. Advancements in imaging and minimally invasive interventional techniques combine to rapidly diagnose, stage, and in certain cases, treat various forms of cancer. Physicians treating patients with cancer are confronted with many challenges beginning with the initial diagnosis. Imaging plays an integral role in every step of caring for the patient with cancer. Advances in imaging allow the earlier detection and staging of the disease and aid in decision making and treatment planning.

Solid tumors of the pancreas encompass a variety of diagnoses with treatments ranging from observation to major abdominal surgery. Pancreatic ductal adenocarcinoma remains one of the most common and most lethal of these differential of diagnoses and requires a multimodality approach through a multidisciplinary team of specialists. This article reviews the classification, clinical presentation, and workup in differentiating solid tumors of the pancreas and serves as an additional tool for general surgeons faced with such a clinical finding, from a surgical oncology perspective.

This article outlines the principles behind the management of pancreatic cystic lesions. We outline what the general surgeon needs to know in managing and triaging these patients. It is our feeling that the general surgeon is often the first line of evaluation of these complex patients and a working knowledge of the different types of cysts is critical to safe care of the patient.

Cytoreductive surgery followed by hyperthermic intraperitoneal chemotherapy is an aggressive, potentially curative approach used to treat locoregional disease associated with primary and secondary malignancies of the peritoneum. It involves resection of all macroscopic disease larger than 2.5 mm, followed by instillation of hyperthermic chemotherapy directly into the peritoneum for higher drug exposure to microscopic disease. In select patients with primary peritoneal mesothelioma, pseudomyxoma peritonei, colorectal adenocarcinoma, appendiceal adenocarcinoma, or ovarian cancer, with no extra-abdominal metastasis and limited involvement of the peritoneum, the procedure can be performed to increase overall survival.

Rectal cancer is often presented with a dizzying array of treatment recommendations. This article clarifies and simplifies this common clinical problem from the surgical perspective. Treatment of rectal cancer requires an understanding of presenting stage (early or advanced) and location (high or low) to provide oncologic sound treatment decisions. Surgical treatment requires a minimum of 1 cm distal margin, careful clearance of the mesorectum and radial margin using total mesorectal excision technique, and 12 or more regional lymph nodes harvested and analyzed. Appropriate and effective multimodality treatments exist and must be used based on sound guidelines as outlined.

SURGICAL CLINICS
OF NORTH AMERICA

FORTHCOMING ISSUES

August 2020
Wound Management
Michael D. Caldwell and Michael J. Harl,
Editors

October 2020
Rural Surgery
Tyler G. Hughes, *Editor*

December 2020
Endoscopy
John H. Rodriguez and Jeffrey L. Ponsky,
Editors

RECENT ISSUES

April 2020
Robotic Surgery
Julio A. Teixeira, *Editor*

February 2020
Contemporary Melanoma Management:
A Surgical Perspective
Rohit Sharma, *Editor*

December 2019
Inflammatory Bowel Disease
Sean J. Langenfeld, *Editor*

SERIES OF RELATED INTEREST

Advances in Surgery
https://www.advancessurgery.com/
Surgical Oncology Clinics
https://www.surgonc.theclinics.com/
Thoracic Surgery Clinics
http://www.thoracic.theclinics.com/

Foreword

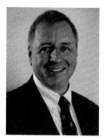

Ronald F Martin, MD, FACS
Consulting Editor

As I write this foreword for this issue of the *Surgical Clinics of North America*, I am the only person in the administrative wing of our hospital. We are on the steep part of the ascending curve of the COVID-19 pandemic, and the hospital at which I work is preparing as best it can for the worst.

This issue, devoted to oncology and aimed at surgeons whose entire practice is *not* isolated to oncology, could in some ways be distilled to "we work in teams." Furthermore, it could be said that if one wants to be an effective member of a team, one needs to be not only truly expert on his/her areas but also extremely conversant and aware of the capabilities and needs of the other members of the team. Perhaps, above all, effective real-time communication is the most important aspect of team functionality. We have left the days of isolated giants in their fields (some time ago now) and entered the era of effective teams of people dedicated to a purpose to gain best outcomes.

It may seem a bit of a stretch to some but COVID pandemics and cancer may have some similarities. At the molecular basis they function at the genetic level—clearly by dissimilar mechanisms, though. Both diseases carry some significant degree of lethality. Both are very resource intensive and consumptive. Both could clearly bankrupt health care systems and economies. And, for both, we have substantial ability to mitigate but not eliminate the consequences of the disease burden.

Of course, the dissimilarities are substantial as well, most notably communicability and timescale. That timescale piece is not to be trivialized as the difference of one side, the pace of cancer, to the other side, the pace of virus transmission, has been the difference between creating an economy (oncologic health care) and crippling all economies.

Perhaps the more important comparator between oncologic care and pandemic response on the larger scale is that they both force us to consider how to use resources when they are limited in some fashion. This pandemic will probably force our community as a whole to reevaluate how it wishes to prepare for future challenges. I say "probably" as I am constantly amazed by our inability to learn from our past errors. Still, we

https://doi.org/10.1016/j.suc.2020.04.002
0039-6109/20/© 2020 Published by Elsevier Inc.
surgical.theclinics.com

should examine this carefully when all is settled down enough and do our best to evaluate where we could have done better while doing our best to avoid recrimination.

I would hope that one day everyone will learn that when it comes to infectious disease of this scale, it is an "everyone's problem." Communicable disease in the era of fast travel respects no geographic, political, or national boundaries. I would also hope that we learn that being prepared allows us to be proactive rather than struggling to react quickly and/or less effectively. We also need to learn how to fund preparation and supply in a time that values just-in-time nearly everything. Most importantly, I hope people realize we are all in this together and that it takes coordinated and effective effort to resolve some problems. For that, we need community in the true sense.

Which brings me back to how I find myself alone here in "admin." As those of you who have followed this series for a while may have observed, we have tried to emphasize the importance of collegiality and community among surgeons to effectively serve our constituencies. Serving as Consulting Editor for this series for many years now has allowed me to work with some of the best thinkers and collaborators in our surgical community. It is through those global surgery community connections that I find myself working here in Montana. As to the alone part, I am not alone here in admin today because I am the only one working; quite the contrary. I am alone here today because of social distancing. We are all doing whatever we can remotely for as long as it takes.

I would like to ask our readership their indulgence for my acknowledging and thanking my colleagues here in Montana. Among them are our Guest Editors, Dr Randy Zuckerman and Dr Neal Wilkinson. Also, Dr John Federico and Dr David Sheldon from the surgical group. Dr Jeff Tjaden, our infectious disease specialist and virology guru, Dr Doug Nelson, our CMO, and Dr Craig Lambrecht, our CEO, are my physician partners on the administrative team and incident command team. I would very much like to thank them all as well as the excellent staff of our facility here that has done extraordinary things to help us prepare for what will come.

We are deeply indebted to Drs Zuckerman, Wilkinson, and their colleagues for their excellent contributions to this series. We also greatly appreciate their efforts to complete this issue under immense pressure to respond to other extraordinary needs. I am hoping by the time this issue physically gets to you, social distancing will be a memory. I hope that is not forgotten, however, and we learn to do better and be better prepared next time. All of us at *Surgical Clinics of North America* wish good health and safety for you, your families, and your communities. We thank you for your support as always.

Ronald F. Martin, MD, FACS
Colonel (retired)
United States Army Reserve
Kalispell Regional Healthcare
Kalispell Regional Medical Group
Division of HPB Surgery and Surgical Oncology
310 Sunnyview Lane
Kalispell, MT 59901, USA

E-mail address:
rfmcescna@gmail.com

Preface

Surgical Oncology for the General Surgeon

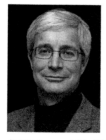 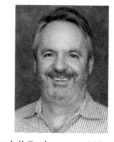

Neal Wilkinson, MD, FACS   Randall Zuckerman, MD, FACS
Editors

The practice of general surgery is dynamic and ever-changing. A well-trained general surgeon is able to handle a wide array of surgical problems with excellent outcomes. Even with increasing specialization, a large percentage of cancer operations in the United States are done by general surgeons. This includes largely breast, colon, and skin cancers, as there has been regionalization of liver, pancreas, and esophageal cancer surgery. Of note, there are only about 10% of counties in the United States that have a surgical oncologist. Most surgical oncologists are concentrated in high-population areas with high-density availability contrasting with large regions of areas served primarily by the general surgeon.

Surgical oncology is a rapidly changing field. Keeping up with advancements and changes in therapies can be very difficult. The core surgical principles in caring for cancer are a constant, but often paradigm shifts occur that change our management of these complex patients. We would very much like to thank all of the authors who contributed to this issue and were able to distill the intricacies of cancer care into a highly readable and useful issue.

Patients across America deserve the best in cancer care. In this issue, we cover a broad array of surgical oncology topics geared for a general surgeon. Our hope is to

Surg Clin N Am 100 (2020) xv–xvi
https://doi.org/10.1016/j.suc.2020.04.001
0039-6109/20/© 2020 Published by Elsevier Inc.

surgical.theclinics.com

provide clear and concise information to help with the efficient management and/or referral of surgical oncology patients.

Neal Wilkinson, MD, FACS
Kalispell Regional Healthcare
1333 Surgical Services Drive
Kalispell, MT 59937, USA

Randall Zuckerman, MD, FACS
Kalispell Regional Healthcare
1333 Surgical Services Drive
Kalispell, MT 59937, USA

E-mail addresses:
nwilkinson@krmc.org (N. Wilkinson)
rzuckerman@krmc.org (R. Zuckerman)

Cancer Incidence and Trends

Melissa C. Hulvat, MD

KEYWORDS

- Cancer incidence • Cancer trends • Modifiable risk factors for cancer
- Cancer survivors • Financial toxicity

KEY POINTS

- The global burden of cancer is unequally distributed, and the propensity toward a higher incidence in high-income countries is evident in North America.
- The types of cancer seen in North America have changed with time, as have the survival rates.
- Modifiable risk factors, such as tobacco use, alcohol, obesity, diet, and lack of physical activity, seem to drive many of the trends seen in cancer incidence in North America.
- Cancer survivors are becoming a larger part of the population, and their needs for ongoing care must be considered in health care and public policy.

INTRODUCTION

Cancer is the second leading cause of death worldwide and in North America, behind only ischemic heart disease.[1,2] However, a recent prospective, population-based cohort study of individuals aged 35 to 70 years who have been enrolled from 21 countries across five continents in the Prospective Urban Rural Epidemiology (PURE) study shows that this may be in transition. In high-income countries, deaths from cancer are now more common than those from cardiovascular disease. The higher a country's gross domestic product, the lower the incidence of deaths from cardiovascular disease compared with those from cancer.[3] Although public health initiatives in high-income countries (eg, United States and Canada), such as smoking cessation and cancer screening, have had positive effects on some cancer incidences and mortality statists, ground is being lost because of other modifiable risk factors. Overall, a combination of screening, prevention, and successful treatment has resulted in a huge number of cancer survivors. Between 1991 and 2015, the overall cancer death rate in the United States fell by 26%. In the United States alone, this amounts to nearly 16 million current cancer survivors, expected to increase to 20.3 million by 2026.[4] An examination of cancer incidences and trends should be with an eye toward gaining knowledge of successes; areas where more work must be done; and creating policies and programs that not only prevent, screen for, and treat disease, but also support cancer survivors to their fullest potential.

Bass Breast Center, Kalispell Regional Healthcare, 310 Sunnyview Lane, Kalispell, MT 59901, USA
E-mail address: mhulvat@krmc.org

Surg Clin N Am 100 (2020) 469–481
https://doi.org/10.1016/j.suc.2020.01.002
surgical.theclinics.com

CANCER INCIDENCE
World

The global cancer burden is estimated to have risen to 18.1 million new cases and 9.6 million deaths in 2018. GLOBOCAN (the World Health Organization's International Agency for Research on Cancer Global Cancer Observatory) predicts there will be 27.5 million new cancer cases worldwide each year by 2040, an increase of 61.7%. Much of this projected increase is caused by demographic factors, such as population growth and aging, but the increasing prevalence of certain cancers linked to social and economic development is also a factor. There is expected to be a shift from cancers associated with infections to cancers associated with Western lifestyle choices. Currently, the most frequently diagnosed cancer and the leading cause of cancer death vary across countries and within each country depending on the degree of economic development and associated social and lifestyle factors.[5]

Examining cancer incidence and mortality data as it relates to the income level of different countries further illustrates this trend. High-income countries have the highest incidence rates for all cancers (including lung, colorectal, breast, and prostate cancer). However, mortality rates are declining. Low- and middle-income countries have higher rates of stomach, liver, esophageal, and cervical cancer, representing a disproportionate burden of infection-related cancers, and mortality rates remain high because of lack of access to effective screening and treatment (**Figs. 1** and **2**).[6]

Canada

Cancer incidence in Canada is consistent with the trends seen in other high-income countries around the globe, with trends in incidence rates variable across cancer types. The age-standardized incidence rate for all cancers combined is decreasing in males and is no longer increasing in females, and there has been a consistent decline in cancer mortality rates since 1988. However, the absolute number of cancer

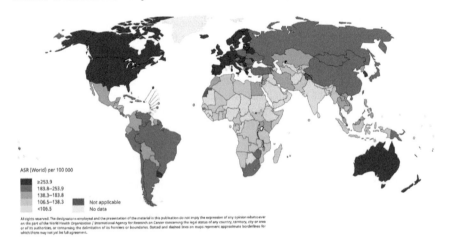

ASR (World) per 100 000

≥253.9
183.8–253.9
138.3–183.8
106.5–138.3
<106.5

Not applicable
No data

Fig. 1. Estimated age-standardized incidence rates (world) in 2018; all cancers, both sexes, all age groups. (*Courtesy of* World Health Organization. International Agency for Research on Cancer and data from GLOBOCAN 2018. Available at: http://gco.iarc.fr/today/online-analysis-map?v=2018&mode=population&mode_population=continents&population=900&populations=900&key=asr&sex=0&cancer=39&type=0&statistic=5&prevalence=0&population_group=0&ages_group%5B%5D=0&ages_group%5B%5D=17&nb_items=5&group_cancer=1&include_nmsc=1&include_nmsc_other=1&projection=natural-earth&color_palette=default&map_scale=quantile&map_nb_colors=5&continent=0&rotate=%255B10%252C0%255D.)

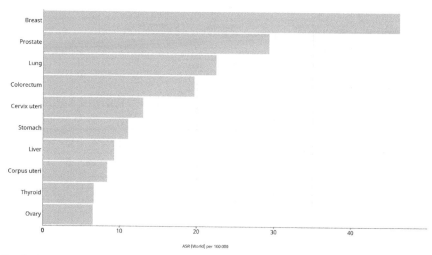

Fig. 2. By cancer type: estimated age-standardized incidence rates (world) in 2018; all cancers, both sexes, all age groups. (*Courtesy of* World Health Organization. International Agency for Research on Cancer and data from GLOBOCAN 2018. Available at: http://gco. iarc.fr/today/online-analysis-multi-bars?v=2018&mode=cancer&mode_population=countries& population=900&populations=900&key=asr&sex=0&cancer=39&type=0&statistic=5& prevalence=0&population_group=0&ages_group%5B%5D=0&ages_group%5B%5D=17&nb_ items=10&group_cancer=1&include_nmsc=1&include_nmsc_other=1&type_multiple=%257B% 2522inc%2522%253Atrue%252C%2522mort%2522%253Afalse%252C%2522prev%2522%253Afalse% 257D&orientation=horizontal&type_sort=0&type_nb_items=%257B%2522top%2522%253Atrue%252C% 2522bottom%2522%253Afalse%257D&population_group_globocan_id=.)

diagnoses is increasing because of the growing and aging Canadian population. Much progress has been made in cancer control in Canada as a result of advances in prevention, screening, early detection, and treatment (**Fig. 3**).[7]

United States

More than 1.7 million new cancer cases are expected to be diagnosed in the United States in 2019, and approximately 606,880 Americans are expected to succumb to cancer in 2019. Cancer is the second most common cause of death in the United States, second only to cardiac disease. Examining cancer death rates, as opposed to incidence, is the best measure of progress against the disease because it is less affected by population growth and methods of detection. The overall age-adjusted cancer death rate rose during most of the twentieth century, mostly because of tobacco as a causative agent. As of 2016, the rate had dropped to 156 per 100,000 (a decline of 27%) because of reductions in smoking, and improvements in early detection and treatment.[8] African American citizens do shoulder a disproportionate share of the cancer burden, but substantial progress is being made. Among men, the overall cancer death rate was 47% higher for blacks than for whites in 1990 versus 19% higher in 2016; among females, the disparity decreased from 19% to 13% over the same period.[9]

SPECIFIC CANCER TYPES IN NORTH AMERICA AND TRENDS
Breast Cancer

Worldwide, female breast cancer incidence rates vary greatly, but it is clear that the highest rates exist in Western Europe and the United States (plus Israel) and the

	New cases (2019 estimates)			Cases per 100,000		
	Total[a]	Males	Females	Both sexes	Males	Females
All cancers[b]	**220,400**	**113,000**	**107,400**	**518.8**	**559.0**	**489.5**
Lung and bronchus	29,300	14,900	14,500	62.1	66.0	59.6
Breast	27,200	230	26,900	66.8	1.2	128.0
Colorectal	26,300	14,600	11,700	60.6	71.7	50.9
Prostate	22,900	22,900	—	—	118.1	—
Bladder	11,800	9,100	2,700	25.0	42.1	10.6
Non-Hodgkin lymphoma	10,000	5,600	4,400	24.2	29.0	20.0
Thyroid	8,200	2,100	6,100	21.8	11.2	32.1
Melanoma	7,800	4,300	3,500	21.7	25.1	19.1
Kidney and renal pelvis	7,200	4,700	2,500	17.0	23.2	11.3
Uterus (body, NOS)	7,200	—	7,200	—	—	34.5
Leukemia	6,700	4,000	2,700	16.4	20.8	12.5
Pancreas	5,800	3,000	2,800	12.9	14.2	11.7
Oral	5,300	3,700	1,600	12.7	18.4	7.4
Stomach	4,100	2,600	1,450	9.3	13.1	6.1
Multiple myeloma	3,300	1,950	1,400	7.7	9.6	6.0
Brain/CNS	3,000	1,650	1,300	7.1	8.3	6.0
Ovary	3,000	—	3,000	—	—	14.2
Liver	3,000	2,200	780	6.7	10.5	3.2
Esophagus	2,300	1,800	540	5.6	9.2	2.4
Cervix	1,350	—	1,350	—	—	7.2
Larynx	1,150	980	190	2.4	4.2	0.7
Testis	1,150	1,150	—	—	6.4	—
Hodgkin lymphoma	1,000	560	440	2.6	2.9	2.3
All other cancers	21,300	11,000	10,300	47.7	53.4	43.3

Analysis by: Centre for Surveillance and Applied Research, Public Health Agency of Canada

Fig. 3. Projected new cases and age-standardized incidence rates for cancers, by sex, Canada 2019. —, not applicable; CNS, central nervous system; NOS, not otherwise specified. Rates are age-standardized to the 2011 Canadian population and exclude Quebec. [a] Column totals may not sum to row totals because of rounding. [b] "All cancers" includes *in situ* bladder cancer and excludes nonmelanoma skin cancer (neoplasms, NOS; epithelial neoplasms, NOS; and basal and squamous). (*From* Canadian Cancer Statistics Advisory Committee. *Canadian Cancer Statistics 2019.* Toronto, ON: Canadian Cancer Society; 2019; with permission. Available at: cancer.ca/Canadian-Cancer-Statistics-2019-EN.)

lowest rates in Africa and Asia. There also exists a substantial variability in mortality based on country of origin, and even in populations with countries. In developing countries where early detection is not the norm, 5-year survival rates are low, ranging from 10% to 40%. In settings where early detection and basic treatment are widespread, the 5-year survival rate for early localized breast cancer exceeds 80%.[10]

In the United States, it has been observed and stated many times that the advent of screening mammography in the 1970s led to an increased incidence of breast cancer simply because of early detection. However, the increase in incidence of female breast cancer by 0.4% per year between 2006 and 2015 is less easily explained. It seems that even after the dramatic decrease in the use of postmenopausal hormone-replacement therapy in the early 2000s, the true risk of developing breast cancer is still increasing in American women. The female breast cancer death rate peaked at 33.2 (per 100,000) in 1989, then declined by 40% to 20.0 in 2016 (a 1.8% per year decrease in death rate from 2007–2016). This progress reflects improvements in early detection and treatment, and the relative contribution of each of these factors is the topic of much debate.[6] In the United States, the highest mortality rates are found among black women, whereas the lowest are in Korean women.[6]

In Canada, an increase in breast cancer incidence corresponding to the advent of screening mammography had also been noted, with a plateau in screening mammography and consequent decrease in the prevalent pool of undiagnosed breast cancer cases in 1999.[11] Around that same time in the early 2000s there was a substantial decline in estrogen receptor–positive breast tumors associated with declining use of hormone replacement, and that plus the plateau in rates of mammography use most fully explain the observed decrease in breast cancer incidence.[12] Mortality rate from breast cancer in Canada is declining, which raises the ever-present question regarding how much of this decrease is from early detection and how much is from treatment advances. The finding that breast cancer mortality is decreasing even in a group of women not subjected to screening (those ages 35–39 at diagnosis) would suggest that advances in treatment, not breast cancer screening, are responsible for much of the breast cancer mortality declines.[13]

Postmenopausal breast cancer risk is particularly modifiable with lifestyle choices. Low weight gain after menopause, no alcohol consumption, high physical activity level, history of breastfeeding, and no menopausal hormone therapy use was associated with a 34.6% decrease in risk in one study. Risk factors that are modifiable at menopause account for more than one-third of postmenopausal breast cancers; therefore, a substantial proportion of breast cancer in the United States is preventable.[14]

Colon

Screening colonoscopy has been driving a decrease in the incidence of colon cancer since the mid-1980s because precancerous polyps are removed before they can become malignant. However, the overall trend is driven by older adults (who have the highest rates of colon cancer and for whom screening colonoscopy is recommended) and masks an increasing incidence in younger age groups. From 2006 to 2015, incidence rates declined by 3.7% annually among adults 55 years of age and older, but increased by 1.8% annually among those younger than age 55.[8] Overall, the colorectal cancer death rate in 2016 (13.7 per 100,000) was less than half of that in 1970 (29.2 per 100,000), but yet again this generalization hides an alarming trend in younger adults. From 2007 to 2016, the colon cancer death rate declined by 2.7% per year among individuals ages 55 and older but increased by 1% per year among adults younger than age 55.[8] What is behind this disturbing trend?

Colorectal cancer incidence has been increasing in the United States among adults aged 55 or younger since the mid-1990s. The increase seems to be confined to white men and women. Unfortunately, the increase is also most rapid for metastatic disease because these cancers are not detected by screening.[15] This same increase has been observed in a Canadian cohort, and seems to be accelerating. For Canadian women younger than 50 years, the incidence of colorectal cancer has increased by 4.45% annually since 2010; for men younger than 50 years the incidence is increasing by 3.47% annually from 2006 through 2015. There is a greater risk of colon cancer in individuals born more recently than those born earlier (birth cohort). Increasing incidence and increased prevalence in later birth cohorts taken together suggest a common exposure in North America that may be placing younger adults at higher risk of colorectal cancer. The rising prevalence of obesity in high-income countries is postulated as a possible driver this trend.[16] However, because the increase in colorectal cancer in persons younger than 50 is confined to white persons, obesity cannot be the only factor, because incidence of that disease is similar in white and black individuals.[17]

Because of the increasing incidence of colorectal cancer in individuals younger than 50, the American Cancer Society now recommends colonoscopy beginning at age 45 years for average-risk adults.[18]

Liver

Liver cancer is the most rapidly increasing cancer in the United States in men and women, increasing by about 3% per year. Approximately three-fourths of liver cancers diagnosed in the United States are hepatocellular carcinoma, which have known environmental risk factors. According to the American Cancer Society, approximately 70% of liver cancer cases in the United States could potentially be prevented through the elimination of exposure to these risk factors including excess body weight, type 2 diabetes, chronic infection with hepatitis B and C viruses, excessive alcohol consumption, and tobacco abuse.[8,19]

Hepatitis B virus and hepatitis C virus account for most cases of hepatocellular carcinoma (40%–50%). When infection leads to cirrhosis, there is a 30-fold increase in hepatocellular carcinoma risk.[20] A vaccine against hepatitis B has been available since 1982. There is no vaccine currently available for hepatitis C, but treatment options have rapidly expanded in availability and efficacy. Although hepatitis C causes a large proportion of liver cancers, the actual risk of a person with hepatitis C developing liver cancer at some point in their life is only about 4%. For those who seek treatment of their hepatitis C, it is currently unclear if hepatocellular carcinoma risk declines over time after hepatitis C virus eradication. Patients with cirrhosis before treatment continue to have a high risk for hepatocellular carcinoma (>2% per year) for many years, and therefore the need for diligent surveillance does not diminish after active virus eradication.[21] Attempts to identify what patients remain at greatest risk for developing hepatocellular carcinoma after successful treatment of hepatitis C continues to make lifelong surveillance mandatory in all of these patients according to present general expert opinion.[22]

Lung

New diagnosis of lung cancer in the United States has been declining since the mid-1980s in men, and since the mid-2000s in women largely because of smoking cessation (81% of lung cancer deaths in the United States are caused by smoking).[8] Cigarette smoking prevalence among adolescents and adults has declined steadily since the early 1990s.[23] The lung cancer death rate has also declined by 48% since 1990 in men and by 23% since 2002 in women, but lung cancer remains the most deadly cancer in the United States (American Cancer Society facts and figures 2019, cancer.org).

Unfortunately, uptake of lung cancer screening with low-dose computerized tomography since 2010 has been limited and stagnant. In 2010 and 2015, only 4.5% and 5.9%, respectively, of adults aged 55 to 80 years who meet the US Preventive Services Task Force criteria for lung cancer screening had a low-dose computerized tomography scan to check for lung cancer within the past year.[23]

Even with declining incidence and death rates overall, the worldwide burden of lung cancer is unevenly distributed. When stratified for age, the incidence and mortality from lung cancer are higher in more developed countries than less developed ones by 1.5- to 1.4-fold in men, and by 1.8- to 1.5-fold fold in women. In fact, lung cancer incidence varied more than 31-fold worldwide in 2012. Mortality rates from lung cancer also varied by approximately 32-fold worldwide at the same point in time. In men, the highest death rates occur in Central and Eastern Europe, Eastern Asia, and Micronesia; in women, the highest mortality was reported in Northern America, Micronesia, and Northern Europe. The higher incidence and mortality of lung cancer in more highly developed countries has been explained by tobacco use and air pollution because of industrialization, which are both more common in these more developed nations.[24] As industrialization spreads, along with decreasing air quality, and as increasing prosperity frees up discretionary income to purchase tobacco products, will lung cancer cases and death rates in developing countries increase to the level currently seen in developed countries? This is a concerning trend that deserves attention.

MODIFIABLE RISK FACTORS

It is estimated that 45% of the 607,000 cancer deaths expected to occur in the United States in 2019 will be related to modifiable risk factors.[25] This makes these modifiable risk factors one of the most important incidences and trends that one can monitor when considering how to modify the cancer burden in the population.

Cancers of the lung, breast, prostate, colon, and rectum accounted for more than half of the overall cancer burden in the most developed regions of the world, such as North America. The lifetime cumulative risk of these four cancers were all more than 3% in higher developed than in less developed areas.[24] It is reasonable to assume that a proportion of this disparity could be attributable to ethnic/genetic makeup of this population, but the explanation for most of this disparity is likely environmental exposures. Anything that you are exposed to during your lifetime and not born with is considered a modifiable risk factor, and represents an opportunity for cancer prevention.

Reducing modifiable cancer risk factors along with improving cancer screening requires improved governmental policies, community efforts, and changes in individual behavioral. Many of these strategies have been proven to be effective, but their application thus far has been suboptimal.[25] "It is the responsibility of government and industry and the public health, medical, and scientific communities to work together to invest in and implement a comprehensive cancer control plan at the national level and support and expand ongoing initiatives at the state and local levels. If we fail to do so, we will slow progress in our national efforts to reduce the burden of cancer."[26]

Tobacco

The estimated annual loss in productivity attributable to tobacco use in the US work force is $156 billion annually, and the direct health care costs a staggering $170 billion. There is considerable evidence that tobacco control can prevent more cancer deaths than any other primary prevention strategy.[26]

Obesity, Alcohol, Diet, and Inactivity

After tobacco use, the second most impactful modifiable risk factors for cancer in the United States are dietary and lifestyle related.

Between 1980 and 2014, overweight or obesity prevalence in the United States increased by more than 100% among children and adolescents and by 60% among adults aged 20 to 74 years.[27] A more in-depth analysis shows that in fact the percentage of US men and women who are considered overweight has been stable at least in recent years at 36.5% of men and 26.9% of women. However, the prevalence of obesity has drastically increased, with seven states having obesity rates of at least 35% in 2017, up from zero states in 2012. These rates vary by ethnicity with the highest rates of obesity occurring in African Americans (54.9%) and the lowest in Asian Americans (14.8%).[25] In adults aged 30 years and older in the United States, excess bodyweight could account for up to 60% of all endometrial cancers, 36% of gallbladder cancers, 33% of kidney cancers, 17% of pancreatic cancers, and 11% of multiple myelomas in 2014.[28] There is also growing evidence to support an association between childhood or adolescent obesity and increased risk of colorectal, endometrial, and pancreatic cancers and multiple myeloma later in life.[29] It seems that obesity causes an increases risk of cancer in the end-organ affected via adipose inflammation and associated alterations in the microenvironment, and systemically via circulating metabolic and inflammatory mediators associated with adipose inflammation.[30]

In 2017%, 5.3% of US adults were considered heavier drinkers (more than 14 drinks per week for men and more than 7 drinks per week for women), with a higher prevalence among white persons.[25] The US Centers for Disease Control and Prevention cites alcohol as a risk factor for six kinds of cancer including cancers of the oropharynx, larynx, esophagus, colon and rectum, liver, and female breast.[31] Alcohol consumption directly attributed to an estimated 40.9% of oral cavity/pharynx cancers, 23.2% of larynx cancers, 21.6% of liver cancers, 21% of esophageal cancers, and 12.8% of colorectal cancers. Among women diagnosed with breast cancer in the United States in 2014, alcohol is implicated in 16.4% of all cases, or 39,060 breast cancer diagnoses.[26]

The type of diet consumed, not just its effect on body weight, also seems to be important in carcinogenesis. A study of the French NutriNet-Santé cohort (2009–2017) shows the consumption of sugary drinks was significantly associated with the risk of overall cancer (hazard ratio for a 100 mL/d increase, 1.18; 95% confidence interval, 1.10–1.27; $P < .0001$).[32] Lack of dietary fiber has long been linked to a higher incidence of colorectal cancer. Increased fiber intake may lead to a dilution of fecal carcinogens, reduced transit time, and bacterial fermentation of fiber to short-chain fatty acids with anticarcinogenic properties.[33,34] In one large prospective study, in which all individuals underwent the same colorectal screening, high fiber intake was associated with a reduced risk of precancerous polyps and cancer.[35]

According to the Centers for Disease Control and Prevention, the percent of adults older than 18 in the United States who met the Centers for Disease Control and Prevention Physical Activity Guidelines for aerobic physical activity is only 53.3%.[36] It is estimated that 2.9% of all cancer cases in the United States are attributable to low physical activity, with the contribution greater among women (4.4%) than among men (1.5%). The cancer with the highest percentage of cases related to low physical activity was uterine cancer (26.7%), followed by colorectal cancer (6.3%).[26] Routine physical activity has been found to be associated with a reduced incidence of several of the other most common malignancies, including breast and lung. Physical activity also seems to reduce all-cause mortality and cancer-related mortality among patients with breast and colon cancer.[37] It does seem that for some cancers physical activity has an independent effect on cancer risk, not just via physical activity's ability to lower body mass index and decrease obesity. For adolescents and young adult women aged 15 to 39 years at diagnosis of breast cancer, higher levels of physical activity, lower red meat intake, and higher intake of plants seem to decrease the risk of developing breast cancer, but an association between obesity and breast cancer risk was not apparent in this population.[38]

The contribution of modifiable risk factors to the incidence of cancer in Canada is similar to that seen in the United States. Nearly one in two Canadians are expected to be diagnosed with cancer in their lifetime. However, there are opportunities to reduce the impact of modifiable cancer risk factors through well-informed interventions and policies. One population-based study estimates that between 33% and 37% (up to 70,000 cases) of incident cancer cases among adults aged 30 years and older in 2015 were attributable to preventable risk factors, with tobacco use and a lack of physical activity responsible for the highest proportions of cancer cases. Cancers with the highest number of preventable cases in this Canadian cohort were lung, colorectal, and female breast cancer. If current trends in the prevalence of preventable risk factors continue into the future, the authors project that by 2042 approximately 102,000 incident cancer cases are expected to be attributable to modifiable risk factors annually, accounting for the same one-third of all incident cancers seen in the United States. Through various risk-reduction interventions, policies, and public health campaigns, an estimated 10,600 to 39,700 cancer cases per year in Canadian citizens could be prevented by 2042.[39]

SURVIVORS

The most hopeful and exciting trend in cancer in North America is the trend toward an ever-increasing number of cancer survivors. According to the National Cancer Institute in the United States the length of cancer survival is increasing for all cancers combined, with the 5-year relative survival for all cancer sites currently at 69.3%. This improving survival reflects real changes because of improved early detection and treatment, which can extend life. However, they do note that there may also be an artifactual lengthening of survival associated with detecting cancers earlier and creating lead time bias.[23] Caring for the physical, emotional, social, and financial well-being of these survivors thus becomes an increasingly important priority in the continuum of cancer care.

The sentinel publication in the United States regarding the care of cancer survivors, *From Cancer Patient to Cancer Survivor: Lost in Transition*, published in 2015 sought to address shortfalls in the care currently provided to the more than 10 million cancer survivors in this country.[40] The sponsors aim to raise awareness of the medical, functional, and psychosocial consequences of cancer and its treatment; define and achieve quality health care for cancer survivors; and improve the quality of life through policies to ensure access to psychosocial services, fair employment practices, and health insurance remain as valid in 2019 as they were 14 years ago. Sadly, many of these goals remain unrealized.

Late effects of treatment of cancer are most profound and most commonly experienced by adults who have survived childhood cancer. A 60% to more than 90% of individuals who have been successfully treated for a childhood cancer develop one or more chronic health conditions; and 20% to 80% experience severe or life-threatening complications during adulthood. The common late effects of pediatric cancer encompass several broad domains, including the following: growth and development; organ function; reproductive capacity and health of offspring; secondary carcinogenesis; and psychosocial sequelae related to the primary cancer, its treatment, or maladjustment associated with the cancer experience.[41] In the St. Jude Lifetime Cohort the average adult survivor of childhood cancer experienced an average of 17.1 chronic health conditions, 4.7 of which were severe/disabling, life threatening, or fatal.[42] By age 50 years, the cumulative incidence of a self-reported severe, disabling, life-threatening, or fatal health condition was 53.6% among survivors, compared with 19.8% among a sibling control group.[43] A proposed remedy to these disturbing statistics is to establish and support multidisciplinary long-term follow-up programs that work collaboratively with community physicians to provide care for childhood cancer survivors. This type of shared care is the optimal model to facilitate coordinated survivor care.[44] The Children's Oncology Group has an excellent Resource Guide for those providing long-term care to survivors of pediatric cancers (found at http://www.survivorshipguidelines.org).

The top four concerns across all cancer survivors have been measured to be (1) eating and nutrition, (2) exercise and being physically active, (3) worry about the future and what lies ahead, and (4) feeling too tired to do the things one needs to do. Other things that cause persistent distress to cancer survivors include poor sleep, health insurance and money worries, body image, and inability to think clearly.[45]

One disturbing trend in the United States regarding patients with cancer is the increasing financial effect of this disease. The National Cancer Institute estimates that national expenditures for cancer care in 2018 for the top five cancer sites were $19.7, $16.6, $15.3, $14.6, and $14.2 billion for female breast, colorectal, prostate, lymphoma, and lung, respectively. Even for patients with health insurance, out-of-pocket costs for cancer care often pose a significant financial burden. As the US population ages and newer technologies and treatments become available, national expenditures for cancer will continue to rise, and cancer costs may increase at a faster rate than overall medical expenditures.[23] This causes significant distress to cancer survivors. Survivors admit to delaying acting on recommendations of supportive physical care because of costs, postponing getting prescriptions filled or seeing a counselor, choosing to forgo treatment altogether because of costs, and worrying about the financial burden of their care on the family.[45]

The term "financial toxicity" has been used to describe the harmful personal financial burden faced by patients receiving cancer treatment.[46] As medical debt grows for some with cancer, the downstream effects are catastrophic. Analyzing population-based data from Western Washington State, Bansal and colleagues[47] found that having a cancer diagnosis was associated with a 2.65-times greater likelihood of declaring personal bankruptcy. In addition, when comparing a sample of patients with cancer who declared bankruptcy with a propensity-matched sample of patients with cancer who had not declared bankruptcy, they found that those patients with cancer who declared bankruptcy had a 79% greater mortality risk than those who had not.[47] At least three factors might explain the relationship between extreme financial distress and greater risk of mortality: (1) poorer subjective well-being, (2) impaired health-related quality of life, and (3) subpar quality of care.[48]

With the populations of the United States and Canada aging, with screening programs catching many common cancers earlier, and with continually improving treatments, how to effectively deal with the physical, emotional, social, and financial needs of the ballooning population of cancer survivors will become an ever more important public health priority. Especially urgent is to have policies and programs in place to deal with the "silver tsunami" of baby boomers, many of whom will be cancer survivors. Understanding the impact of a graying nation on cancer prevalence and comorbidity burden is critical in informing efforts to design and implement quality cancer care for this population.[49] This a cancer trend that requires full attention.

DISCLOSURE

The author has nothing to disclose.

REFERENCES

1. Global health estimates 2016: deaths by cause, age, sex by country and region, 2000-2015. World Health Organization; 2018. Available at: https://www.who.int/healthinfo/global_burden_disease/en/. Accessed September 11, 2019.

2. Deaths: leading causes for 2016. CDC/National Center for Health Statistics; 2017. Available at: https://www.cdc.gov/nchs/index.htm. Accessed September 11, 2019.

3. Dagenais G, Leong DP, Rangaraian S, et al. Variations in common diseases, hospital admissions, and deaths in middle-aged adults in 21 countries from five continents (PURE): a prospective cohort study. Lancet 2020;395(10226):785–94.

4. Noone AM, Howlader N, Krapcho M, et al. SEER cancer statistics review, 1975-2015. Bethesda (MD): National Cancer Institute; 2018.

5. Bray F, Ferlay J, Soerjomataram I, et al. "Global cancer statistics 2018: GLOBOCAN estimates of incidence and mortality worldwide for 36 cancers in 185 countries. CA Cancer J Clin 2018;68:394–424.

6. Torre LA, Siegel RL, Ward EM, et al. Global cancer incidence and mortality rates and trends: an update. Cancer Epidemiol Biomarkers Prev 2016;25(1):16–27.

7. Canadian Cancer Statistics Advisory Committee. Canadian cancer statistics 2018. Canadian Cancer Society; 2018.

8. American Cancer Society. Cancer facts & figures 2019. American Cancer Society; 2019.

9. DeSantis CE, Miller KD, Goding Sauer A, et al. Cancer statistics for African Americans. CA Cancer J Clin 2019;69(3):211–33.

10. WHO position paper on mammography screening 2014vol. 13. World Health Organization; 2014. Available at: https://apps.who.int/iris/bitstream/handle/10665/137339/9789241507936_eng.pdf;jsessionid=96997CB73F6426B9403625CFB2137806?sequence=1. Accessed September 11, 2019.

11. Jemal A, Ward E, Thun MJ. Recent trends in breast cancer incidence rates by age and tumor characteristics among U.S. women. Breast Cancer Res 2007;9(3):R28.

12. Zakaria D, Shaw A. Trends in mammography, hormone replacement therapy, and breast cancer incidence and mortality in Canadian women. Cancer Causes Control 2019;30:137–47.

13. Bleyer A, Baines C, Miller AB. Impact of screening mammography on breast cancer mortality. Int J Cancer 2016;138(8):2003–12.

14. Tamimi RM, Spiegelman D, Smith-Warner SA, et al. Population attributable risk of modifiable and nonmodifiable breast cancer risk factors in postmenopausal breast cancer. Am J Epidemiol 2016;184(12):884–93.

15. Siegel RL, Miller KD, Jemal A. Colorectal cancer mortality rates in adults aged 20 to 54 years in the United States, 1970-2014. JAMA 2017;318(6):572–4.

16. Brenner DR. National trends in colorectal cancer incidence among older and younger adults in Canada. JAMA Netw Open 2019;2(7):1–7.

17. Fedewa SA, Sauer AG, Siegel RL, et al. Prevalence of major risk factors and use of screening tests for cancer in the United States. Cancer Epidemiol Biomarkers Prev 2015;24(4):637–52.

18. Wolf AMD, Fontham ETH, Church TR, et al. Colorectal cancer screening for average-risk adults: 2018 guideline update from the American Cancer Society. CA Cancer J Clin 2018;68(4):250–81.

19. Petrick JL, Kelly SP, Altekruse SF, et al. Future of hepatocellular carcinoma incidence in the United States forecast through 2030. J Clin Oncol 2016;34(15):1787–94.

20. Marsarweh NN, El-Serag HB. Epidemiology of hepatocellular carcinoma and intrahepatic cholangiocarcinoma. Cancer Control 2017;24(3):1–11.

21. Ioannou GN, Beste LA, Green PK, et al. Increased risk for hepatocellular carcinoma persists up to 10 years after HCV eradication in patients with baseline cirrhosis or high FIB-4 scores. Gastroenterology 2019. [Epub ahead of print].

22. Galati G, Muley M, Viganò M, et al. Occurrence of hepatocellular carcinoma after direct-acting antiviral therapy for hepatitis C virus infection: literature review and risk analysis. Expert Opin Drug Saf 2019;18(7):603–10.

23. National Cancer Institutes Cancer Trends Progress Report. 2019. Available at: https://progressreport.cancer.gov. Accessed September 11, 2019.

24. Wong MCS, Lao XQ, Ho HF, et al. Incidence and mortality of lung cancer: global trends and association with socioeconomic status. Sci Rep 2017;7:14300.

25. Sauer A, Siegel R, Jemal A, et al. Current prevalence of major cancer risk factors and screening test use in the United States: disparities by education and race/ethnicity. Cancer Epidemiol Biomarkers Prev 2019;28(4):629–42.

26. Gapstur SM, Drope JM, Jacobs EJ, et al. A blueprint for the primary prevention of cancer: targeting established, modifiable risk factors. CA Cancer J Clin 2018;68: 446–70.

27. Centers for Disease Control and Prevention. Prevalence of overweight, obesity, and extreme obesity among adults aged 20 and over: United States, 1960–1962 through 2013–2014. Available at: https://www.cdc.gov. Accessed March 1, 2018.

28. Islami F, Goding Sauer A, Miller KD, et al. Proportion and number of cancer cases and deaths attributable to potentially modifiable risk factors in the United States. CA Cancer J Clin 2018;68:31–54.

29. Sung H, Siegel RL, Torre LA, et al. Global patterns in excess body weight and the associated cancer burden. CA Cancer J Clin 2019;69(2):88–112.

30. Iyengar NM, Gucalp A, Dannenberg AJ, et al. Obesity and cancer mechanisms: tumor microenvironment and inflammation. J Clin Oncol 2016;34(35):4270–6.

31. Division of Cancer Prevention and Control, Centers for Disease Control and Prevention. 2019. Available at: https://www.cdc.gov. Accessed September 11, 2019.

32. Chazelas E, Srour B, Desmetz E, et al. Sugary drink consumption and risk of cancer: results from NutriNet-Santé prospective cohort. Br J Med 2019;366:l240.

33. Sengupta S, Muir JG, Gibson PR. Does butyrate protect from colorectal cancer? J Gastroenterol Hepatol 2006;21:209–18.

34. Lipkin M, Reddy B, Newmark H, et al. Dietary factors in human colorectal cancer. Annu Rev Nutr 1999;19:545–86.

35. Kunzmann AT, Coleman HG, Huang WY, et al. Dietary fiber intake and risk of colorectal cancer and incident and recurrent adenoma in the Prostate, Lung, Colorectal, and Ovarian Cancer Screening Trial. Am J Clin Nutr 2015;102(4):881–90.

36. Exercise or Physical Activity. CDC/National Center for Health Statistics. 2017. Available at: https://www.cdc.gov/nchs/fastats/exercise.htm. Accessed September 11, 2019.

37. Lugo D, Pulido AL, Mihos CG, et al. The effects of physical activity on cancer prevention, treatment and prognosis: a review of the literature. Complement Ther Med 2019;44:9–13.

38. Cathcart-Rake EJ. Modifiable risk factors for the development of breast cancer in young women. Cancer J 2018;24(6):275–84.

39. Brenner DR, Poirier AE, Walter SD, et al. Estimating the current and future cancer burden in Canada: methodological framework of the Canadian population attributable risk of cancer (ComPARe) study. BMJ Open 2018;8(7):e022378.

40. Hewitt M, Greenfield S, Stovall E, editors. From cancer patient to cancer survivor: lost in transition. Committee on Cancer Survivorship: Improving Care and Quality of Life, National Cancer Policy Board; 2006.
41. "Late effects of treatment for childhood cancer (PDQ®): health professional version." PDQ cancer information summaries. National Cancer Institute (US); 2002-2019. Available at: https://www.cancer.gov/types/childhood-cancers/late-effects-hp-pdq. Accessed September 11, 2019.
42. Bhakta N, Liu Q, Ness KK, et al. The cumulative burden of surviving childhood cancer: an initial report from the St Jude Lifetime Cohort Study (SJLIFE). Lancet 2017;390(10112):2569–82.
43. Armstrong GT, Kawashima T, Leisenring W, et al. Aging and risk of severe, disabling, life-threatening, and fatal events in the childhood cancer survivor study. J Clin Oncol 2014;32(12):1218–27.
44. Oeffinger KC, McCabe MS. Models for delivering survivorship care. J Clin Oncol 2006;24(32):5117–24.
45. Cancer Support Community. Insight into the patient experience: caner experience registry report. 2017. Available at: cancersupportcommunity.org. Accessed September 11, 2019.
46. Zafar SY, Peppercorn JM, Schrag D, et al. "The financial toxicity of cancer treatment: a pilot study assessing out-of-pocket expenses and the insured cancer patient's experience. Oncologist 2013;18(4):381–90.
47. Bansal A, Ramsey SD, Fedorenko CR, et al. Financial insolvency as a risk factor for mortality among patients with cancer. J Clin Oncol 2015;33(15):650.
48. Zafar SY. Financial toxicity of cancer care: it's time to intervene. J Natl Cancer Inst 2015;108(5) [pii:djv370].
49. Bluethmann SM, Mariotto AB, Rowland JH. Anticipating the 'Silver Tsunami': prevalence trajectories and co-morbidity burden among older cancer survivors in the United States. Cancer Epidemiol Biomarkers Prev 2016;25(7):1029–36.

Cancer Genetics

Christine Van Cott, MD[a,b,*]

KEYWORDS

- Genetic testing • Hereditary cancer syndromes • Lynch syndrome
- Familial adenomatous polyposis • BRCA

KEY POINTS

- As the understanding of the human genome progresses, so does the understanding of genetic mutations.
- Obtaining a complete individual and family cancer history is crucial to the care of general surgery patients. Recognizing patterns of cancer within a personal and/or family history is vital to ensuring the appropriate patients are offered genetic testing.
- Understanding genetic testing results is important for any provider caring for patients with cancer or those who are high risk for cancer development.
- Accessing updated expert surveillance recommendations for those patients with a deleterious mutation is a necessity for general surgeons.
- Using the expertise of genetic counselors when possible is always recommended.

INTRODUCTION

Medicine has undergone staggering advancement over the past decades. From the discovery of DNA to sequencing the human genome, genetics has, and will continue to have, significant implications on health care. The practice of surgery has, over time, allowed general surgeons to develop a disciplined approach to the diagnosis and treatment of many surgical diseases. The understanding of clinical genetics and the role it plays in the treatment of surgical patients, especially those with cancer diagnoses, has not until recent times been part of medical training or of care algorithms. However, as general surgeons, especially rural general surgeons, continue to provide cancer care for most patients in this country, it is imperative they understand the principles of clinical genetics and its role in a modern surgical practice. Understanding basic genetic principles, practical application of genetics into practice, as well as application of gene-specific recommendations are now necessary to provide complete quality care. When available, the expertise and consultation of a genetic counselor is always advised when a patient meeting criteria for genetic testing is identified.

[a] Department of Surgery, St. Vincent's Medical Center, Bridgeport, CT, USA; [b] Frank H. Netter MD School of Medicine, Quinnipiac University, North Haven, CT, USA
* Corresponding author. Acute Care Trauma Department, St. Vincent's Medical Center, Bridgeport, CT.
E-mail address: cvancott@gmail.com

Surg Clin N Am 100 (2020) 483–498
https://doi.org/10.1016/j.suc.2020.02.012
0039-6109/20/© 2020 Elsevier Inc. All rights reserved.

surgical.theclinics.com

THE GENETICS OF CANCER

Within the human genome there are approximately 21,000 genes, with most coding for specific proteins. The basic principles of mendelian genetics have been the building blocks to a now more complete understanding of the patterns of inheritance of these genes. Although most traits are influenced by multiple genes, a much smaller number of traits are influenced by a single gene. When different versions of a gene (alleles) occur in the germline (ie, egg and sperm), these alleles can pass to offspring. Not all alleles are harmful, with most alleles being clinically insignificant. However, in the case of cancer risk, these differences, or mutations, in a single gene can create variation in the product of the gene; either the protein or regulation of the protein. Between 5% and 10% of all cancers have been found to have germline mutations and are attributable to a hereditary cancer predisposition syndrome.[1] Identifying patients (and potential relatives) at risk of hereditary cancer syndromes and providing evidence-based care for those patients with a known mutation are a necessary part of modern surgical care.

FAMILY HISTORY

Although there has been much scientific advancement in genomics and its role in providing personalized care, its transition into everyday clinical care has been limited at best. Many barriers have been identified to providers incorporating genetics in standard practice, including knowledge of the testing available, clinical utility, and application of testing data.[2] For general surgeons to begin to incorporate genetics into practice, they must start with obtaining a personal and family history. Although all providers have been taught this skill during training, the reality is that they often do not practice as they were taught. A personal and family history of cancer is central to determining whether patients are appropriate for testing or whether they meet criteria for being considered high risk even if genetic testing is not appropriate.

Obtaining a third-degree or fourth-degree family history is the gold standard according to the National Society of Genetic Counselors.[3] Obtaining a family history in this detail can be both labor and time intensive. Guidelines from the National Comprehensive Cancer Network (NCCN), the Society of Gynecologic Oncologists, as well as the American College of Obstetrics and Gynecologists focus on first-degree and second-degree relatives and recently incorporate third-degree relatives.[1,4] The American Society of Clinical Oncology recommends that the minimum adequate family history of patients with cancer be defined as family history of cancer in first-degree and second-degree relatives.[1]

Free or commercially available data collection tools can assist general surgeons in obtaining such robust and detailed information. The Centers for Disease Control and Prevention has a free online tool, My Family Health Portrait (https://phgkb.cdc.gov/FHH/html/index.html) that can be used by patients and information shared with their physicians.[5] Having patients complete such a tool before an appointment can allow general surgeons to spend valuable time focusing on completion of necessary details and creating a true medical pedigree. My Family Health Portrait is also able to be customized and adopted by practices and/or organizations free of charge as part of the United States Surgeon General's tool kit.[5]

When obtaining a complete family history, it is important to customize questions that are matched to each specific patient (**Boxes 1–3**).

Time should be taken to complete a thorough and detailed personal and family history at each patient's initial visit and this should be updated at every subsequent visit. Remembering that both personal and family history are not stagnant data points but are surrogate markers for potential risk that change with time is key.

Box 1
Personal history for a patient without cancer diagnosis

Age

Ethnicity (specifically Jewish or Ashkenazi Jewish ancestry)

Biopsy history/polyp history

History of previous genetic testing and date

Family member with known genetic mutation

CREATING AND UNDERSTANDING A PEDIGREE

With a family and personal history, clinicians can then either complete or interpret a pedigree. The Pedigree Standardization Task Force created the initial standardized pedigree nomenclature in 1995, and it was most recently updated in 2008.[6] This standardized nomenclature is considered the current standard of documentation of personal and family history (**Figs. 1–3**).[6]

GERMLINE TESTING AND THE ADVENT OF THE MULTIGENE PANEL

As previously discussed, hereditary cancers are related to single-gene mutations. With this knowledge, early genetic tests offered to patients tested only for a single or limited number of genes. Some of the early testing criteria used and familiar to general surgeons are *BRCA*pro, and Amsterdam and Bethesda criteria. With advancements in next-generation sequencing, multigene or multipanel tests have become more widely available. As data have become more robust, clinicians have come to realize that many patients carry genetic mutations that are considered unexpected for their clinical profiles. A recent study found that, of 1260 subjects with a Lynch-associated cancer that underwent a 25-gene panel test, 114 patients, or 9%, were found to have a Lynch mutation and 43 or 3.4% of patients had a non-Lynch mutation. Most strikingly, 15 patients, or 10% of mutation carriers, were found to have *BRCA*1 or *BRCA*2 mutations.[7] These findings seem to hold true even for a more diverse patient population.[8,9] In a large cohort of 23,179 patients referred for 30-gene multipanel testing, clinical mutations were identified in 192 individuals or 11.6% of patients. Interestingly, 21.7% of individuals with mutations did not meet current NCCN testing criteria.[10] A smaller study assessed 377 patients previously tested and found negative for *BRCA*1 and *BRCA*2. Retesting on a 25-gene panel found that 14 patients, or 3.7%, had a non-*BRCA*1 or *BRCA*2 deleterious mutation.[9] This finding highlights the risk of

Box 2
Personal history for a patient with cancer diagnosis

Age

Ethnicity (specifically Jewish or Ashkenazi ancestry)

Biopsy history/polyp history

Cancer sites, bilaterally if applicable, pathology, age at time of diagnosis, determine site of metastatic disease versus second primary cancer

History of previous genetic testing and date

Family member with known genetic mutation

Box 3
Family history for all patients

First-degree relatives: parents, children, and full siblings

Second-degree relatives: grandparents, aunts, uncles, nieces, nephews, grandchildren and half siblings

Third-degree relatives: great-grandparents, cousins, great-grandchildren, great-aunts, great-uncles
   Noting maternal or paternal for all of the above

If cancers identified: cancer sites, bilaterally if applicable, pathology, age at time of diagnosis
   Determine site of metastatic disease versus second primary cancer

Note any unknown cause of death

Note any early deaths

Note any surgery at young ages

Polyp history of relatives that have undergone colonoscopy

---

single-gene or limited-gene testing in that it does not account for overlap in hereditary cancer syndromes or variability in the presentation of hereditary cancer syndromes.[11,12] These limitations account for the recent increased use of multigene testing as well as opening the door for increased gene testing in the future.[13,14] For general surgeons to refer patients to a genetic counselor; offer testing themselves; or to understand single, limited, and most recently multigene panel testing, it is imperative they understand what genes are available for testing as well as associated risks and recommendations.

GENES

Although genes associated with hereditary cancer syndromes are numerous, general surgeons are advised to focus on those genes with established and accepted data as well as clinical care guidelines supported by the NCCN.[4] Using an already familiar resource can allow general surgeons to remain informed and up to date with consensus and professional organization recommendations without having to scour multiple data sources. The NCCN provides evidence-based risks associated with certain genes as well as providing clinical management recommendations.[4,11] These genes are considered to be clinically actionable. **Table 1** lists some clinically actionable genes present at the time of publication.[4,11]

TESTING RESULTS

Once a patient has been counseled on the option of genetic testing, ideally by a genetic counselor, and chooses to undergo testing (via either blood or sputum sample) results will be released within a few weeks. Expedited results can often be obtained if the patient is pending a surgical procedure. Possible results of single-gene, limited-gene, and multigene testing are limited but important for general surgeons to understand. Results are more complicated than just positive or negative. In general, with slight variation per testing company, results are reported in the simplest of terms as no mutation detected, variant of unknown significance (VUS) or positive for pathogenic mutation.

No mutation detected, although helpful, should not lull general surgeons into a false sense of security for their patients. A result is only as good as the data behind it. It was

Instructions:
— Key should contain all information relevant to interpretation of pedigree (eg. define fill/shading)
— For clinical (non-published) pedigrees include:
  a) name of proband/consultand
  b) family names/initials of relatives for identification, as appropriate
  c) name and title of person recording pedigree
  d) historian (person relaying family history information)
  e) date of intake/update
  f) reason for taking pedigree (eg. abnormal ultrasound, familial cancer, developmental delay, etc.)
  g) ancestry of both sides of family
— Recommended order of information placed below symbol (or to lower right)
  a) age; can note year of birth (eg. b.1978) and/or death (eg. d. 2007)
  b) evaluation (see Figure 4)
  c) pedigree number (eg. I-1, I-2, I-3)
— Limit identifying information to maintain confidentiality and privacy

	Male	Female	Gender not specified	Comments
1. Individual	b. 1925	30y	4 mo	Assign gender by phenotype (see text for disorders of sex development, etc.). Do not write age in symbol.
2. Affected individual				Key/legend used to define shading or other fill (eg. hatches, dots, etc.). Use only when individual is clinically affected.
				With ≥2 conditions, the individual's symbol can be partitioned accordingly, each segment shaded with a different fill and defined in legend.
3. Multiple individuals, number known	5	5	5	Number of siblings written inside symbol. (Affected individuals should not be grouped).
4. Multiple individuals, number unknown or unstated	n	n	n	"n" used in place of "?".
5. Deceased individual	d. 35	d. 4 mo	d. 60's	Indicate cause of death if known. Do not use a cross (†)to indicate death to avoid confusion with evaluation positive (+).
6. Consultand				Individual(s) seeking genetic counseling/ testing.
7. Proband	P	P		An affected family member coming to medical attention independent of other family members.
8.Stillbirth (SB)	SB 28 wk	SB 30 wk	SB 34 wk	Include gestational age and karyotype, if known.
9. Pregnancy (P)	LMP: 7/1/2007 47,XY,+21	20 wk 46,XX	P	Gestational age and karyotype below symbol. Light shading can be used for affected; define in key/legend.

Pregnancies not carried to term	Affected	Unaffected	
10. Spontaneous abortion (SAB)	17 wks female cystic hygroma	<10 wks	If gestational age/gender known, write below symbol. Key/legend used to define shading.
11. Termination of pregnancy (TOP)	18 wks 47,XY,+18		Other abbreviations (eg. TAB, VTOP) not used for sake of consistency.
12. Ectopic pregnancy (ECT)		ECT	Write ECT below symbol.

Fig. 1. Common pedigree symbols, definitions, and abbreviations. (*From* Bennett RL, French KS, Resta RG, et al. Standardized human pedigree nomenclature: update and assessment of the recommendations of the national society of genetic counselors. J Genet Couns. 2008; 17(5):424 – 433; with permission.)

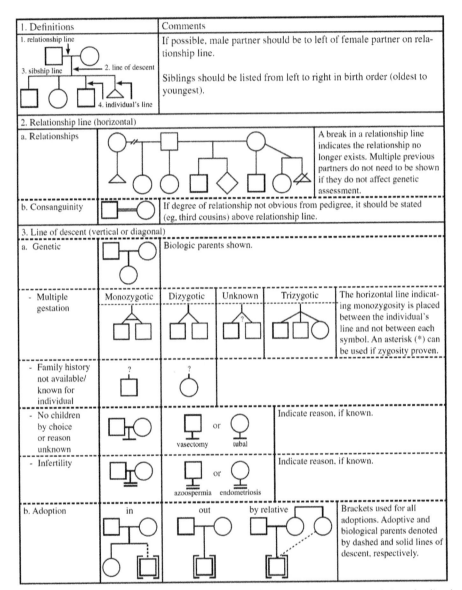

Fig. 2. Pedigree line definitions. (*From* Bennett RL, French KS, Resta RG, et al. Standardized human pedigree nomenclature: update and assessment of the recommendations of the national society of genetic counselors. J Genet Couns. 2008; 17(5):424 – 433; with permission.)

not long ago that a woman with a *BRCA* rearrangement would have been given a result of no mutation detected who now would be positive for a *BRCA* mutation. It is important to understand that a clinical profile may be related to a gene yet to be understood or realized. Using clinical judgment to still consider certain patients high risk even with a result of no mutation detected is an important concept.

A VUS is reported when an alteration in a gene sequence is detected but it is unknown whether that alteration is clinically significant. As the number of individuals,

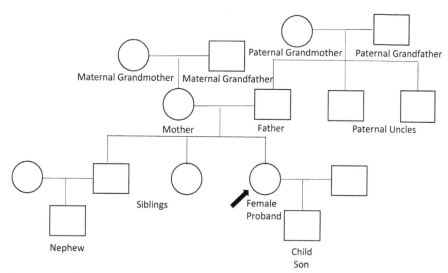

Fig. 3. Example pedigree. Proband - patient to whom genetic testing is being discussed (arrow).

and therefore genes, tested increases, so does the number of VUSs.[12] Over time and with more data points many VUSs will eventually be reclassified to either no mutation detected or positive for pathogenic mutation. A review of 1.45 million individuals tested showed that, of those with VUSs, 24.9% were reclassified in a median of 1.87 years; 91.2% were downgraded to benign or likely benign and 8.7% were upgraded to pathogenic or likely pathogenic.[15] It is important that practitioners do not make recommendations based on VUSs and do not treat patients as if they have a deleterious mutation but one based on personal/family history.

A result of positive for a pathogenic mutation is the most significant of results, leading general surgeons to better understand increased cancer development risk in individual patients. With that knowledge, general surgeons are able to discuss, treat, and refer patients based on expert surveillance/care recommendations such as those from the NCCN.[4] For patients with cancer, the finding of a positive mutation can, in some cases, lead to the opportunity for targeted surgical or medical therapy, such as a risk-reducing mastectomy or the use of PARP (poly-ADP ribose polymerase) inhibitors in patients with specific *BRCA*-positive breast cancers. A positive for a pathogenic mutation would also allow testing to be offered to at-risk relatives, with the goal being to improve outcomes to those with cancer and those without cancer, as well as to use health care resources in a more effective and efficient manner.

Cancer Specifics

Colorectal cancer

Colorectal cancer (CRC) is the third most common malignant tumor in the United States according to the American Cancer Society 2019 data.[16] As such, it is one of the most common cancers general surgeons encounter in daily practice. Studies have shown that approximately 30% of CRCs developed from genetic factors.[17] However, only 5% to 10% of colorectal cases related to inherited mutations are understood and fully or partially characterized.[18] The most common CRC syndromes that general surgeons encounter are hereditary nonpolyposis colorectal cancer (HNPCC), familial adenomatous polyposis (FAP), attenuated familial adenomatous polyposis,

Table 1
Clinically actionable genes and associated cancers

Gene and Associated Risks	Breast Cancer	Ovarian Cancer	Endometrial Cancer	Colorectal Cancer	Gastric Cancer	Pancreatic Cancer	HB Cancer	Small Bowel Cancer	Melanoma	Prostate Cancer	Renal and Urinary Tract Cancer	Endocrine Cancer	Brain Cancer	Other
APC	–	–	–	X	X	X	X	X	–	–	–	X	–	–
ATM	X	–	–	X	–	X	–	–	–	–	–	–	–	–
BARD1	X	–	–	–	–	–	–	–	–	–	–	–	–	–
BLM	–	–	–	X	–	–	–	–	–	–	X	–	–	–
BMPRIA	–	–	–	X	X	–	–	–	–	–	–	–	–	–
BRCA1	X	X	–	–	–	X	–	–	X	X	–	–	–	–
BRCA2	X	X	–	–	–	X	–	–	X	X	–	–	–	–
BRIP1	–	X	–	–	–	–	–	–	–	–	–	–	–	–
CDH1	X	–	–	–	X	–	–	–	–	–	–	–	–	–
CDKN2A	–	–	–	–	–	X	–	–	X	–	–	–	–	–
CHEK2	X	–	–	X	–	–	–	–	–	–	–	–	–	–
EPCAM	X	X	X	X	X	–	X	X	–	X	X	–	–	X
GREM1	–	–	–	X	–	–	–	–	–	–	–	–	–	–
MEN1	–	–	–	–	–	–	–	–	–	–	–	X	–	–
MLH1	X	X	X	X	X	X	X	X	–	X	X	–	X	X

Gene												
MSH2	X	X	X	X	X	X	—	X	X	X	—	X	X
MSH6	X	X	X	X	X	—	X	X	X	—	X	X	—
MUTYH	—	X	X	X	—	—	—	X	—	—	—	—	—
NBN	X	—	—	—	—	—	—	—	—	—	—	X	—
NF1	X	—	—	—	—	X	X	—	—	—	X	X	X
PALB2	X	—	—	X	X	—	—	X	—	—	X	—	—
PMS2	—	X	X	X	—	—	—	—	—	—	—	—	—
POLD1	—	—	X	—	—	—	—	—	—	—	—	—	—
POLE	—	—	X	—	—	—	—	—	X	—	—	—	—
PTEN	X	—	X	X	—	—	—	—	—	X	X	X	X
RAD51C	—	X	—	—	—	—	—	—	—	—	—	—	—
RAD51D	—	X	—	—	—	—	—	—	—	—	—	—	—
RET	—	—	—	—	—	—	—	—	—	—	X	—	—
SDHB	—	—	—	—	—	—	—	—	—	—	X	—	—
SDHD	—	—	—	—	—	—	—	—	—	—	X	—	—
SMAD4	—	—	X	X	—	—	—	—	—	—	—	—	—
STK11	X	X	X	X	X	X	—	X	—	—	—	X	X
TP53	X	—	—	—	—	—	—	—	—	—	—	X	X
VHL	—	—	—	—	X	X	—	—	—	X	—	X	—

Not all associated cancers have clinical recommendations.
Abbreviation: HB, hepatobiliary.

and MUTYH-associated polyposis. For each of these syndromes, it is important for clinicians to partner with gastroenterology colleagues to better identify, treat, and surveil their patients.

Hereditary nonpolyposis colorectal cancer

HNPCC, otherwise known as Lynch syndrome (LS), is an autosomal dominant disorder with a germline mutation in mismatch repair (MMR) genes (MLH1, MSH2, MSH6, PMS2, EPCAM). LS is characterized with increased lifetime risk of developing a multitude of cancers. In patients with LS, the risk of colon cancer is greater than 52% depending on specific gene mutation. LS is also related to an increased risk of developing endometrial, ovarian, urinary tract, bladder, gastric, small bowel, hepatobiliary tract, pancreas, and brain/central nervous system cancer.[4] It is impossible for general surgeons to keep abreast of literature related to updates on individual genes. Therefore, relying on consensus guidelines such as those published by the NCCN can be helpful.[4] Using guidelines such as the Amsterdam I and II criteria (**Box 4** from Guidelines on Genetic Evaluation and Management of Lynch Syndrome: A Consensus Statement by the US Multi-Society Task Force on Colorectal Cancer), surgeons can identify patients meeting clinical criteria for LS.[19] All patients meeting these guidelines should be offered germline genetic testing.[4,19,20]

In addition to traditional paper guidelines, there are computational models such as MMRpro and PREMM models that have been found to be equivalent, if not superior, for detection of high-risk patients.[21,22] Using both guidelines and prediction resources, general surgeons can provide comprehensive risk assessment.

For patients with CRC, the Revised Bethesda Guidelines (**Box 5** from Guidelines on Genetic Evaluation and Management of Lynch Syndrome: A Consensus Statement by the US Multi-Society Task Force on Colorectal Cancer) provide direction as to which patients should be offered genetic testing.[4,19,20,23]

For those patients with sufficient tumor, the NCCN advises universal testing using either immunohistochemistry or microsatellite instability testing.[4,24] This approach is one that general surgeons are advised to discuss with their departments of pathology and cancer committees.

Management of patients with LS are aimed at risk reduction, including, but not limited to, increased frequency of annual examinations, surveillance testing, and in some cases prophylactic surgery. Because these guidelines are updated regularly,

---

Box 4
Amsterdam I and II criteria for diagnosis of hereditary nonpolyposis colorectal cancer

Amsterdam I criteria
1. Three or more relatives with histologically verified colorectal cancer, 1 of which is a first-degree relative of the other 2. FAP should be excluded.
2. Two or more generations with colorectal cancer.
3. One or more colorectal cancer cases diagnosed before the age of 50 years.

Amsterdam II criteria
1. Three or more relatives with histologically verified HNPCC-associated cancer (colorectal cancer; cancer of the endometrium, small bowel, ureter, or renal pelvis), 1 of which is a first-degree relative of the other 2. FAP should be excluded.
2. Cancer involving at least 2 generations.
3. One or more cancer cases diagnosed before the age of 50 years.

From Giardiello FM, Allen JI, Axibund JE, et al. Guidelines on genetic evaluation and management of Lynch syndrome: a consensus statement by the US Multi-Society Task Force on colorectal cancer. Gastroenterology. 2014;147(2):502 – 526; with permission.

Box 5
Revised Bethesda guidelines

1. CRC diagnosed at younger than 50 years.

2. Presence of synchronous or metachronous CRC or other LS-associated tumors.[a]

3. CRC with microsatellite instability testing–high pathologic-associated features (Crohn-like lymphocytic reaction, mucinous/signet cell differentiation, or medullary growth pattern) diagnosed in an individual younger than 60 years old.

4. Patient with CRC and CRC or LS-associated tumor[a] diagnosed in at least 1 first-degree relative younger than 50 years old.

5. Patient with CRC and CRC or LS-associated tumor[a] at any age in 2 first-degree or second-degree relatives.

[a] LS-associated tumors include tumor of the colorectum, endometrium, stomach, ovary, pancreas, ureter, renal pelvis, biliary tract, brain, small bowel, sebaceous glands, and keratoacanthomas.
From Giardiello FM, Allen JI, Axibund JE, et al. Guidelines on genetic evaluation and management of Lynch syndrome: a consensus statement by the US Multi-Society Task Force on colorectal cancer. Gastroenterology. 2014;147(2):502 – 526; with permission.

---

it is important for general surgeons to reference updated consensus guidelines such as those published by the NCCN.[4]

Familial adenomatous polyposis, attenuated familial adenomatous polyposis

FAP and attenuated familial adenomatous polyposis (AFAP) are autosomal dominant disorders related to a germline mutation in the APC genes. FAP is characterized by the development of more than 100 polyps, often even hundreds to thousands, starting in childhood. The risk of malignant degeneration is almost 100% by age 50 years. This hereditary disorder also has an increased risk for the development of duodenal cancer, small bowel cancer, thyroid cancer, hepatoblastoma, and medulloblastoma.[4] FAP also increases the risk of nonmalignant conditions, namely osteomas, dental anomalies, lesions of the retina, cutaneous lesions, and desmoid tumors. In patients found to have a deleterious mutation in the APC gene, the general surgeon's priority is to evaluate the colon, offering a proctocolectomy or colectomy to those affected. A total proctocolectomy with ileal pouch–anal anastomosis is the preferred surgery endorsed by the American Society of Colon and Rectal Surgeons.[25] Guidelines, such as those published by the NCCN, for surveillance and care of patients with the FAP mutation should begin after colectomy.[4] For unaffected patients with an APC mutation, recommendations are for colonoscopy to begin as young as 10 years of age.[4] It is for this reason that general surgeons should advise patients with an APC mutation who have children to discuss the matter with the child's pediatrician to avoid delay in both diagnosis and possible treatments.

AFAP is also related to the development of polyps but fewer (<100) and/or later onset of polyp development. Management of these individuals depends on tumor burden and can range from frequent colonoscopy and endoscopic removal of polyps to undergoing surgical resection. A total abdominal colectomy with ileorectal anastomosis is the preferred surgery endorsed by the American Society of Colon and Rectal Surgeons.[25] Patients with AFAP are also at an increased risk of developing thyroid cancer, and consensus guidelines should be followed once a diagnosis of mutation is made.[4]

Germline genetic testing for an APC mutation should be recommended for patients that have a personal history of 20 or more adenomas in a lifetime, known as polyposis syndrome, in a family member or a personal history of extracolonic manifestations.[4,25]

MUTYH-associated polyposis

Unlike the previous polyposis syndromes, MUTYH-associated polyposis is an autosomal recessive disorder from a germline mutation in the MYH gene. The same recommendations for germline genetic testing apply, including testing people with a personal history of 20 or more adenomas in a lifetime, or known polyposis syndrome in a family member.[4] With the increased use of limited gene or gene panel testing, often all polyposis syndromes are tested for simultaneously. Management of these individuals depends on tumor burden and can range from frequent colonoscopy and endoscopic removal of polyps to undergoing surgical resection. MUTYH-associated polyposis has a later age of onset so, for patients with an MYH gene mutation, screening is advised to begin in their 20s. MUTYH-associated polyposis also carries an increased risk of development of duodenal cancer and, as such, guidelines should be followed for appropriate surveillance.[4,25]

BREAST CANCER

Breast cancer is the most common malignant tumor diagnosed in women in the United States according to the American Cancer Society 2019 data.[16] Many general surgeons actively treat patients with breast cancer, but all will encounter patients with past personal history and/or family history of breast cancer. Between 5% and 10% of all breast cancers and 36% of breast cancers in women less than 35 years of age are thought to be related to an underlying genetic mutation.[26,27]

The most frequent mutations encountered by general surgeons that increase breast cancer susceptibility include BRCA1, BRCA2, PALB2, TP53, PTEN, and STK111.

For years, practitioners have been guided by the NCCN guidelines to determine what subgroup of patients should be offered genetic testing.[4] This paradigm has recently been challenged by research published in December 2018. The results showed no statistical difference in positive for a pathogenic mutation in women with breast cancer who met and those who did not meet NCCN guidelines.[28] With evidence that nearly half of patients with breast cancer with a mutation are missed by current guidelines, The American Society of Breast Surgeons has taken immediate action. They released Consensus Guidelines on Genetic Testing for Hereditary Breast Cancer in July 2019.[29] These guidelines recommend that genetic testing should be made available to all patients with a personal history of breast cancer and that all patients who had genetic testing previously may benefit from updated testing.[29]

This recommendation dramatically simplifies general surgeons' decisions of whom, at minimum, to offer and discuss testing with[4]:

Any patient with breast cancer, current or historical
A known mutation in a cancer susceptibility gene within the family
A first-degree or second-degree relative with any of the following:
- Breast cancer at age less than or equal to 45 years
- Male breast cancer
- Ovarian cancer, pancreatic cancer, metastatic prostate
- Two or more breast cancer primaries in a single individual
- Two or more individuals with breast cancer on the same side of family with at least 1 diagnosed at less than or equal to 50 years
- Same-side family history of 3 or more of the following: breast cancer, sarcoma, adrenocortical carcinoma, brain cancer, leukemia, colon cancer, endometrial

cancer, thyroid cancer, kidney cancer, gastric cancer, dermatologic manifestations, macrocephaly or gastrointestinal hamartomatous polyps, ovarian sex chord tumors, pancreatic cancer, testicular Sertoli cell tumors, and childhood skin pigmentation

Management of patients with a genetic mutation for hereditary breast cancer can include, but is not limited to, increased frequency of annual examinations, use of alternative radiological imaging for surveillance, risk-reducing surgery, and chemoprevention.[30] These guidelines are updated regularly but, in general, are more aggressive with a higher penetrant gene than with a lower penetrate gene. It is important for general surgeons to reference updated guidelines such as those published by the NCCN.[4]

BRCA1 and BRCA2 Genes: Hereditary Breast and Ovarian Cancer Syndrome

Hereditary breast and ovarian cancer syndrome is the name given to the constellation of cancer risk associated with the BRCA1 and BRCA2 germline mutations and accounts for 15% to 20% of all hereditary breast cancers.[31] BRCA1 and BRCA2 are inherited in an autosomal dominant fashion but both show dramatic variation in penetrance. The risk of developing breast cancer by age 80 years is 72% with a BRCA1 mutation or 69% with a BRCA2 mutation.[32] Hereditary breast and ovarian cancer syndrome is also related to an increased risk of developing male breast cancer, ovarian cancer, prostate cancer, and pancreas cancer, as well as melanoma. Risk of development differs on specific BRCA1 and BRCA2 gene mutation; for example, the risk of developing ovarian cancer by age 80 years is 44% with a BRCA1 mutation or 17% with a BRCA2 mutation.[32]

PALB2 Gene

PALB2 mutations are the most common of the non-BRCA mutations. Biallelic mutations are present in a subset of patients with Fanconi anemia but, in addition, a pathogenic mutation is related to hereditary risk for developing breast cancer. Breast cancer risk increases with age, with a 14% risk by age 50 years and a 35% risk by age 70 years.[33] Although there are some studies that increase concern for increased risk of pancreatic and/or ovarian cancer, there are no expert guidelines.

TP53 Gene and Li-Fraumeni Syndrome

Although TP53 somatic mutations are related to increased risks of many cancers, Li-Fraumeni syndrome is the only cancer syndrome related to a hereditary mutation. It accounts for approximately 1% of all hereditary breast cancers. Patients with Li-Fraumeni have a nearly 100% risk of developing cancer: breast cancer, soft tissue sarcoma, osteosarcoma, colon cancer, adrenocortical carcinoma, and brain cancer. The cumulative risk of developing female breast cancer by age 70 years is 54% and for men 22%.[34]

PTEN Gene

Inherited germline mutations in PTEN are also called Cowden syndrome: development of benign tumors as well as multiple cancers. Individuals with Cowden syndrome develop many cancers, including, but not limited to, breast cancer, endometrial cancer, thyroid cancer, and brain cancer. Fifty percent of patients with Cowden syndrome develop breast cancer.[35]

SK111 Gene

Inherited germline mutations in STK111 are otherwise known as Peutz-Jeghers syndrome. It is inherited in an autosomal dominant fashion. It is related to the development of mucocutaneous pigmentation, colonic polyps, gastrointestinal cancer, and breast and ovarian cancers. There is a 31% risk of developing breast cancer by age 60 years.[36]

As general surgeons encounter these mutations and others, it is important to use expert guidelines such as those updated regularly by the NCCN.[4]

GASTRIC CANCER
CDH1 Gene and Hereditary Diffuse Gastric Cancer

There were 27,510 new cases of gastric cancer diagnosed in the United States last year.[16] A subset of these patients have what is referred to as hereditary diffuse gastric cancer, a hereditary syndrome related to a germline mutation in the CDH1 gene. This mutation is related to the development of a diffuse-type gastric cancer, often at very young ages.[37] The NCCN and hereditary diffuse gastric cancer consensus guidelines recommend screening if[4,38]:

- Two or more gastric cancers, with 1 being diffuse gastric cancer at less than 50 years of age
- Three confirmed cases of diffuse gastric cancer regardless of age in first-degree or second-degree relative
- Personal history of diffuse gastric cancer at less than 40 years of age
- Personal or family history of diffuse gastric cancer and lobular breast cancer, 1 at less than 50 years of age

In the largest reported case series of those affected by a CDH1 mutation, the risk of developing gastric cancer by age 80 years was 70% for men and 56% for women. CDH1 is also related to an increased risk of developing lobular breast cancer.[39] All at-risk relatives should be tested starting at age 14 years, because most investigators advocate gastrectomy in mutation carriers by age 16 years.[40]

AT-RISK RELATIVES

General surgeons can only be responsible for the care of the patients they are treating, but it is important to recommend (and document that recommendation) that patients with any genetic mutation share their results with all first-degree and second-degree relatives. For those patients of childbearing age, it is important to communicate the risk of passing the mutation to their children. Patients should be encouraged to speak to their obstetricians before conception and they may consider referral to a tertiary care center for preimplantation testing.

DISCLOSURE

The author has nothing to disclose.

REFERENCES

1. Lu KH, Wood ME, Daniels M, et al. American Society of Clinical Oncology expert statement: collection and use of a cancer family history for oncology providers. J Clin Oncol 2014;32:833–40.
2. Delaney SK, Hultner ML, Jacob HJ, et al. Toward clinical genomics in everyday medicine: perspectives and recommendations. Expert Rev Mol Diagn 2016;16: 521–32.
3. Riley BD, Culver JO, Skrynia C, et al. Essential elements of genetic cancer risk assessment, counseling, and testing: updated recommendations of the National Society of Genetic Counselors. J Genet Couns 2012;21:151–61.

4. National Comprehensive Cancer Network. 2019. Available at: www.ncc.org. Accessed April 8, 2020.

5. My Family Health Portrait A tool from the Surgeon General. 2019. Available at: https://phgkb.cdc.gov/FHH/html/index.htm. Accessed April 8, 2020.

6. Bennett RL, French KS, Resta RG, et al. Standardized human pedigree nomenclature: update and assessment of the recommendations of the National Society of Genetic Counselors. J Genet Couns 2008;17:424–33.

7. Yurgelun M, Allen B, Kaldate RR, et al. Multi-Gene Panel Testing in Patients Suspected to Have Lynch Syndrome. Poster Presented at American Society of Clinical Oncology ASCO Annual Meeting, Chicago (IL), May 30 – June 3, 2014.

8. Ricker C, Culvera JO, Lowstuter K, et al. Increased yield of actionable mutations using multi-gene panels to assess hereditary cancer susceptibility in an ethnically diverse clinical cohort. Cancer Genet 2016;209:130–7.

9. Allen B. Prevalence of Gene Mutations Among Hereditary Breast and Ovarian Cancer Patients Using a 25-Gene Panel. Poster Presented at Annual Clinical Genetics ACMG Meeting, Nashville (TN), March 25-29, 2014.

10. Neben CL, Zimmer AD, Stedden W, et al. Multi-gene panel testing of 23,179 individuals for hereditary cancer risk identifies pathogenic variant carriers missed by current genetic testing guidelines. J Mol Diagn 2019;21:646–57.

11. Okur V, Chung WK. The impact of hereditary cancer gene panels on clinical care and lessons learned. Cold Spring Harb Mol Case Stud 2017;3(6) [pii:a002154].

12. Domchek SM, Bradbury A, Garber JE, et al. Multiplex genetic testing for cancer susceptibility: out on the high wire without a net? J Clin Oncol 2013;31:1267–70.

13. Susswein LR, Marshall ML, Nusbaum R, et al. Pathogenic and likely pathogenic variant prevalence among the first 10,000 patients referred for next-generation cancer panel testing. Genet Med 2016;18:823–32.

14. Yurgelun MB, Allen B, Kaldate RR, et al. Identification of a variety of mutations in cancer predisposition genes in patients with suspected lynch syndrome. Gastroenterology 2015;149:604–13.

15. Mersch J, Brown N, Pirzadeh-Miller S, et al. Prevalence of variant reclassification following hereditary cancer genetic testing. JAMA 2018;320:1266–74.

16. American Cancer Society Cancer Facts and Figures 2019. 2019. Available at: https://www.cancer.org/content/dam/cancer-org/research/cancer-facts-and-statistics/annual-cancer-facts-and-figures/2019/cancer-facts-and-figures-2019.pdf. Accessed April 8, 2020.

17. Lichtenstein P, Holm NV, Verkasalo PK, et al. Environmental and heritable factors in the causation of cancer–analyses of cohorts of twins from Sweden, Denmark, and Finland. N Engl J Med 2000;343:78–85.

18. Jasperson KW, Tuohy TM, Neklason DW, et al. Hereditary and familial colon cancer. Gastroenterology 2010;138:2044–58.

19. Giardiello FM, Allen JI, Axibund JE, et al, US Multi-Society Task Force on Colorectal Cancer. Guidelines on genetic evaluation and management of lynch syndrome: a consensus statement by the US multi-society task force on colorectal cancer. Am J Gastroenterol 2014;147:502–26.

20. Syngal S, Brand RE, Church JM, et al. ACG clinical guideline: Genetic testing and management of hereditary gastrointestinal cancer syndromes. Am J Gastroenterol 2015;110:223–63.

21. Balmaña J, Balaguer F, Castellví-Bel S, et al, Gastrointestinal Oncology Group of the Spanish Gastroenterological Association. Comparison of predictive models, clinical criteria and molecular tumor screening for the identification of patients

with Lynch syndrome in a population-based cohort of colorectal cancer patients. J Med Genet 2008;45:557–63.

22. Monzon JG, Cremin C, Armstrong L, et al. Validation of predictive models for germline mutations in DNA mismatch repair genes in colorectal cancer. Int J Cancer 2010;126:930–9.

23. Stoffel EM, Koeppe E, Everett J, et al. Germline genetic features of young individuals with colorectal cancer. Gastroenterology 2018;154:897–905.e1.

24. Moreira L, Balaguer F, Lindor N, et al. Identification of lynch syndrome among patients with colorectal cancer. J Am Med Assoc 2012;308:1555–65.

25. Herzig D, Hardiman K, Weiser M, et al. The American Society of Colon and Rectal Surgeons clinical practice guidelines for the management of inherited polyposis syndromes. Dis Colon Rectum 2017;60:881–94.

26. Goldberg JI, Borgen PI. Breast cancer susceptibility testing: past, present and future. Expert Rev Anticancer Ther 2006;6:1205–14.

27. Claus EB, Risch N, Thompson WD. Genetic analysis of breast cancer in the cancer and steroid hormone study. Am J Hum Genet 1991;48:232–42.

28. Beitsh PD, Whitmorth PW, Hughes K, et al. Under diagnosis of hereditary breast cancer: are genetic testing guidelines a tool or an obstacle? J Clin Oncol 2018;37:453–60.

29. Manahan ER, Kuerer HM, Sebastian M, et al. Consensus guidelines on genetic' testing for hereditary breast cancer from the American Society of Breast Surgeons. Ann Surg Oncol 2019;26:3025–31.

30. Krontiras H, Farmer M, Whatley J. Breast cancer genetics and indications for prophylactic mastectomy. Surg Clin North Am 2018;98:677–85.

31. Balmain A, Gray J, Ponder B. The genetics and genomics of cancer. Nat Genet 2003;33 Suppl:238–44.

32. Kuchenbaecker KB, Hopper JL, Barnes DR, et al. Risks of breast, ovarian, and contralateral breast cancer for *BRCA*1 and *BRCA*2 mutation carriers. J Am Med Assoc 2017;317:2402–16.

33. Antoniou AC, Casadei S, Heikkinen T, et al. Breast-cancer risk in families with mutations in PALB2. N Engl J Med 2014;371:497–506.

34. Mai PL, Best AF, Peters JA, et al. Risks of first and subsequent cancers among TP53 mutation carriers in the National Cancer Institute Li-Fraumeni syndrome cohort. Cancer 2016;122:3673–81.

35. Starink TM, van der Veen JP, Arwert F, et al. The Cowden syndrome: a clinical and genetic study in 21 patients. Clin Genet 1986;29:222–33.

36. Hearle N, Schumacher V, Menko FH, et al. Frequency and spectrum of cancers in the Peutz-Jeghers syndrome. Clin Cancer Res 2006;12:3209–15.

37. Seevaratnam R, Coburn N, Cardoso R, et al. A systematic review of the indications for genetic testing and prophylactic gastrectomy among patients with hereditary diffuse gastric cancer. Gastric Cancer 2012;15 Suppl 1:153–63.

38. Fitzgerald RC, Hardwick R, Huntsman D, et al. Hereditary diffuse gastric cancer: updated consensus guidelines for clinical management and directions for future research. J Med Genet 2010;47:436–44.

39. Hansford S, Kaurah P, Li-Chang H, et al. Hereditary diffuse gastric cancer syndrome CDH1 mutations and beyond. JAMA Oncol 2015;1:23–32.

40. Moslim MA, Heald B, Tu C, et al. Early genetic counseling and detection of CDH1 mutation in asymptomatic carriers improves survival in hereditary diffuse gastric cancer. Surgery 2018;164:754–9.

Imaging and Interventional Radiology for Cancer Management

Benjamin J. Pomerantz, MD

KEYWORDS

- Radiology • Interventional radiology and oncology • MRI • Computed tomography
- Ultrasound

KEY POINTS

- Advanced imaging is central to the appropriate management of patients with cancer.
- Imaging is used for diagnosis, staging, and evaluating treatment response.
- Interventional oncology is an emerging field offering many new and novel cancer treatments.

IMAGING

Worldwide, medical imaging is used as both a screening tool for various forms of cancer as well as the initial investigative modality when cancer is suspected. Many societal guidelines include imaging recommendations for cancer screening, most notably for breast and lung cancer. With the significant advancements in medical imaging over the past 20 years, imaging has become more sensitive, allowing earlier and more accurate diagnosis, ultimately leading to improved outcomes in patients with cancer.[1]

Not only is imaging essential for the detection and diagnosis of a neoplastic process, imaging is essential to determine the appropriate therapy or therapies for the patient. In addition, imaging is crucial for the evaluation of treatment response and for posttreatment surveillance. Cross-sectional imaging, computed tomography (CT), and MRI, are the most common modalities used for initial evaluation or in certain instances, screening.

The National Comprehensive Cancer Network (NCCN) publishes guidelines for the treatment of cancer based on the site of the cancer. In addition, NCCN guidelines are available for the detection, prevention, and risk reduction of cancer that are also based on the location of the cancer. NCCN guidelines provide detailed decision-making

Department of Radiology, Vascular and Interventional Radiology, University of Michigan, University Hospital, UH B1 D530A, 1500 E. Medical Center Drive, SPC 5030, Ann Arbor, MI 48109-5030, USA
E-mail address: pomerabe@med.umich.edu

Surg Clin N Am 100 (2020) 499–506
https://doi.org/10.1016/j.suc.2020.02.002
surgical.theclinics.com
0039-6109/20/© 2020 Elsevier Inc. All rights reserved.

algorithms based on scientific evidence that is applicable to over 97% of cancers.[2] The guidelines are continuously updated and revised as new evidence becomes available for the diagnosis, treatment, and management of patients diagnosed with cancer. An integral component of the NCCN guidelines is imaging. The NCCN guidelines contain imaging appropriate use criteria (NCCN imaging AUC), which consist of recommendations for screening, diagnosis, staging, and treatment response related to cancer. The NCCN imaging AUC are available via a Web-based interface designed to guide clinicians through the virtual maze of imaging studies available with recommendations to accurately diagnose, stage, and treat patients with malignancies.

Virtually all clinical practice guidelines for the evaluation of patients with suspected or confirmed malignancies rely on the extensive use of imaging. Plain film radiography, ultrasound (US), CT, MRI, and functional imaging using various radioisotopes are included in the NCCN imaging AUC. In addition, research is being conducted with the goal of further characterizing tumors using radiomics. Radiomics combines artificial intelligence with large datasets, which may render a biopsy unnecessary. Each imaging modality has inherent advantages and disadvantages that need to be taken into account when trying to determine what form of imaging will give you the most information in a single examination. It is very common that multiple types of imaging are necessary to completely evaluate patients with suspected malignancies.

RADIOGRAPHIC IMAGING

Radiography-based imaging systems have been central to screening, evaluation, diagnosis, and surveillance of oncologic patients. With the implementation of digital radiography and picture archiving and communication systems have streamlined the use, sharing, and evaluation of images. Computed radiography and digital radiography (CR and DR) are the digital equivalents of plain film radiography. CR and DR are predominantly used to evaluate structures with relatively increased density, that is, calcium-containing tissues, and have the ability to characterize bony lesions including lytic, sclerotic, and blastic processes. In addition, calcified pleural plaques and nodal calcifications are easily identified with CR and DR.

Mammographic systems also use X-rays to image breast tissue. The introduction and implementation of digital-based mammographic imaging have resulted in decreasing patient dose, increasing the sensitivity of the examination and allowing computer-assisted detection to aid radiologists in image analysis.[3] Technological advances have led to the widespread adoption of digital tomosynthesis. Tomosynthesis uses multiple images taken from different projections, which are then compiled to make a 3D image of the breast for review.[4] This technology increases the sensitivity and specificity of mammography. Screening and diagnostic mammography are the standard imaging studies for the evaluation of breast cancer.

COMPUTED TOMOGRAPHY

CT imaging systems are currently in widespread uses throughout the United States with an estimated 42.64 CT scanners per 1,000,000 people.[5] Advances in both hardware and software have made CT scanning extremely fast, while providing exquisite soft tissue detail in a noninvasive fashion. Powerful postprocessing software is available to allow manipulation of the dataset to further improve analysis by enhancing areas of interest. CT imaging is beginning to be used as a screening tool for lung cancer as recommended by the United States Preventive Services Task Force in a certain subset of patients who use tobacco.[6] **Fig. 1.**

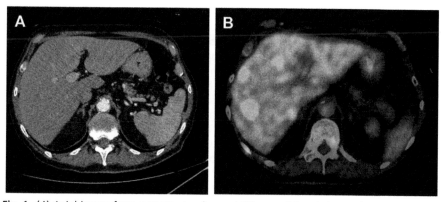

Fig. 1. (*A*) Axial image from a contrast-enhanced CT scan of the abdomen in a patient with lung cancer with liver metastases. (*B*) Axial PET-CT image from the same patient showing multiple areas of increased activity corresponding to hepatic metastases, not well seen on contrast-enhanced scan.

The current generation of CT scanners use multidetector arrays, up to 640 and counting, with a fan-shaped X-ray beam for image acquisition, giving the ability to cover large volumes of tissue in a single rotation. The X-ray source and detectors rotate around the patient while the gantry and patient are moving along the z axis, resulting in spiral or helical imaging. Data are gathered based on the attenuation the X-ray beam by the tissues. Complex computer algorithms create images from the data acquired during the scan. Technologic advances have made CT scanning extremely fast allowing 4D imaging. Powerful computers and software permit the manipulation of the acquired data and postprocessing to create highly detailed images including 3D reconstruction of the area of interest.

Advantages of CT scanning include image acquisition speed, widespread availability, postprocessing capabilities, high spatial resolution and high tissue contrast. Disadvantages of CT scanning include exposure to ionizing radiation, and the need for iodinated contrast, which carries the risk of nephrotoxicity and allergic reactions. In addition, metallic implants may cause significant streak artifact reducing the sensitivity of the examination. CT is also well suited for guiding interventional procedures.

MRI

MRI is a powerful tool used to characterize biologic tissue by using strong magnetic fields and radiofrequency (RF) energy to generate images. The physics behind MRI is beyond the scope of this article. However, it is important to have some background to apply MRI to clinical practice. This section provides a gross oversimplification of MRI but is necessary to understand the images.

MRI is based on atomic nuclei, namely hydrogen or ^1H most abundantly in water. It is helpful to think of atomic particles as "spinning" around a central axis, similar to a top. As the particles spin around its axis, a static gravitational field, Earth's gravity, acts on the particle resulting in perturbation of the axis around which the particle is spinning, causing the axis to deflect into a circular motion akin to a spinning top beginning to wobble. The circular motion of the central axis is known as precession. Particles with an odd number of protons will precess, which generates a magnetic "moment" with north and south poles, analogous to a bar magnet with north and south poles. It is this magnetic moment produced by spinning protons, ^{1}H, that is used to generate the images.[7] At a basal state the protons are freely precessing randomly. When a strong magnetic field is applied by an MRI magnet, the nuclei align with this magnetic field. This is followed by the application of an RF pulse perpendicular to the axis of the magnetic field causing the nuclei to come out of alignment with the magnetic field. When the RF pulse stops, the nuclei realign themselves with the magnetic field, returning to equilibrium. During the return to equilibrium or relaxation, the protons emit a small signal (RF energy). The signal emitted during the relaxation phase is detected using a receiver or coil. Complex computing and mathematical formulas are used to process the data to construct images. The varying amount of water or protons produce the contrast between tissues on MR images. MRI sequences differ by manipulating the magnetic field, RF pulses, and varying the timing of data acquisition.[7]

MRI produces images with extremely high soft tissue contrast making it well suited for oncologic imaging. Numerous imaging sequences are used to further characterize soft tissue lesions based on different characteristics[7] (**Fig. 2**). Certain types of cancer have such a characteristic appearance on MRI that a biopsy may not be necessary. In addition, there is no exposure to ionizing radiation and no iodinated contrast material is required. Gadolinium-based contrast agents are used as an adjunct to MRI and are generally not a concern with regard to patient allergies. These contrast agents are associated with nephrogenic systemic fibrosis (NSF), a rare fibrosing disease involving the skin and often internal organs occurring in patients with renal insufficiency or renal failure who have received gadolinium contrast agents. These agents are contraindicated in this subset of patients. Investigators continue to create imaging sequences to obviate the need for IV contrast. MR images require interpretation by radiologists familiar with the modality.

Although MRI is widely used for oncologic imaging there are several disadvantages and drawbacks. MRI equipment is often very expensive but this is decreasing with advances in technology. Image acquisition time can be lengthy and is sensitive to patient motion. MRI scanners are not suitable for patients with claustrophobia or for patients with certain metallic implants. In addition, MRI does not evaluate compact bone or calcified lesions.

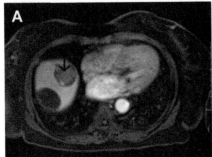 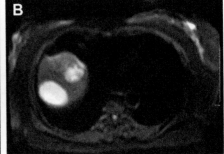

Fig. 2. (*A*) Contrast-enhanced MRI of the abdomen showing 2 right lobe liver lesions. Patchy enhancement of the anterior lesion (*black arrow*) with no enhancement of the posterior lesion. (*B*). Axial diffusion-weighted image of the same patient showing diffusion restriction in both lesions. Diffusion restriction combined with contrast enhancement are characteristic of tumors, in this case hepatocellular carcinoma. The posterior lesion is a simple hepatic cyst.

ULTRASOUND IMAGING

US imaging is one of the most common diagnostic imaging modalities used in current day practice. US is noninvasive, fast, relatively inexpensive, and safe. However, it is only suitable for more superficial soft tissue structures and is operator dependent. Contrast-enhanced ultrasound (CEUS) may be used as an adjunct to further characterize soft tissue lesions including lesion perfusion. CEUS uses intravenous microbubble contrast combined with dedicated imaging processing software to evaluate lesions. This technique has shown the most promise in evaluating liver masses.[8] The greatest strength of US is when it is used for guidance for interventional procedures.

RADIOPHARMACEUTICAL IMAGING

Nuclear medicine has been integral in oncologic imaging for decades and may be considered functional imaging in that this form of imaging often involves incorporation of the radiopharmaceutical into a metabolic pathway followed by imaging. Radiopharmaceutical imaging provides more of a physiologic or functional image as opposed to an image with fine anatomic detail. Numerous gamma-emitting isotopes are available and are chosen depending on the area of interest. Using a disease-specific target, focal uptake in the location of the disease is possible. Patient management often relies on this form of imaging, which also may predict response to treatment.[9]

In the most basic form, a radiopharmaceutical is administered followed by imaging using a gamma camera. This type of imaging produces only 2D images with poor spatial resolution. Three-dimensional images are obtained by rotating the detector around the patient during image acquisition and are known as single-photon emission computerized tomography images.

PET imaging has become the standard for oncologic imaging.[9] PET uses the radiopharmaceutical [^{18}F]fluorodeoxyglucose (FDG), which is beta emitter for imaging. FDG is a glucose analog that accumulates in metabolically active tissues, such as tumors that have an overexpression of membrane transport proteins.[9] **Fig. 3**. Several additional radiopharmaceuticals are available and are used for PET imaging depending on the biology of the target tissue. PET imaging suffers from poor spatial resolution and the inability to precisely localize lesions within a patient's anatomy. By coregistering the PET images with CT images, spatial resolution and the ability to localize lesions is greatly improved. Research is being conducted in an attempt to combine MR and PET images to take advantage of the ability of MRI to visualize soft tissue lesions and the ability of PET to determine metabolic activity with the hope of further improvement in noninvasive tumor characterization.

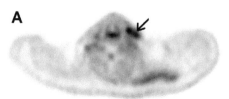
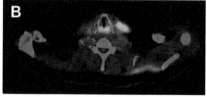

Fig. 3. (A) Axial image from a PET scan. Area of increased activity in the left neck (*black arrow*). (B) Axial PET-CT image from the same patient showing area of increased activity corresponding to a cervical lymph node.

RADIOMICS

Radiomics is a developing field combining large volumes of clinical images and data to create reliable models to determine diagnosis and prognosis in a noninvasive fashion. Radiomics uses large image datasets and dedicated software to extract qualitative and quantitative features from images to accurately characterize tumor biology and heterogeneity; ultimately using the data to customize treatment to the individual as well as monitor for treatment resistance.[10] It is likely that radiomics will be an integral part of the growing trend of precision/personal medicine for treatment of patients with cancer.

INTERVENTIONAL RADIOLOGY AND THE MANAGEMENT OF PATIENTS WITH CANCER

Paralleling the advancement in diagnostic imaging, the past decade has brought about significant technologic advances in interventional radiology. Although diagnostic imaging can accurately characterize most lesions, the ultimate diagnosis and treatment are based on pathologic analysis of the tumor tissue. Tissue analysis will likely play a bigger role in determining treatment given the rapid incorporation of agents with specific molecular targets. Interventional radiologists play an important role in obtaining a tissue sample for pathologic analysis. Image-guided biopsy is one of the most common procedures performed by interventional radiologists. There are very few locations that are not amenable to an image-guided biopsy. Core biopsies are preferred because there is a larger volume of tissue when compared with a fine needle aspiration, and the cellular morphology and overall architecture of the tumor are preserved.

Image-guided core biopsies are generally performed using a coaxial biopsy system. A coaxial system uses a guide needle with a removable stylet through which a core biopsy device is passed and is used to sample the tissue. Coaxial systems range from 16 to 20 gauge with a spring-loaded mechanism that is used for the biopsy. The coaxial technique allows multiple samples to be obtained through a single introducer needle and, if necessary, the same introducer needle can be used for fine-needle aspiration.

Image-guided biopsies may be performed using US, CT, MRI or X-ray guidance depending on the location of the target lesion. US guidance allows real-time imaging of the biopsy device and the lesion making US guidance efficient and safe. CT may be used for lesions that are not seen with US, and MRI-guided biopsy may be used when lesions are not visible by other modalities (**Figs. 4 and 5**). MRI-guided biopsies require specialized equipment and are predominantly used for soft tissue biopsy.

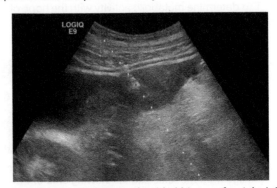

Fig. 4. Ultrasound image from an ultrasound-guided biopsy of a right lobe liver lesion.

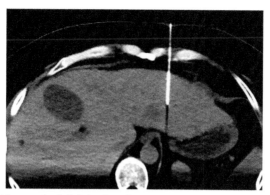

Fig. 5. CT-guided biopsy of a left lobe liver lesion.

Most patients with cancer need long-term venous access for frequent blood tests, contrast administration, and administration of chemotherapy. A large part of an interventional practice is venous access. Interventional radiologists are adept in placing long-term venous access devices, such as subcutaneous central venous ports and tunneled central venous catheters. Many interventionalists are able to obtain central venous access using nontraditional routes such as trans-lumbar, trans-hepatic, and via the azygous system.

Most procedures performed in interventional radiology are done using conscious sedation monitored by interventional radiology nursing staff including central venous access and most biopsies. These procedures have been proven to be safe with very little associated morbidity and can be performed on an outpatient basis.

With the increasing involvement of interventional radiologists in the diagnosis and treatment of patients with cancer, there is a growing subset of interventional radiologists specializing in the care of oncologic patients and have been termed interventional oncologists. Recently, interventional oncology had been referred to as the "fourth pillar of oncology" alongside medical, surgical, and radiation oncologists.[11] Interventional radiologists in some cases are becoming the primary therapy provider for patients with certain types of cancer with a shift to minimally invasive therapies.

INTERVENTIONAL TREATMENTS

The rapid growth of interventional oncology is largely the result of the development of minimally invasive image-guided treatments, many with similar clinical outcomes to surgery. A comprehensive discussion of the available therapies is beyond the scope of this article. Being aware of available treatments is important for oncologic patient management.

Image-guided ablation of solid organ tumors is one of the most common procedures performed by interventional oncologists. Various forms of thermal energy are currently available for use in ablation, including RF, microwave, and extreme cold (cryoablation). Tumors in multiple sites are routinely treated with ablation including the liver, kidney, and lung. In addition, research is being conducted in ablating thyroid and breast lesions. Generally, ablation is used to treat smaller tumors with excellent results.

Catheter-based therapies are also in widespread use throughout the world, primarily for the treatment of hepatic tumors, both tumors of hepatic origin as well as for hepatic metastatic disease. These therapies are based on the dual blood supply of the liver with hepatic tumors receiving arterial blood supply and the portal vein supplying most normal liver parenchyma. Transcatheter arterial therapies involve embolization of the tumor with small particles, which may be loaded with chemotherapy or a radioisotope.

Interventional radiology/interventional oncology is undergoing rapid changes with continual refinement of techniques as well as development of novel, minimally invasive therapies.

As the population ages and life expectancy increases, health care providers are increasingly confronted with patients with cancer. Imaging and interventional radiology are often central to the evaluation, diagnosis, and monitoring of oncology patients. Understanding the available resources as well as when and how to use them will help expedite care and treatment for patients with cancer. In addition, the early detection of a malignancy often leads to better outcomes.

DISCLOSURE

The authors have nothing to disclose.

REFERENCES

1. Fass L. Imaging and cancer: a review. Mol Oncol 2008;2:115–52.
2. National Comprehnsive Cancer Network. Available at: NCCN.org. Accessed September 18, 2019.
3. Pisano ED, Gatsonis C, Hendrick E, et al. Diagnostic performance of digital versus film mammography for breast-cancer screening. N Engl J Med 2005; 353:1773–83.
4. Rafferty EA. Digital mammography: novel applications. Radiol Clin North Am 2007;45:831–43, vii.
5. OECD. Number of computer tomography (CT) scanners in selected countries as of 2017 (per million population). Statista; 2018. Available at;. https://www.statista.com/statistics/266539/distribution-of-equipment-for-computer-tomography/. Accessed September 18, 2019.
6. Humphrey LL, Deffebach M, Pappas M, et al. Screening for lung cancer with low-dose computed tomography: a systematic review to update the US Preventive services task force recommendation. Ann Intern Med 2013;159:411–20.
7. Westbrook C, Talbot J. MRI in practice. London: John Wiley & Sons, Inc; 2011.
8. Wilson SR, Greenbaum LD, Goldberg BB. Contrast-enhanced ultrasound: what is the evidence and what are the obstacles? AJR Am J Roentgenol 2009;193:55–60.
9. Kundra V, Schellingerhout D, Jackson EF. Targeted and functional imaging. Totowa (NJ): Humana Press; 2008.
10. Rizzo S, Botta F, Raimondi S, et al. Radiomics: the facts and the challenges of image analysis. Eur Radiol Exp 2018;2:36.
11. Kim HS, Chapiro J, Geschwind JH. From the guest editor: interventional oncology: the fourth pillar of oncology. Cancer J 2016;22:363–4.

Esophagus and Gastrointestinal Junction Tumors

Saba Kurtom, MD, MS[a], Brian J. Kaplan, MD[b],*

KEYWORDS

- Esophageal cancer • Gastroesophageal junction cancer
- Esophageal squamous cell carcinoma • Esophageal adenocarcinoma

KEY POINTS

- Esophageal squamous cell carcinoma (ESCC) and esophageal adenocarcinoma (EADC) account for more than 95% of all esophageal malignancies.
- Most ESCC arises in the thoracic esophagus, with tobacco and alcohol use being major risk factors.
- Most EADC arises in the distal esophagus, with the presence of gastroesophageal reflux disease leading to Barrett esophagus as the primary risk factor.
- Low-grade tumors can be managed with endoscopic resection in conjunction with radio-frequency ablation.
- Minimally invasive approaches for esophagectomy are viable treatment options.

INTRODUCTION

In the United States, esophageal cancer accounts for approximately 18,000 new cases annually, with an estimated 16,000 deaths.[1] It comprises 1% of new cancer diagnoses and 2.6% of all cancer deaths. Rates for new esophageal cancer cases have been declining an average 1.2% per year over the last 10 years. Globally, an estimated 572,000 cases occurred in 2018, with the highest rates seen in Asia and eastern and southern Africa, and lowest in western Africa.[2] There is also a varied distribution of the type of esophageal cancer (squamous cell carcinoma vs adenocarcinoma) based on geographic location. Squamous cell carcinoma is predominant in the area known as the esophageal cancer belt, which extends from northern Iran, through central Asia

[a] Department of Surgery, Virginia Commonwealth University, West Hospital, 1200 East Broad Street, Box 980135, Richmond, VA 23298, USA; [b] Department of Surgery, Division of Surgical Oncology, West Hospital, Virginia Commonwealth University, 1200 East Broad Street, Box 980011, Richmond, VA 23298, USA
* Corresponding author.
E-mail address: Brian.Kaplan@VCUHealth.org

Surg Clin N Am 100 (2020) 507–521
https://doi.org/10.1016/j.suc.2020.02.003
0039-6109/20/© 2020 Elsevier Inc. All rights reserved.
surgical.theclinics.com

to central China. Men are 3 to 4 times more likely to be diagnosed with esophageal cancer than women.

Esophageal squamous cell carcinoma (ESCC) and esophageal adenocarcinoma (EADC) comprise more than 95% of all esophageal malignancies. Sixty years ago, squamous cell carcinoma accounted for more than 90% of all esophageal cancers; however, over time, the incidence of EADC has increased in Western countries. EADC now accounts for more than 60% of esophageal cancer in the United States.[3]

ANATOMY/PATHOLOGY

The adult esophagus extends from the hypopharynx to the stomach and is between 18 and 25 cm in length. The 3 anatomic regions are the cervical region (pharyngoesophageal junction to suprasternal notch), thoracic (suprasternal notch to the diaphragmatic hiatus), and abdominal (hiatus to the orifice of the cardia of the stomach). Esophageal cancer can spread through direct extension, lymphatic spread, and hematogenous metastasis. The lack of serosa in the wall plays a crucial role in the direct and local extension of esophageal cancer.

Squamous Cell Carcinoma

Most ESCC arises in the thoracic esophagus, with the minority in the cervical esophagus (5%). Squamous cell carcinoma develops from the stratified squamous epithelial lining in the upper and middle esophagus secondary to chronic inflammation and mucosal damage. Early lesions that present as small polypoid excrescences, denuded epithelium, or plaques can be missed on endoscopy. Advanced lesions are shown by infiltrating and ulcerated masses. Squamous cell carcinoma starts as epithelial dysplasia, which progresses to carcinoma in situ and subsequently into invasive carcinoma.[4] The most common distant sites of metastases are lung, liver, and bone, which can be seen in almost 30% of patients. Bone marrow involvement can also be found in up to 40% of patients.[5]

Several risk factors have been found to be associated with ESCC. Tobacco and alcohol use have been identified as major risk factors. Individuals who smoke have a 5-fold risk of developing ESCC compared with nonsmokers.[6] The relative risk of ESCC with increases with the amount of alcohol consumption, varying between 1.8 and 7.4 depending on the weekly ingested volume.[7] Yerba mate tea has also been shown to be linked to an increase risk, in terms of both amount consumed and the temperature of the beverage. Chewing areca nut (which is often mixed with tobacco) is a practice common in Southeast Asia and India and is linked to the development of ESCC. Consumption of foods containing N-nitroso compounds has been shown to induce alkyl adducts in DNA. Other dietary factors that have been shown to be risk factors for ESCC include red meat intake and deficiency or low levels of selenium, zinc, and folate.[8–10] Certain genetic factors have also been linked with the development of ESCC. Tylosis, an autosomal dominant disorder characterized by hyperkeratosis of the palms and souls, is associated with an increased risk of ESCC in the middle and distal esophagus.[11,12] Bloom syndrome, associated with increased sister chromatid exchange rates in all cells, is also associated with an increased risk of ESCC.[13] Four genome-wide association studies have shown genetic susceptibility factors, which include several single nucleotide polymorphisms, enzymes responsible for metabolizing alcohol (alcohol dehydrogenase and acetyl dehydrogenase), and loci present on phospholipase C and chromosome 20.[14]

Adenocarcinoma

Esophageal adenocarcinoma is the most rapidly increasing type of cancer in certain populations. The male predilection of EADC is higher than that of any other non–sex-specific cancer across several populations.[15] Approximately 75% of EADCs occur in the distal esophagus. EADC is characterized by glandular differentiation that most commonly arises in the setting of Barrett esophagus (BE). Adenocarcinoma that arises from BE may present as an ulcer, nodule, an alteration in the normal mucosal pattern, or with no visual abnormalities on endoscopy.[16] Similar to ESCC, lymph nodes metastases occur early to adjacent or regional lymph nodes. Celiac and perihepatic node involvement in EADC is more common because of the more distal location of most tumors.[17]

The prevalence of gastroesophageal reflux disease (GERD) in the Western population is approximately 10% to 20%, amounting to 30 million to 60 million people in the United States.[7] A meta-analysis showed that weekly symptoms of GERD increased the odds of EADC 5-fold, whereas daily symptoms increased the odd by 7-fold.[18] GERD can directly lead to EADC, but more commonly progresses through the intermediate preneoplastic lesion, BE. BE is defined as columnar metaplasia that has replaced the normal stratified squamous epithelium of the distal esophagus. In the United States, intestinal-type goblet cells (intestinal metaplasia) are required for diagnosis of BE, whereas the inclusion of goblet cells is not required for diagnosis in other parts of the world.[19] American Gastroenterological Association guidelines state that BE should be diagnosed when there is extension of salmon-colored mucosa located greater than or equal to 1 cm proximal to the gastroesophageal junction (GEJ) on endoscopy, in addition to intestinal metaplasia on endoscopy.[20] Patients diagnosed with BE have a 30-fold increased risk of EADC compared with the general population, although the absolute risk of developing cancer is low (estimated annual incidence, 0.12%).[21] The risk is increased to 7% in the presence of high-grade dysplasia.[22] Investigation into EADC risk increase in low-grade dysplasia yields disparate results, because establishing the diagnosis on pathologic review is not always uniform.[23] One study examined 147 patients diagnosed with low-grade dysplasia at community hospitals. Expert pathologists reviewing these biopsy slides confirmed the diagnosis in only 15% of cases. Among the patients with confirmed disease, the cumulative risk of progression was 85% at 109 months.[24] In contrast, another study examining patients with low-grade dysplasia found the annual rate of neoplastic progression to be only 1.8%.[25] Smoking in itself is considered a risk factor for EADC, but this risk is also increased in patients with existing BE. One analysis found the risk of adenocarcinoma of the esophagus or GEJ was 2.08 times greater in smokers, with the risk increasing with increase in total dose (pack-years of smoking).[26] In contrast with ESCC, there has not been a documented association between alcohol use and EADC.[27] Obesity has been linked to an increased risk for esophageal and gastric cardia adenocarcinomas, and to BE, with the relative risk of carcinoma of 1.71 for a body mass index (BMI) between 25 and 30 kg/m^2 and 2.34 for BMI greater than or equal to 30 kg/m^2.[28] Nitrosamine-rich foods have also been implicated in the propagation of EADC formation, but the mechanism is poorly understood. In contrast with the aforementioned drugs, nonsteroidal antiinflammatory drugs may play a protective role against the development of EADC, particularly in the setting of BE.[29] Genetic factors that may have the propensity for an increased risk for adenocarcinoma include epidermal growth factor polymorphisms, which lead to an increased in serum levels of epidermal growth factor.[30] Familial BE, inherited in an autosomal dominant fashion, also places patients at a high risk of EADC.[31] Endoscopic screening is recommended in these patients after the age of 40 years. In contrast with gastric adenocarcinoma, colonization with *Helicobacter pylori* may be protective against EADC, although conflicting evidence has been published.[32,33]

CLINICAL MANIFESTATIONS

Patients with early esophageal carcinoma may be asymptomatic. More advanced cases typically present with progressive dysphagia (from solids to difficulty with liquids as well), odynophagia, and unintentional weight loss. Other presenting symptoms include epigastric pain and regurgitation of saliva or food. Patients may also have chronic gastrointestinal blood loss from esophageal or GEJ cancers, resulting in iron deficiency anemia.[34] However, it is uncommon for patients to complain of melena or hematemesis. An acute upper gastrointestinal bleed is rare. Patients presenting with intractable coughing, especially after eating, or recurrent pneumonias may have secondary tracheobronchial fistulas, which are a late complication of esophageal cancer. Some patients also present with signs or symptoms attributable to metastatic disease. The most common locations for metastases in esophageal cancer are the liver, lungs, bone, and adrenal glands.[35] EADCs frequently metastasize to intraabdominal locations (peritoneum, liver), whereas ESCCs most frequently metastasize to intrathoracic sites. Cervical esophageal tumors are usually locally advanced at the time of diagnosis, sometimes with extension into the hypopharynx. The most common symptoms in these patients are unintentional weight loss and dysphagia.[36]

SCREENING AND DIAGNOSIS

Cross-sectional imaging, such as computed tomography (CT), is unable to accurately identify localized esophageal cancer. Barium esophagrams are able to identify irregular strictures; however, histologic examination of tissue obtained from endoscopy is the standard for diagnosis. During upper endoscopy, esophageal cancer can appear as a stricture, mass, raised nodule, ulceration, or a subtle irregularity in the mucosa. Although patients with GERD undergo frequent endoscopies for surveillance for BE, less than 15% of EADCs are detected on surveillance endoscopies.[37] During endoscopy, it is important to document the proximal and distal extents of the tumor and their relation to the incisors and GEJ, because it can have implications for surgical management.[38] Smaller lesions that meet the following criteria may be amenable to endoscopic resection (ER): diameter less than or equal to 2 cm, involves less than one-third of the circumference of the esophageal wall, and is limited to the mucosa.

Screening of BE-associated adenocarcinoma by endoscopy is a global clinical practice. Current guidelines from the American College of Gastroenterology dictate that, in patients with suspected BE, at least 8 random biopsies must be obtained to maximize the yield of intestinal metaplasia on histology. In patients with short-segment BE (1–2 cm), at least 4 biopsies per centimeter of circumferential BE are needed. Endoscopic screening for patients should be considered in men with chronic (>5 years) and/or frequent symptoms of gastroesophageal reflux and 2 or more risk factors for BE or EADC. These risk factors include age greater than 50 years, white race, central obesity, current or past history of smoking, and confirmed family history of BE or EADC in a first-degree relative. Screening for women with chronic GERD is generally not recommended, given the substantially lower risk of EADC in women. However, screening for women can be considered in individual cases as determined by the risk factors listed earlier. For patients diagnosed with BE without dysplasia, endoscopic surveillance should be performed every 3 to 5 years. Patients with evidence of high-grade dysplasia should be managed with endoscopic therapy, as should patients with low-grade dysplasia (for those without life-limiting comorbidities). Patients with low-grade dysplasia who have comorbidities that preclude them from ER may alternatively undergo endoscopic surveillance every 12 months.[39]

STAGING

Once the diagnosis of esophageal cancer has been established from endoscopic biopsy, the next diagnostic step involves evaluation for locoregional disease extent and distant metastases. The preferred and most accurate method for locoregional evaluation is endoscopic ultrasonography (EUS). EUS uses a high-frequency ultrasound transducer to provide images of the mass and its relationship to the layers of the esophageal wall. EUS has a sensitivity of 0.85 (95% confidence interval [CI], 0.82–0.88) for T1a staging and 0.86 (95% CI, 0.82–0.89) for T1b staging.[40] There have been recent studies showing that EUS has a limited role for staging superficial esophageal cancers, concluding that patients with suspected superficial tumors should undergo endomucosal resection as the first diagnostic, staging, and therapeutic option.[41] However, a meta-analysis has shown that EUS has overall good sensitivity and specificity for detecting mucosal or submucosal invasion in superficial cancers.[40] A caveat for EUS T staging is that the transducer cannot traverse tumor-induced stenosis (which can be present in up to 30% of cases). Regional node staging can also be achieved by EUS. Criteria used to determine malignant involvement in the nodes include width greater than 10 mm, round shape, smooth border, and echo-poor pattern. When all 4 criteria are met, there is an 80% to 100% chance of metastatic involvement.[42]

The National Comprehensive Cancer Network (NCCN) guidelines advocate the use of bronchoscopy with biopsy and brush cytology in staging work-up for patients who have locally advanced tumors located at or above the level of the carina (in the esophagus). For cervical ESCC, flexible laryngoscopy can be used to assess local disease.

Evaluation for the presence of distant metastases is completed through different imaging modalities. Helical CT scans are often the first imaging studies that patients undergo after diagnosis; however, they are limited in being able to identify locally advanced disease (T4) as well as subclinical metastatic spread (particularly in the peritoneal cavity).[43] Integration of PET with CT has become increasingly favored because of better spatial resolution; however, to be most accurate in identifying metastases, intravenous contrast must be used. Whole-body fluorodeoxyglucose (FDG)-PET is more sensitive than using contrast-enhanced CT or EUS for detecting distant metastases. Addition of PET to preoperative assessment of patients alters the treatment strategy in 5% to 20% of patients, mainly by decreasing the number of patients that undergo surgery because of the finding of occult metastatic disease.[44,45] PET/CT may also be beneficial when used for clinically restaging patients following initial induction therapy. Occult metastases may be identified in about 8% of patients after induction chemoradiation therapy.[46] One study that examined the ability of PET/CT to predict complete pathologic response found that a standardized uptake value of less than 45% on PET/CT was associated with patients having residual disease but not complete pathologic response.[47] Another study found no significant association between metabolic imaging and prognosis of patients with locally advanced esophageal cancer undergoing neoadjuvant chemoradiotherapy and esophagectomy.[48] Use of laparoscopy or thoracoscopy for staging remains controversial, and the NCCN considers it an optional procedure for patients with esophageal and GEJ tumors.[49]

MANAGEMENT AND TREATMENT
Management of Barrett Esophagus

Patients with BE should receive once-daily proton pump inhibitor therapy. If nodularity is present in the BE segment, endoscopic mucosal resection (EMR) of the lesion should be performed as a diagnostic and therapeutic maneuver. If low-grade or high-grade dysplasia is present on EMR, patients should proceed to have endoscopic ablative therapy, with radiofrequency ablation (RFA) being the most cost-effective method.[22,50] Following successful endoscopic treatment and complete elimination of intestinal metaplasia, endoscopic surveillance should be continued to detect recurrent intestinal metaplasia/and or dysplasia. For patients with high-grade dysplasia (or intramucosal carcinoma), repeat endoscopy should be performed every 3 months for the first year, every 6 months the second year, and annually thereafter. In patients with low-grade dysplasia (present before ablation), repeat endoscopy should be performed every 6 months in the first year, and annually thereafter. Antireflux surgery can be considered in patients who have incomplete control of their reflux symptoms on optimal medical therapy, although it should not be performed as an antineoplastic measure. According to the Society of American Gastrointestinal Endoscopic Surgery (SAGES), surveillance for BE does not change after antireflux surgery. There is no evidence to suggest that surveillance is more challenging or less effective after antireflux surgery.[51–53]

Early-Stage/Superficial Carcinoma

Appropriate management of superficial carcinoma requires an accurate diagnosis of the extent of disease. Involvement of the submucosa is an important prognostic determinant for early carcinomas because of the presence of lymphatic vessels. In order to more closely identify mucosal and submucosal extension of the tumor, a subclassification system was created in which Tis is classified as M1 (limited to epithelial layer), T1a lesions divided as M2 (invade lamina propria) and M3 (invades into but not through muscularis mucosa). T1b is further divided as SM1 (penetrates the superficial one-third of the submucosa), SM2 (penetrates into the intermediate one-third of the submucosa), and SM3 (penetrates the deepest one-third of the submucosa).[54] Multiple studies have shown no association with lymph node metastases in M1 and M2 tumors, and therefore EMR or endoscopic submucosal dissection of these tumors is an appropriate curative treatment strategy, although there are no randomized control trials comparing EMR versus esophagectomy.[55–57] M3 tumors have a varying risk of nodal metastases based on several studies, with some showing a risk of 0%, and 1 showing a risk as high as 18%.[55,58] Submucosal tumors (SM1–SM3) have a high risk of lymph node metastases. EMR should not be performed in these patients, because they have an increased risk of recurrence.[59]

Outcomes of ER versus esophagectomy for superficial cancers are mostly available from retrospective reviews. Overall, procedure-related morbidity and mortality were higher after esophagectomy in some studies.[60] Although recurrence risk was higher in ER-treated groups, repeat endoscopic treatment was possible in all patients and the long-term response rates were similar after esophagectomy and ER. Based on the National Cancer Institute Surveillance, Epidemiology, and End Results (SEER) registry review, of 742 patients undergoing ER or esophagectomy for superficial ESCC (Tis or T1), there was no difference in cancer-specific mortality between the 2 groups.[61] Complications associated with ER include perforation, bleeding, and delayed esophageal strictures. Cryotherapy, photodynamic therapy, or RFA may be added to treatment in addition to ER. Photodynamic therapy and RFA have been associated with esophageal stenosis.

An alternative approach for treatment of superficial invasive cancers involves use of external beam radiation therapy (with or without concurrent chemotherapy) and brachytherapy. However, data for this approach are limited. Patients who would be best suited for this treatment modality are those who would be candidates for treatment with ER but have contraindications to this approach (eg, patients with extensive liver disease and esophageal varices, previous history of perforation, or severe cervical spinal disease).[62–64]

Management of Locoregional and Advanced Tumors

Esophagectomy is indicated as the initial treatment of patients with clinical T1bN0M0 lesions; however, if there is no evidence of nodal involvement, ER can alternatively be performed in patients who may not be candidates for esophagectomy. Patients with T2 disease without nodal involvement are candidates for primary esophagectomy, with adjuvant chemoradiation for selected patients (NCCN). Patients with T2 tumors with nodal metastases, and T3 to T4a tumors (thoracic or GEJ) with or without nodal spread, should undergo neoadjuvant chemotherapy or chemoradiotherapy, followed by esophagectomy if they have resectable disease. Patients with T4b tumors or with tumor present less than 5 cm from the cricopharyngeus muscle are considered to have unresectable disease and should therefore have definitive chemoradiation. Patients that undergo neoadjuvant chemoradiation should have response assessment through imaging (FDG-PET/CT preferred). Based on the response, patients should have continued surveillance or esophagectomy (with esophagectomy being the preferred management strategy). Those who develop localized, resectable esophageal cancer after undergoing definitive chemoradiation can be considered for esophagectomy if there is no evidence of distant recurrence.[65]

Gastroesophageal Junction Tumors

The GEJ is anatomically located at the level of the angle His; however, the definitions differ based on endoscopic visualization and histologic evaluation. The Siewert classification was published in 1987[66] and describes the following categories based on anatomic location: type I (located between 5 and 1 cm proximal to the anatomic squamocolumnar junction or Z line) is EADC arising from the distal esophagus, type II (located between 1 cm proximal and 2 cm distal to the anatomic Z line) is true carcinoma of the cardia arising from cardiac epithelium with segments of intestinal metaplasia, and type III (located between 2 and 5 cm distal to the anatomic Z line) is subcardial gastric carcinoma. Per the most recent American Joint Committee on Cancer (AJCC) classification, tumors involving the GEJ with the tumor epicenter no more than 2 cm into the proximal stomach are staged as esophageal cancers, whereas those with their epicenters located more than 2 cm into the proximal stomach are considered gastric cancers. Therefore, all esophageal cancers that have an epicenter more than 2 cm distal from the GEJ (even if the GEJ is involved) are staged and treated as gastric cancers. Therefore, Siewert types I and II tumors are treated as esophageal/GEJ tumors, whereas Siewert type III are considered gastric tumors and should follow gastric cancer treatment guidelines.

Systemic therapy

Combined modality therapy has been shown to significantly increase survival in patients with esophageal and GEJ cancer with locoregional disease compared with resection alone.[67] Preoperative chemoradiation is associated with improved overall survival, disease-free survival, and pathologic complete response compared with preoperative chemotherapy or surgery alone. Results from the Chemoradiotherapy for

Oesophageal Cancer followed by Surgery Study (CROSS; a multicenter phase III clinical trial) showed that preoperative chemoradiation with paclitaxel and carboplatin significant improved overall survival and disease-free survival compared with surgery alone in patients with resectable (T2–T3, N0–1, M0) esophageal or GEJ cancers.[68] R0 resection rate was also higher in the preoperative chemoradiation group. Definitive chemoradiation therapy with paclitaxel and carboplatin is also recommended for patients with unresectable esophageal cancer.[69] Other regimens that can be used for preoperative chemoradiation include use of folinic acid, fluorouracil (5-fu), oxaliplati,[70] fluorouracil and cisplatin,[71] irinotecan and cisplatin,[72] or paclitaxel and flouropyrmidine.[73] The cancer and leukemia group B 9781 prospective phase III trial found that patients receiving preoperative chemoradiation with fluorouracil and cisplatin followed by surgery had increased overall survival, and improved 5-year overall survival, indicating the long-term survival advantage of this approach.[71]

The Intergroup-0116 (INT-0116) trial investigated the effectiveness of postoperative chemoradiation in GEJ and gastric cancers.[74,75] Patients were randomized to receive fluorouracil plus leucovorin before and after concurrent chemoradiation. After 5 years of follow-up, the median overall survival was higher in the postoperative chemoradiation group (36 months vs 27 months in the surgery-only group). Survival was also higher at more than 10 years of follow-up in the postoperative chemoradiation group. The results of this trial established the efficacy for the use of postoperative chemoradiation in patients with resected GEJ cancers; however, the recommended doses have been changed because of high rates of hematologic and gastrointestinal toxicities in the initial trial. Another trial evaluated the use of cisplatin and fluorouracil for postoperative chemoradiation in patients with poor-prognosis esophageal and GEJ adenocarcinoma, which showed that 4-year overall survival was significantly higher in the adjuvant therapy group compared with surgery only in patients with node-positive T3 or T4 tumors.[76]

There are currently 3 drugs that are US Food and Drug Administration approved for use in esophageal and GEJ cancers: trastuzumab, pembrolizumab, and ramucirumab. Trastuzumab is used based on testing of human epidermal growth factor receptor 2 (HER2) status and pembrolizumab for microsatellite instability and/or programmed death-ligand 1 (PD-L1) expression. Ramucirumab is a vascular endothelial growth factor receptor 2 (VEGFR-2) antibody used in patients with previously treated advanced or metastatic gastroesophageal cancers. The trastuzumab for gastric cancer trial was a randomized prospective phase III trial that evaluated the use of trastuzumab in HER2-positive patients with gastric and GEJ adenocarcinoma. Patients with HER2-positive locally advanced, recurrent, or metastatic GEJ or gastric cancer were randomized to receive trastuzumab plus chemotherapy (cisplatin plus fluorouracil or capecitabine) or chemotherapy alone. The results showed significant improvement in median overall survival in the trastuzumab group. The study established trastuzumab in combination with cisplatin and a fluoropyrimidine as the standard therapy for patients with HER2-positive metastatic gastroesophageal adenocarcinoma.[77] Pembrolizumab is a monoclonal programmed cell death protein 1 (PD-1) antibody against PD-1 receptors that is approved for use in patients with unresectable or metastatic tumors with MSI-H (high levels of microsatellite instability) or dMMR (deficient mismatch repair) that have progression despite initial treatment (NCCN). Ramucirumab has shown positive results in patients with previously treated advanced or metastatic gastroesophageal cancer in 2 phase II clinical trials.[78,79]

ESCC has been shown to have a higher sensitivity to chemoradiotherapy, with pathologic complete response rates as high as 46% to 49%.[68,80] As with EADC, the NCCN guidelines recommend a trimodal treatment approach to locally advanced ESCC with neoadjuvant chemoradiotherapy. Patients who undergo neoadjuvant chemoradiation should undergo subsequent esophagectomy so long as there is no evidence of unresectable or metastatic disease. Patients who are treated with definitive chemoradiation may be followed with surveillance if there is no evidence of residual disease per the NCCN guidelines. Despite the NCCN guidelines, an analysis performed of the SEER-Medicare linked database found that only 5% of patients with locally advanced ESCC received neoadjuvant therapy followed by surgery; most patients (49%) were treated with definitive chemoradiation therapy, with the most common reason for exclusion being that surgical management was not recommended.[81] Analysis from a Memorial Sloan Kettering Cancer Center institutional database of locally advanced ESCC (stage II–III) revealed that recurrence rates for patients treated with definitive chemoradiation were as high as 38% at 5 years, compared with 0% for patients treated with neoadjuvant chemoradiation followed by surgery.[81]

Surgical Approaches

The type of esophageal resection performed is determined by the location of the tumor as well as the choices available for conduit. The 4 main options available for resection are Ivor Lewis esophagectomy (right thoracotomy and laparotomy), transhiatal esophagectomy (laparotomy and cervical anastomosis), McKeown esophagectomy (right thoracotomy with laparotomy and cervical anastomosis), and left thoracoabdominal esophagectomy. The selected approach should also include an R0 resection (indicating no cancer present at the resection margins), an adequate lymphadenectomy (at least 15 lymph nodes[82]), and consideration of placement of a feeding tube (most commonly a jejunostomy tube).

The Ivor Lewis transthoracic esophagectomy can be used for resection of tumors in the lower third of the esophagus but is not an ideal choice for cancers located in the middle third because of limited access to the proximal margin. This approach involves a laparotomy with a right thoracotomy and an intrathoracic esophagogastric anastomosis. The procedure allows direct visualization of the thoracic esophagus and a full thoracic lymphadenectomy. The stomach is mobilized for use as the conduit, the celiac and left gastric lymph nodes are dissected, the left gastric artery is divided, and the gastroepiploic and right gastric arteries are preserved. Disadvantages of the transthoracic approach include the limitation to the length of the proximal esophagus that be reached for an R0 resection, the intrathoracic location of the esophagogastric anastomosis, and a higher risk of severe bile reflux (seen in 3%–20% of patients).[83] Leaks occurring at the intrathoracic anastomosis also have morbidity and mortality as high as 64%; however, use of current surgical techniques (using linear or curved staplers) has decreased the incidence of leaks.[84] A modified version of the Ivor Lewis esophagectomy includes a left thoracoabdominal incision with gastric pull-up and esophagogastric anastomosis in the left chest. This approach can be used for tumors involving the GEJ.

A transhiatal esophagectomy can be performed to resect cervical, thoracic, and GEJ carcinomas. This approach uses an upper midline laparotomy incision and left neck incision. The thoracic esophagus is dissected through the diaphragmatic hiatus and the neck. A cervical esophagogastric anastomosis is created with a gastric pull-up. Disadvantages of this approach include the inability to perform a full thoracic lymphadenectomy and inability to visualize the midthoracic dissection.

The McKeown or 3-hole esophagectomy combines the transhiatal and transthoracic approaches into a transthoracic total esophagectomy with thoracic lymphadenectomy and cervical esophagogastric anastomosis. This approach is ideal for tumors in the middle or upper third of the esophagus and allows a complete 2-field (mediastinal and upper abdominal) lymphadenectomy under direct visualization. A thoracoscopic approach can also be used instead of a thoracotomy. A right postero-lateral thoracotomy or thoracoscopy is first performed with en bloc resection of the esophagus and mediastinal and upper abdominal lymph nodes. Subsequently a lap-arotomy is performed to exclude metastatic disease and the stomach is mobilized for use as conduit and a left cervical incision is used. The advantage of the esophagogas-tric anastomosis in the neck includes potentially easier management of a possible anastomotic leak, lower incidence of reflux, and more extensive resection of the prox-imal margin.

A left thoracoabdominal esophagectomy uses a contiguous abdominal and left thoracic incision through the eighth intercostal space.[85] This approach is best suited for lesions in the distal esophagus, particularly bulky tumors around the hiatus, because it allows optimal visualization of the anatomy. Esophagogastric anastomosis is performed in the left chest (and the stomach is mobilized for the conduit).

Minimally invasive approaches include modified approaches to the traditional Ivor Lewis, McKeown, and transabdominal esophagectomies. Minimally invasive strate-gies using thoracoscopy and or laparoscopy may be associated with decreased morbidity and faster recovery times. The Traditional Invasive Versus Minimally Inva-sive Esophagectomy (TIME) trial found that patients who had a total minimally invasive Ivor Lewis esophagectomy had a better perioperative hospital course, with a lower rate of in-hospital pulmonary infections (12% for minimally invasive vs 34% for open esophagectomy) and lower postoperative (within 2 weeks of surgery) rate of pulmo-nary infections (9% vs 29% for open esophagectomy).[86]

SUMMARY

ESCC and EADC account for more than 95% of all esophageal malignancies. ESCC arises from the stratified epithelial lining of the esophagus secondary to repeat inflammation and damage to the mucosa. EADC arises from BE, with intestinal meta-plasia and goblet cells replacing the normal stratified squamous epithelium of the distal esophagus. Tobacco and alcohol use are significant risk factors for ESCC, whereas GERD is a major risk factor for EADC. Treatment of both types of esopha-geal cancer has shifted to a less invasive approach using endoscopic mucosal or submucosal resection with ablation for superficial cancers, whereas esophagec-tomy (with preoperative chemoradiation) remains the mainstay for locally advanced tumors. Minimally invasive techniques can be used for surgical resection. Definitive chemoradiation is reserved for patients with unresectable disease or those who refuse surgery.

DISCLOSURE

The authors have nothing to disclose.

REFERENCES

1. Howlader N, Noone AM, Krapcho M, et al, editors. SEER Cancer Statistics Review, 1975–2016. Bethesda (MD): National Cancer Institute; 2019.
2. American Cancer Society. Global Cancer Facts & Figures 4th Edition. Atlanta (GA): American Cancer Society; 2018.
3. Thrift AP. The epidemic of oesophageal carcinoma: where are we now? Cancer Epidemiol 2016;41:88–95.

4. Kuwano H, Saeki H, Kawaguchi H, et al. Proliferative activity of cancer cells in front and center areas of carcinoma in situ and invasive sites of esophageal squamous-cell carcinoma. Int J Cancer 1998;78(2):149–52.

5. Thorban S, Roder JD, Nekarda H, et al. Immunocytochemical detection of disseminated tumor cells in the bone marrow of patients with esophageal carcinoma. J Natl Cancer Inst 1996;88(17):1222–7.

6. Domper Arnal MJ, Ferrandez Arenas A, Lanas Arbeloa A. Esophageal cancer: risk factors, screening and endoscopic treatment in Western and Eastern countries. World J Gastroenterol 2015;21(26):7933–43.

7. Wheeler JB, Reed CE. Epidemiology of esophageal cancer. Surg Clin North Am 2012;92(5):1077–87.

8. Cross AJ, Freedman ND, Ren J, et al. Meat consumption and risk of esophageal and gastric cancer in a large prospective study. Am J Gastroenterol 2011;106(3): 432–42.

9. Mark SD, Qiao YL, Dawsey SM, et al. Prospective study of serum selenium levels and incident esophageal and gastric cancers. J Natl Cancer Inst 2000;92(21): 1753–63.

10. Abnet CC, Lai B, Qiao YL, et al. Zinc concentration in esophageal biopsy specimens measured by x-ray fluorescence and esophageal cancer risk. J Natl Cancer Inst 2005;97(4):301–6.

11. Lindor NM, Greene MH. The concise handbook of family cancer syndromes. Mayo Familial Cancer Program. J Natl Cancer Inst 1998;90(14):1039–71.

12. Lindor NM, McMaster ML, Lindor CJ, et al, National Cancer Institute, Division of Cancer Prevention, Community Oncology and Prevention Trials Research Group. Concise handbook of familial cancer susceptibility syndromes - second edition. J Natl Cancer Inst Monogr 2008;(38):1–93.

13. Ellis NA, German J. Molecular genetics of Bloom's syndrome. Hum Mol Genet 1996;5 Spec No:1457–63.

14. Zhang HZ, Jin GF, Shen HB. Epidemiologic differences in esophageal cancer between Asian and Western populations. Chin J Cancer 2012;31(6):281–6.

15. Xie SH, Lagergren J. The Male Predominance in Esophageal Adenocarcinoma. Clin Gastroenterol Hepatol 2016;14(3):338–347 e331.

16. Paraf F, Flejou JF, Pignon JP, et al. Surgical pathology of adenocarcinoma arising in Barrett's esophagus. Analysis of 67 cases. Am J Surg Pathol 1995;19(2): 183–91.

17. Lieberman MD, Shriver CD, Bleckner S, et al. Carcinoma of the esophagus. Prognostic significance of histologic type. J Thorac Cardiovasc Surg 1995;109(1): 130–8 [discussion: 139].

18. Rubenstein JH, Taylor JB. Meta-analysis: the association of oesophageal adenocarcinoma with symptoms of gastro-oesophageal reflux. Aliment Pharmacol Ther 2010;32(10):1222–7.

19. Sampliner RE. Practice guidelines on the diagnosis, surveillance, and therapy of Barrett's esophagus. The Practice Parameters Committee of the American College of Gastroenterology. Am J Gastroenterol 1998;93(7):1028–32.

20. Naini BV, Chak A, Ali MA, et al. Barrett's oesophagus diagnostic criteria: endoscopy and histology. Best Pract Res Clin Gastroenterol 2015;29(1):77–96.

21. Hvid-Jensen F, Pedersen L, Drewes AM, et al. Incidence of adenocarcinoma among patients with Barrett's esophagus. N Engl J Med 2011;365(15):1375–83.

22. Rastogi A, Puli S, El-Serag HB, et al. Incidence of esophageal adenocarcinoma in patients with Barrett's esophagus and high-grade dysplasia: a meta-analysis. Gastrointest Endosc 2008;67(3):394–8.

23. Spechler SJ, Souza RF. Barrett's esophagus. N Engl J Med 2014;371(9):836–45.
24. Curvers WL, ten Kate FJ, Krishnadath KK, et al. Low-grade dysplasia in Barrett's esophagus: overdiagnosed and underestimated. Am J Gastroenterol 2010; 105(7):1523–30.
25. Wani S, Falk GW, Post J, et al. Risk factors for progression of low-grade dysplasia in patients with Barrett's esophagus. Gastroenterology 2011;141(4):1179–86, 1186.e1.
26. Cook MB, Kamangar F, Whiteman DC, et al. Cigarette smoking and adenocarcinomas of the esophagus and esophagogastric junction: a pooled analysis from the international BEACON consortium. J Natl Cancer Inst 2010;102(17):1344–53.
27. Tramacere I, Pelucchi C, Bagnardi V, et al. A meta-analysis on alcohol drinking and esophageal and gastric cardia adenocarcinoma risk. Ann Oncol 2012; 23(2):287–97.
28. Turati F, Tramacere I, La Vecchia C, et al. A meta-analysis of body mass index and esophageal and gastric cardia adenocarcinoma. Ann Oncol 2013;24(3):609–17.
29. Liao LM, Vaughan TL, Corley DA, et al. Nonsteroidal anti-inflammatory drug use reduces risk of adenocarcinomas of the esophagus and esophagogastric junction in a pooled analysis. Gastroenterology 2012;142(3):442–52.e5 [quiz: e422–3].
30. Lanuti M, Liu G, Goodwin JM, et al. A functional epidermal growth factor (EGF) polymorphism, EGF serum levels, and esophageal adenocarcinoma risk and outcome. Clin Cancer Res 2008;14(10):3216–22.
31. Sun X, Elston R, Barnholtz-Sloan J, et al. A segregation analysis of Barrett's esophagus and associated adenocarcinomas. Cancer Epidemiol Biomarkers Prev 2010;19(3):666–74.
32. Ye W, Held M, Lagergren J, et al. Helicobacter pylori infection and gastric atrophy: risk of adenocarcinoma and squamous-cell carcinoma of the esophagus and adenocarcinoma of the gastric cardia. J Natl Cancer Inst 2004;96(5):388–96.
33. Xia HH, Talley NJ. Helicobacter pylori infection, reflux esophagitis, and atrophic gastritis: an unexplored triangle. Am J Gastroenterol 1998;93(3):394–400.
34. Schatz RA, Rockey DC. Gastrointestinal bleeding due to gastrointestinal tract malignancy: natural history, management, and outcomes. Dig Dis Sci 2017; 62(2):491–501.
35. Meltzer CC, Luketich JD, Friedman D, et al. Whole-body FDG positron emission tomographic imaging for staging esophageal cancer comparison with computed tomography. Clin Nucl Med 2000;25(11):882–7.
36. Zhang P, Xi M, Zhao L, et al. Clinical efficacy and failure pattern in patients with cervical esophageal cancer treated with definitive chemoradiotherapy. Radiother Oncol 2015;116(2):257–61.
37. Verbeek RE, Leenders M, Ten Kate FJ, et al. Surveillance of Barrett's esophagus and mortality from esophageal adenocarcinoma: a population-based cohort study. Am J Gastroenterol 2014;109(8):1215–22.
38. Rubenstein JH, Shaheen NJ. Epidemiology, diagnosis, and management of esophageal adenocarcinoma. Gastroenterology 2015;149(2):302–317 e301.
39. Shaheen NJ, Falk GW, Iyer PG, et al, American College of Gastroenterology. ACG clinical guideline: diagnosis and management of Barrett's esophagus. Am J Gastroenterol 2016;111(1):30–50 [quiz: 51].
40. Thosani N, Singh H, Kapadia A, et al. Diagnostic accuracy of EUS in differentiating mucosal versus submucosal invasion of superficial esophageal cancers: a systematic review and meta-analysis. Gastrointest Endosc 2012;75(2):242–53.

41. Pouw RE, Heldoorn N, Alvarez Herrero L, et al. Do we still need EUS in the workup of patients with early esophageal neoplasia? A retrospective analysis of 131 cases. Gastrointest Endosc 2011;73(4):662–8.
42. Catalano MF, Sivak MV Jr, Rice T, et al. Endosonographic features predictive of lymph node metastasis. Gastrointest Endosc 1994;40(4):442–6.
43. Romagnuolo J, Scott J, Hawes RH, et al. Helical CT versus EUS with fine needle aspiration for celiac nodal assessment in patients with esophageal cancer. Gastrointest Endosc 2002;55(6):648–54.
44. van Westreenen HL, Heeren PA, van Dullemen HM, et al. Positron emission tomography with F-18-fluorodeoxyglucose in a combined staging strategy of esophageal cancer prevents unnecessary surgical explorations. J Gastrointest Surg 2005;9(1):54–61.
45. Block MI, Patterson GA, Sundaresan RS, et al. Improvement in staging of esophageal cancer with the addition of positron emission tomography. Ann Thorac Surg 1997;64(3):770–6 [discussion: 776–7].
46. Bruzzi JF, Swisher SG, Truong MT, et al. Detection of interval distant metastases: clinical utility of integrated CT-PET imaging in patients with esophageal carcinoma after neoadjuvant therapy. Cancer 2007;109(1):125–34.
47. Kukar M, Alnaji RM, Jabi F, et al. Role of repeat 18F-fluorodeoxyglucose positron emission tomography examination in predicting pathologic response following neoadjuvant chemoradiotherapy for esophageal adenocarcinoma. JAMA Surg 2015;150(6):555–62.
48. Vallbohmer D, Holscher AH, Dietlein M, et al. [18F]-Fluorodeoxyglucose-positron emission tomography for the assessment of histopathologic response and prognosis after completion of neoadjuvant chemoradiation in esophageal cancer. Ann Surg 2009;250(6):888–94.
49. NCCN Clinical Practice Guidelines in Oncology. 2019. Available at: https://www.nccn.org/professionals/physician_gls/default.aspx. Accessed September 1, 2019.
50. Hur C, Choi SE, Rubenstein JH, et al. The cost effectiveness of radiofrequency ablation for Barrett's esophagus. Gastroenterology 2012;143(3):567–75.
51. Abbas AE, Deschamps C, Cassivi SD, et al. Barrett's esophagus: the role of laparoscopic fundoplication. Ann Thorac Surg 2004;77(2):393–6.
52. Peters JH, Hagen JA, DeMeester SR. Barrett's esophagus. J Gastrointest Surg 2004;8(1):1–17.
53. Oberg S, Johansson J, Wenner J, et al. Endoscopic surveillance of columnar-lined esophagus: frequency of intestinal metaplasia detection and impact of anti-reflux surgery. Ann Surg 2001;234(5):619–26.
54. Japanese Society for Esophageal Diseases. Guidelines for clinical and pathologic studies on carcinoma of the esophagus, ninth edition: Preface, general principles, part I. Esophagus 2004;1(2):61–88.
55. Ancona E, Rampado S, Cassaro M, et al. Prediction of lymph node status in superficial esophageal carcinoma. Ann Surg Oncol 2008;15(11):3278–88.
56. Holscher AH, Bollschweiler E, Schroder W, et al. Prognostic impact of upper, middle, and lower third mucosal or submucosal infiltration in early esophageal cancer. Ann Surg 2011;254(5):802–7 [discussion: 807–8].
57. Shimada H, Nabeya Y, Matsubara H, et al. Prediction of lymph node status in patients with superficial esophageal carcinoma: analysis of 160 surgically resected cancers. Am J Surg 2006;191(2):250–4.
58. Eguchi T, Nakanishi Y, Shimoda T, et al. Histopathological criteria for additional treatment after endoscopic mucosal resection for esophageal cancer: analysis of 464 surgically resected cases. Mod Pathol 2006;19(3):475–80.

59. Akutsu Y, Uesato M, Shuto K, et al. The overall prevalence of metastasis in T1 esophageal squamous cell carcinoma: a retrospective analysis of 295 patients. Ann Surg 2013;257(6):1032–8.
60. Pech O, Bollschweiler E, Manner H, et al. Comparison between endoscopic and surgical resection of mucosal esophageal adenocarcinoma in Barrett's esophagus at two high-volume centers. Ann Surg 2011;254(1):67–72.
61. Das A, Singh V, Fleischer DE, et al. A comparison of endoscopic treatment and surgery in early esophageal cancer: an analysis of surveillance epidemiology and end results data. Am J Gastroenterol 2008;103(6):1340–5.
62. Nemoto K, Yamada S, Nishio M, et al. Results of radiation therapy for superficial esophageal cancer using the standard radiotherapy method recommended by the Japanese Society of Therapeutic Radiology and Oncology (JASTRO) Study Group. Anticancer Res 2006;26(2B):1507–12.
63. Maingon P, d'Hombres A, Truc G, et al. High dose rate brachytherapy for superficial cancer of the esophagus. Int J Radiat Oncol Biol Phys 2000;46(1):71–6.
64. Okawa T, Tanaka M, Kita-Okawa M, et al. Superficial esophageal cancer: multicenter analysis of results of definitive radiation therapy in Japan. Radiology 1995;196(1):271–4.
65. Swisher SG, Wynn P, Putnam JB, et al. Salvage esophagectomy for recurrent tumors after definitive chemotherapy and radiotherapy. J Thorac Cardiovasc Surg 2002;123(1):175–83.
66. Siewert JR, Holscher AH, Becker K, et al. Cardia cancer: attempt at a therapeutically relevant classification. Chirurg 1987;58(1):25–32 [in German].
67. Coccolini F, Nardi M, Montori G, et al. Neoadjuvant chemotherapy in advanced gastric and esophago-gastric cancer. Meta-analysis of randomized trials. Int J Surg 2018;51:120–7.
68. van Hagen P, Hulshof MC, van Lanschot JJ, et al. Preoperative chemoradiotherapy for esophageal or junctional cancer. N Engl J Med 2012;366(22):2074–84.
69. Ruppert BN, Watkins JM, Shirai K, et al. Cisplatin/Irinotecan versus carboplatin/paclitaxel as definitive chemoradiotherapy for locoregionally advanced esophageal cancer. Am J Clin Oncol 2010;33(4):346–52.
70. Leichman LP, Goldman BH, Bohanes PO, et al. S0356: a phase II clinical and prospective molecular trial with oxaliplatin, fluorouracil, and external-beam radiation therapy before surgery for patients with esophageal adenocarcinoma. J Clin Oncol 2011;29(34):4555–60.
71. Tepper J, Krasna MJ, Niedzwiecki D, et al. Phase III trial of trimodality therapy with cisplatin, fluorouracil, radiotherapy, and surgery compared with surgery alone for esophageal cancer: CALGB 9781. J Clin Oncol 2008;26(7):1086–92.
72. Sharma R, Yang GY, Nava HR, et al. A single institution experience with neoadjuvant chemoradiation (CRT) with irinotecan (I) and cisplatin (C) in locally advanced esophageal carcinoma (LAEC). J Clin Oncol 2009;27(15_suppl):e15619.
73. Ajani JA, Winter K, Okawara GS, et al. Phase II trial of preoperative chemoradiation in patients with localized gastric adenocarcinoma (RTOG 9904): quality of combined modality therapy and pathologic response. J Clin Oncol 2006;24(24):3953–8.
74. Smalley SR, Benedetti JK, Haller DG, et al. Updated analysis of SWOG-directed intergroup study 0116: a phase III trial of adjuvant radiochemotherapy versus observation after curative gastric cancer resection. J Clin Oncol 2012;30(19):2327–33.

75. Macdonald JS, Smalley SR, Benedetti J, et al. Chemoradiotherapy after surgery compared with surgery alone for adenocarcinoma of the stomach or gastro-esophageal junction. N Engl J Med 2001;345(10):725–30.
76. Adelstein DJ, Rice TW, Rybicki LA, et al. Mature results from a phase II trial of postoperative concurrent chemoradiotherapy for poor prognosis cancer of the esophagus and gastroesophageal junction. J Thorac Oncol 2009;4(10):1264–9.
77. Bang YJ, Van Cutsem E, Feyereislova A, et al. Trastuzumab in combination with chemotherapy versus chemotherapy alone for treatment of HER2-positive advanced gastric or gastro-oesophageal junction cancer (ToGA): a phase 3, open-label, randomised controlled trial. Lancet 2010;376(9742):687–97.
78. Fuchs CS, Tomasek J, Yong CJ, et al. Ramucirumab monotherapy for previously treated advanced gastric or gastro-oesophageal junction adenocarcinoma (RE-GARD): an international, randomised, multicentre, placebo-controlled, phase 3 trial. Lancet 2014;383(9911):31–9.
79. Wilke H, Muro K, Van Cutsem E, et al. Ramucirumab plus paclitaxel versus placebo plus paclitaxel in patients with previously treated advanced gastric or gastro-oesophageal junction adenocarcinoma (RAINBOW): a double-blind, randomised phase 3 trial. Lancet Oncol 2014;15(11):1224–35.
80. Molena D, Sun HH, Badr AS, et al. Clinical tools do not predict pathological complete response in patients with esophageal squamous cell cancer treated with definitive chemoradiotherapy. Dis Esophagus 2014;27(4):355–9.
81. Barbetta A, Hsu M, Tan KS, et al. Definitive chemoradiotherapy versus neoadjuvant chemoradiotherapy followed by surgery for stage II to III esophageal squamous cell carcinoma. J Thorac Cardiovasc Surg 2018;155(6):2710–21.e3.
82. Rizk NP, Ishwaran H, Rice TW, et al. Optimum lymphadenectomy for esophageal cancer. Ann Surg 2010;251(1):46–50.
83. Orringer MB, Marshall B, Iannettoni MD. Transhiatal esophagectomy: clinical experience and refinements. Ann Surg 1999;230(3):392–400 [discussion: 400–3].
84. Price TN, Nichols FC, Harmsen WS, et al. A comprehensive review of anastomotic technique in 432 esophagectomies. Ann Thorac Surg 2013;95(4):1154–60 [discussion 1160–1].
85. Forshaw MJ, Gossage JA, Ockrim J, et al. Left thoracoabdominal esophagogastrectomy: still a valid operation for carcinoma of the distal esophagus and esophagogastric junction. Dis Esophagus 2006;19(5):340–5.
86. Biere SS, van Berge Henegouwen MI, Maas KW, et al. Minimally invasive versus open oesophagectomy for patients with oesophageal cancer: a multicentre, open-label, randomised controlled trial. Lancet 2012;379(9829):1887–92.

Management of Gastric Adenocarcinoma for General Surgeons

Hisakazu Hoshi, MD

KEYWORDS

- Gastric cancer • Staging • Diagnostic imaging • Endoscopy • Laparoscopy
- Multimodality treatment • Neoadjuvant chemotherapy • Radiation therapy

KEY POINTS

- Gastric cancer should be suspected for patients with persistent vague abdominal symptoms.
- Precise staging with various imaging techniques knowing strength and weakness of each imaging modality is extremely important to select appropriate treatment strategy.
- Most of the resectable gastric cancers diagnosed in the United States are advanced stage and neoadjuvant chemotherapy is indicated.
- Diagnostic laparoscopy with peritoneal cytology should be performed preoperatively for resectable advanced disease.
- Surgical resection should be performed with at least D1, preferably D2 nodal dissection to aim at least 15 lymph nodes harvested for pathology examination.

INTRODUCTION

Gastric adenocarcinoma is one of the most common cancers in the world, although the incidence of that in the United States is declining about 1.5% per year over the last 10 years.[1] The American Cancer Society estimates that 27,510 cases will be diagnosed and 11,140 patients will die from this disease in 2019.[2] Because of the rare occurrence of the disease in the United States, there is significant treatment variance in use of diagnostic modalities, neoadjuvant/adjuvant therapies, and surgical techniques.[3] The survival of patients with gastric cancer in the United States is significantly lower than those of Asian countries, where the diagnosis is made at an earlier stage and uniform high-quality treatment is delivered.[4,5] This article reviews pearls and pitfalls of multidisciplinary management of the gastric adenocarcinoma for best outcomes.

Division of Endocrine and Surgical Oncology, Department of Surgery, University of Iowa Hospitals and Clinics, 200 Hawkins Drive, 4637 JCP, Iowa City, IA 52242, USA
E-mail address: Hisakazu-hoshi@uiowa.edu

Surg Clin N Am 100 (2020) 523–534
https://doi.org/10.1016/j.suc.2020.02.004
surgical.theclinics.com

DIAGNOSIS AND STAGING
Endoscopy

The cornerstone of the diagnosis of gastric cancer is an upper endoscopy examination. The symptoms of gastric cancer are typically vague and nonspecific. In Asia, where the gastric cancer incidence is high, there is a very low threshold to perform upper endoscopy to rule out the diagnosis. Any nonresolving vague upper gastrointestinal (GI) symptoms, including indigestion, epigastric pain, and excessive belching, could be a symptom of gastric cancer and a high index of suspicion needs to be maintained.

In the United States general surgeons are involved in the diagnostic process of this disease and it is vital to have knowledge of endoscopic features of suspicious gastric lesions. Particularly in early gastric cancer, which is highly curable, the diagnosis depends on the ability of operators of endoscopy to recognize subtle changes of mucosa.[6] A well-demarcated lesion either elevated or depressed, or the irregularity of color/surface pattern is a sign of suspicious lesions and magnifying endoscopy with narrow-band imaging should be used to further evaluate the lesion.[7]

When biopsies are performed on suspicious ulcerated lesion, they should be taken from the far edge (not near edge) of the ulcer and the base of the ulcer. Malignant tissue typically exists at the margin of the ulceration and biopsy of near edge creates a higher rate of false-negative results caused by the angle of forceps to obtain the tissue. When linitis plastica type cancer is suspected from the stiffness of the wall/thick folds, biopsies of the superficial mucosa typically do not confirm the diagnosis. Either boring biopsy (repeat biopsy of the same area for deep biopsy) and/or endoscopic ultrasound–guided core needle biopsy of the wall of the stomach is necessary to make a diagnosis. Single biopsy of the lesion confirms the diagnosis in only 70% of gastric cancer. A total of seven biopsies increases the diagnostic accuracy to 98%.[8]

Endoscopic ultrasound is necessary if early versus more advanced disease cannot be determined by gross endoscopic appearances or other imaging modalities, or if endoscopic treatment is planned for suspected T1 cancer. Gastric cancer higher than or equal to T2 (involving muscular layer) should be treated with neoadjuvant chemotherapy (discussed later). T1 cancer is treated by an endoscopic resection and needs to be referred to endoscopic specialists who have significant experience treating this disease.

Endoscopy is also a necessary component of the preoperative planning. Information about the extent of involvement of the gastric wall is used to determine if the patient needs a total versus distal gastrectomy. Also, esophageal extension, which makes complexity and morbidities of operation much higher, should be carefully assessed. It is important to do an inflation-deflation examination to evaluate the stiffness of the gastric wall for advanced disease. Involved portion of the gastric wall typically loses pliability and becomes stiff. This creates conversion/thickening of the gastric folds and relative fixed appearances of the area. If the large portion of the stomach is diffusely involved then the affected portion of the stomach does not insufflate or collapse and mucosal fold remains fixed and thick with air insufflation. This finding strongly suggests presence of diffuse gastric cancer even in the absence of a mucosal lesion. Precise documentation of extent of the disease by the endoscopic examination is extremely important and helpful for assessment of the tumor response to preoperative chemotherapy and for procedure planning.

Cross-sectional Imaging

Contrast-enhanced computed tomography

Although contrast-enhanced computed tomography (CT) is a gold standard for preoperative staging, there are a few pitfalls of which general surgeons should be aware. At the time of staging CT, chest and pelvis should be included in the image. For the chest CT, particular attention should be directed to mediastinal and supraclavicular adenopathy. These nodes are not regional lymph nodes of stomach and if these turn out to be positive for a metastatic disease then they should be staged as M1 disease. Also, lung metastases could occur without nodal or liver metastatic disease and any noncalcified nodules should raise the suspicion of a metastatic disease. For the abdomen and pelvis images, presence of periceliac/para-aortic adenopathy, peritoneal nodules/ascites/increased omental density, involvement of pancreatic head in the distal gastric cancer, and pancreatic tail/spleen/distal esophagus/diaphragmatic crus in the proximal one should be noted. These findings are potential signs of marginally resectable/nonresectable cancers and further investigation with PET, endoscopic ultrasound, or laparoscopy is warranted. Overall accuracy of CT staging is only 53% because of low accuracy in T stage (43%–82%); however, it is an effective tool to stage regional and distant extent of the disease. One possible way to enhance the accuracy of T staging on CT is use of CT gastrography.[9,10] CT gastrography is a modification technique of CT colonoscopy and the stomach is distended to create virtual gastroscopy images. CT gastrography adds information of mucosal surface irregularity and stiffness/thickness of the gastric wall, which is used to estimate the depth and the extent of the disease.

PET/computed tomography scan

In recent years PET scan is used more often for staging; however, fluorodeoxyglucose (FDG)-PET itself has low sensitivity (58%–94%) in making diagnosis of this disease.[11] This means FDG-PET cannot be used to confirm the diagnosis of gastric cancer. Combination of FDG-PET/CT has better accuracy on staging (66%) than PET (47%) or CT (51%) alone.[12] FDG-PET has low accuracy particularly in poorly differentiated (diffuse signet ring cell) or mucinous adenocarcinoma.[13] In these histologic types of gastric cancer, PET grossly underestimates the extent of the disease and negative uptake does not rule out presence of metastatic disease or response to the treatment. Contrast-enhanced CT and FDG-PET/CT are considered as complementary tests.

Diagnostic laparoscopy with wash cytology

In gastric adenocarcinoma about 20% to 30% of patients have peritoneal disseminated disease at the time of initial diagnosis.[14] Proximal or whole stomach cancer and poorly differentiated histologic type have higher risk of associated peritoneal carcinomatosis. Once diagnosed, peritoneal disease carries extremely poor prognosis and it is staged as stage IV disease.[15,16] Because of this surgical resection is not recommended outside of clinical trial setting. Also peritoneal carcinomatosis is the most difficult metastatic disease to be detected by cross-sectional imaging. Thus, diagnostic laparoscopy is recommended for initial staging of any resectable gastric adenocarcinoma except T1 disease. At the time of diagnostic laparoscopy, all of the peritoneal surface should be carefully examined and any suspicious lesion should be biopsied. Also, wash cytology should be obtained by installing a few hundred milliliters of normal saline into the peritoneal cavity and collected into a suction trap after agitating abdominal contents. Typically, cytologic examination consumes a significant amount of time and diagnostic laparoscopy is scheduled separate from a definitive resection to avoid false-negative results. Cytology-positive peritoneal disease has a much worse prognosis than gross (peritoneal nodule) positive peritoneal disease.

MULTIDISCIPLINARY TREATMENT
Neoadjuvant/Perioperative Chemotherapy

In 2006 MAGIC trial was published from the MRC England, which randomized resectable gastric and gastroesophageal junction adenocarcinoma to either perioperative chemotherapy (epirubicin, cisplatin, and 5FU) followed by surgery or surgery alone.[17] A small number of T1 or N0 patients were included in the study but most patients had disease stage higher than or equal to T2 or N1. The results showed significant downstaging effect with improved disease-free survival and overall survival (5-year, 36.3 vs 23.0) in the perioperative chemotherapy group. In the perioperative chemotherapy group, 90.7% of randomized patients who started preoperative chemotherapy competed intended three cycles but only 49.5% patients completed three more cycles of chemotherapy following surgical resection. It is highly likely that surgical resection of the stomach has significant impact on GI function and its associated morbidity, which made delivery of postoperative chemotherapy difficult. Because of this it is generally accepted that the effect of perioperative chemotherapy is largely derived from preoperative chemotherapy.

In recent years German-AIO published a randomized phase II/III trial comparing perioperative chemotherapy with epirubicin, cisplatin, and 5FU regimen versus 5FU, leucovorin, oxaliplatin, docetaxel (FLOT) regimen for disease stage higher than or equal to T2 or N1.[18] The results showed better downstaging and higher R0 resection rate with improved median (35 vs 50 months) and 5-year overall survival (36% vs 45%) in FLOT group. Toxicity profiles of each regimen were different but rates of grade III and VI toxicity were similar. With this result FLOT became a first-choice regimen of perioperative chemotherapy.

Because patients with gastric cancer are most likely seen by surgeons first, it is vitally important for surgeons to realize that most patients with resectable gastric cancer (except T1b tumor, which is rare in the United States) receive benefits from preoperative chemotherapy and medical oncology should be involved in patient care before the operation.

Surgical Resection

The principle of oncologic resection is to gain maximum locoregional control of the disease while minimizing tissue/functional loss, morbidity, and mortality. Well-planned, high-quality surgery is one of the most important factors that impacts overall outcome of the cancer treatment; however, it is extremely difficult to measure surgical quality directly and hence to improve individual technical quality of the operation. In gastric cancer operation, two factors that have significant effect on locoregional control of disease are negative margin resection and clearance of nodal disease.

Negative Margin Resection

Margin-positive (R1 or R2) resection is a significant prognostic indicator for poor survival outcome from the resection.[19] One could argue this is merely an expression of biologic aggressiveness; however, a few principles should be followed to ensure the highest possibilities of negative margin resection with maximum preservation of stomach. Preoperative assessment of tumor extension by CT gastrography or endoscopy plays a significant role on selection of the extent of the resection and method of reconstruction. Intraoperatively initial transection margin should be grossly 3 cm from tumor margin for well to moderately differentiated adenocarcinoma and 5 cm for poorly differentiated adenocarcinoma.[20] The former histologic type typically shows less infiltrative nature compared with the latter and distal or subtotal gastrectomy is appropriate for antral or body cancer if histologic negative margin can be achieved.[21] Proximal gastric cancer most likely requires total gastrectomy not because of the distal margin but because of the associated postoperative bile reflux esophagitis complication of proximal gastrectomy. Frozen section of proximal and distal margins should be sent. Additional 3 to 5 cm of abdominal esophagus from gastroesophageal junction could be resected by abdominal approach to achieve negative margin but further proximal extension necessitates approach through either thoracotomy or cervical incision with subtotal or total esophagectomy, which increases morbidities of the operation and creates significant problems in reconstruction. A gastric cancer requiring resection of significant length of esophagus to achieve negative margin typically is an advanced cancer and risk-benefit balance should be carefully assessed before proceeding with esophagogastrectomy, particularly in T3/4 tumor, node-positive disease, or poorly differentiated adenocarcinoma. Duodenal microscopic positive margin is difficult to manage because of lack of additional resectable tissue to achieve negative margin and it is likely related to aggressive biology with poor resection outcome. Pancreaticoduodenectomy is rarely indicated in this situation.

A T4b tumor invading adjacent organs requires multiorgan resection to obtain negative margin.[22] Common adjacent organs involved by the gastric cancer are spleen, pancreas, liver, and transverse colon. A metanalysis of more than 1300 patients undergoing en bloc resection for T4 disease showed significantly higher morbidity (11%–90%) and mortality (2%–15%) with R0 resection rate of 38% to 100% and 5-year overall survival of 11% to 45%.[23] These patients were highly selected patients. For the best outcome, staging, operative risks, and tumor biology should be carefully assessed. For these cases diagnostic laparoscopy is a must to rule out peritoneal disseminated disease or small liver metastasis and neoadjuvant chemotherapy should be given to eliminate biologically aggressive disease, which is refractory to chemotherapy. Outcome of R1/R2 resection is extremely poor and should be avoided by meticulous preoperative planning.

Clearance of Nodal Disease

Effectiveness and optimal extent of nodal dissection have been a focus of debate for the last several decades. All the randomized trials comparing D1 with D2 nodal dissection have failed to prove the effect of survival improvement; however, two important facts should be considered to interpret these results.

The first fact is that no randomized study exists comparing no nodal dissection with nodal dissection (D0 vs D1). Historically many patients with gastric cancer in the United States were treated with no nodal dissection or limited nodal dissection. Even in 1990s most of the operations were categorized D0 as seen in the results of Intergroup 0116.[24] It has been demonstrated that more than 15 lymph nodes need to be examined for accurate staging of this disease and failure to do so associates with lower survival.[25,26] If less than a D1 dissection is performed then it is highly unlikely to harvest even a minimum of 15 lymph nodes, which leads to understaging and R1 resection (residual nodal disease). The consequence of this is clinically significant with increased locoregional recurrence and nondelivery of adjuvant treatment (particularly radiation therapy), which could potentially salvage these patients with limited regional disease (discussed later). Surgical undertreatment creates understaging with high risk of locoregional recurrence and poor long-term outcome. These results led the Commission on Cancer to adapt quality metric of 15 lymph nodes for gastric cancer in the fall of 2014 for Commission on Cancer accredited cancer pro-grams. Despite this as of July 2019 only 65.9% of the patients treated at Commission on Cancer accredited hospitals met this metric (2019 unpublished data National Cancer Database). Although specimen processing may be a factor for noncompli-ance, considering the historical low adaption rate of nodal dissection, it is suspected that the surgical nodal dissection quality plays a significant role.

Although technical details of nodal dissection are beyond the scope of this article, a few points need to be emphasized. D1 nodal dissection must include infrapyloric node (station 6), right paracardiac (station 1), and left gastric nodes (station 7) regardless of the location of the tumor.[27] These are the nodal stations with high rate of involvement.

The infrapyloric nodes are located in front of the uncinate process of the pancreatic head surrounding insertion point of the right gastroepiploic vein to gastrocolic trunk (then superior mesenteric vein) and origin of right gastroepiploic artery. If the dissec-tion is done properly, one should see the surface of the pancreatic head exposed caudal to the first portion of duodenum (**Fig. 1**).

Left gastric nodes are located around the origin of the left gastric artery from the ce-liac axis. Complete removal of left gastric nodes typically requires ligation and transec-tion of the left gastric artery at its origin (**Fig. 2**). If a left replaced/accessory hepatic artery is branching off of the left gastric artery then the left gastric artery can be skel-etonized from the origin to the branching point of the left hepatic artery ligating all branches supplying the stomach and the dissected soft tissue containing lymph nodes should be included in the specimen.

Right paracardial nodes are located between proximal lesser curvature of the stom-ach and diaphragmatic crus. If a total gastrectomy is the procedure then after ligating left gastric artery at its origin, the soft tissue covering the anterior surface of the crus should be completely dissected off toward esophageal hiatus. This ensures entire lesser curvature and right paracardial nodes within the specimen. If the procedure is a distal gastrectomy, after dissecting soft tissue from diaphragmatic crus, the soft tissue containing nodal tissue in lesser curvature needs to be separated from the

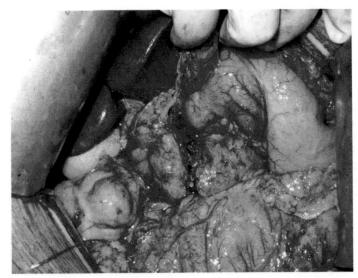

Fig. 1. Infrapyloric nodal dissection (station 6). Note ligated stumps of left gastroepiploic vein and artery and exposed pancreatic uncinate process.

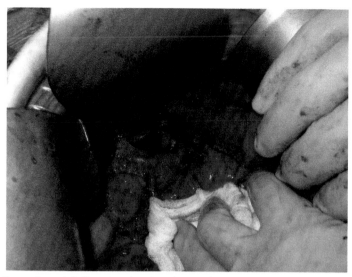

Fig. 2. Left gastric nodal dissection (station 7). Note ligated left gastric artery stump at the celiac axis and mobilized soft tissue from the surface of diaphragmatic crus.

wall of lower esophagus and proximal stomach to the point of gastric transection line by ligating terminal branches of the left gastric artery (**Fig. 3**).

The second fact that needs to be realized is that nodal dissection surgery is a regional therapy and has little systemic treatment effect. This means if the disease is advanced and has high risk of systemic or peritoneal disease then nodal dissection will likely not have an effect on improving outcome. However, if a tumor is early stage and no nodal metastasis is present then removing normal nodes will not improve

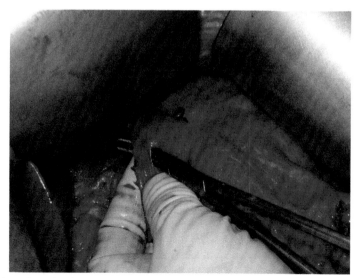

Fig. 3. Dissection of right paracardial (station 1) and lesser curvature node (station 3) from lower esophagus and upper lesser curvature.

outcome. Pathologic T1a carcinoma has only about a 10% chance of nodal metastasis and formal D2 nodal dissection is not recommended by the Japanese gastric cancer treatment guideline.[20] This is likely the reason why nearly all the retrospective studies and randomized trials of D1 versus D2 nodal dissection show benefit of D2 nodal dissection on survival for stage II and IIIa subgroups even though there are negative results of the entire cohort.[25] On the Dutch D1 versus D2 trial, at least a quarter of enrolled patients had T1 disease, which dilutes the true therapeutic effect of nodal dissection. Despite this, 15-year follow-up analysis shows superior disease-specific survival in D2 patients' group; however, the overall survival benefit was canceled out by the high postoperative mortality from pancreaticosplenectomy in D2 nodal dissection patients.[28] Because routine splenectomy is no longer a part of the D2 nodal dissection procedure with the result of the JCOG trial[29] and elimination of distal pancreatectomy for nodal retrieval in current standard D2 nodal dissection procedure, recent series of D2 nodal dissection patients enjoy significantly lower mortality (0%–2.2%) in even western series.[30,31] Currently D2 nodal dissection is standard of care in Asia and Europe and the National Comprehensive Cancer Network guidelines recommend D1 or modern D2 (no pancreaticosplenectomy) nodal dissection, with a goal of examining 15 or more lymph nodes for resectable cancer. Also the guidelines emphasize that D2 nodal dissection should be performed by experienced surgeons in high-volume centers (discussed next).

Learning Curve of the D2 Nodal Dissection and Surgical Quality Control

The D2 nodal dissection is a technically challenging procedure that calls for detailed anatomic understanding of the nodal structures around the stomach. Both UK and Netherland D1 versus D2 randomized trials suffered from high morbidity and mortality of D2 arm patients and underdissection of nodal stations (noncompliance).[32,33] The Dutch trial had more rigorous surgical quality control than the UK trial but in the end they experienced 81.5% noncompliance rate.[34]

Typically Japanese surgical trainees observe a large number of D2 gastrectomy procedures early in their training. They start performing the procedure under direct supervision of gastric cancer specialists as early as postgraduate year 2 or 3. Lee and colleagues[35] published the Korean experience of learning curve on the D2 nodal dissection technique. They used node retrieval of more than 25 as a quality measure and studied two junior staff members who joined their National Cancer Center. Their conclusion is that at least 23 cases or 8 months of training is required to produce 92.5% successful node retrieval rate. Of note, these two junior staff members were not novices and had been trained in gastric cancer surgery for 2 years at their respective university hospitals. They assisted in more than 200 gastrectomies per year before they join National Cancer Center and they performed the gastric cancer surgery as first assistants for 3 months after joining. In western institutions it is rare to have this volume of cases and the result may not be directly applicable.

McCulloch published in 1996 his own learning curve of this procedure.[36] He began to perform this procedure unsupervised after spending 4 months in Japan undergoing intensive training under the supervision. He used physiologic score (POSSUM) and morbidity for quality measures. His conclusion was that 18 to 24 months or 15 to 25 procedures are required to reach plateau on his learning curve. He did not report any changes in the number of nodal retrieval during the study period; however, the study mainly addresses the learning curve of safety aspect and not that of quality aspect.

From the author's personal experience, to master this procedure requires some form of preparation (video instruction, assistant experience) and at least 20 to 30 supervised hands-on experiences, which is difficult to achieve in most western institutions. Furthermore, the procedure becomes technically more challenging once the patient's body mass index is greater than 30 to 35. Previous Japanese randomized D2 versus D3 trial showed body mass index greater than 25 is associated with decreased nodal retrieval in the D2 nodal dissection.[37] The quality control of the procedure is even more difficult in western institutions because of these reasons.

Role of Radiation Therapy

Radiation therapy is another form of locoregional treatment that does not have an effect on distant metastatic disease. The role of radiation therapy for gastric cancer is controversial despite the positive results of the Intergroup trial (INT-0116).[24] This trial published 2001 randomized patients with resectable gastric cancer into surgery only versus adjuvant chemoradiation therapy. The results showed significantly lower locoregional recurrence and improved overall survival in the adjuvant chemoradiation group. The trial was criticized for low survival in the surgery only group with most of the patients treated with D0 nodal dissection. It was thought that the benefit of the radiation therapy was largely derived from controlling residual locoregional disease from inadequate resections.

The recently published CRITICS trial from the Netherland randomized stage IB-IVA patients into perioperative chemotherapy versus preoperative chemotherapy and postoperative chemoradiation therapy groups.[38] Most of the patients received at least D1+ resection. The result showed identical median overall survival of 43 versus 37 months for chemotherapy versus chemoradiation. The trial was criticized for low compliance rate (59% for postoperative chemotherapy and 62% for postoperative chemoradiation) of postresection treatment in both arms, which makes distinction of two arms ambiguous.

A smaller Korean trial (ARTIST) comparing adjuvant chemotherapy with chemoradiation in patients who underwent D2 gastrectomy also failed to show a difference in disease-free and overall survival.[39] These results led to investigating neoadjuvant radiation combined with perioperative chemotherapy approach. Currently two large randomized trials (TOPGEAR[40,41] and CRITCS II[42]) are ongoing.

SPECIAL ISSUES
Nutritional Assessment/Education

Nutritional assessment and education are important components of surgical care but particular attention should be paid for gastrectomy patients. Gastrectomy has a much larger impact on postoperative oral intake than other abdominal operations. Gastrectomy patients, particularly total gastrectomy patients, typically lose significant amount of weight postresection and they slowly or even never gain back their weight.[43] Also, they tend to have nausea/vomiting from maladaptation of their eating habits with occasional dumping symptoms. This tenuous nutritional status poses significant difficulty for oncologists to deliver planned postoperative treatment.[44]

Nutritional intervention should start preoperatively recognizing presence or absence of their nutritional deficit and educating about upcoming changes on their dietary habits. Involvement of nutritional specialists from the beginning is highly recommended.

Feeding jejunostomy is placed during the resection for selected patients. The author does not place it for distal gastrectomy patients and selectively places it for total gastrectomy patients.

Education for postoperative diet modification should start preoperatively and emphasis should be placed on chewing food thoroughly, small frequent meals, no concentrated sweets, separate solids and fluids, and stopping eating with 80% full. A food diary is an important tool for assessment of progress in oral intake and identifying problematic food creating GI symptoms.

DISCLOSURE

No disclosure.

REFERENCES

1. Torre LA, Bray F, Siegel RL, et al. Global cancer statistics, 2012. CA Cancer J Clin 2015;65(2):87–108.
2. Miller KD, Nogueira L, Mariotto AB, et al. Cancer treatment and survivorship statistics, 2019. CA Cancer J Clin 2019;69(5):363–85.
3. Ikoma N, Cormier JN, Feig B, et al. Racial disparities in preoperative chemotherapy use in gastric cancer patients in the United States: analysis of the National Cancer Data Base, 2006-2014. Cancer 2018;124(5):998–1007.
4. Suh YS, Yang HK. Screening and early detection of gastric cancer: east versus west. Surg Clin North Am 2015;95(5):1053–66.
5. Chan WL, Lam KO, Lee VHF, et al. Gastric cancer: from aetiology to management: differences between the east and the west. Clin Oncol (R Coll Radiol) 2019;31(8):570–7.
6. Ngamruengphong S, Abe S, Oda I. Endoscopic management of early gastric adenocarcinoma and preinvasive gastric lesions. Surg Clin North Am 2017; 97(2):371–85.
7. Yao K. The endoscopic diagnosis of early gastric cancer. Ann Gastroenterol 2013;26(1):11–22.
8. Graham DY, Schwartz JT, Cain GD, et al. Prospective evaluation of biopsy number in the diagnosis of esophageal and gastric carcinoma. Gastroenterology 1982;82(2):228–31.
9. Kim JW, Shin SS, Heo SH, et al. Diagnostic performance of 64-section CT using CT gastrography in preoperative T staging of gastric cancer according to 7th edition of AJCC cancer staging manual. Eur Radiol 2012;22(3):654–62.
10. Kim JW, Shin SS, Heo SH, et al. The role of three-dimensional multidetector CT gastrography in the preoperative imaging of stomach cancer: emphasis on detection and localization of the tumor. Korean J Radiol 2015;16(1):80–9.
11. Dassen AE, Lips DJ, Hoekstra CJ, et al. FDG-PET has no definite role in preoperative imaging in gastric cancer. Eur J Surg Oncol 2009;35(5):449–55.
12. Chen J, Cheong JH, Yun MJ, et al. Improvement in preoperative staging of gastric adenocarcinoma with positron emission tomography. Cancer 2005; 103(11):2383–90.
13. Stahl A, Ott K, Weber WA, et al. FDG PET imaging of locally advanced gastric carcinomas: correlation with endoscopic and histopathological findings. Eur J Nucl Med Mol Imaging 2003;30(2):288–95.
14. Sarela AI, Lefkowitz R, Brennan MF, et al. Selection of patients with gastric adenocarcinoma for laparoscopic staging. Am J Surg 2006;191(1):134–8.
15. Bentrem D, Wilton A, Mazumdar M, et al. The value of peritoneal cytology as a preoperative predictor in patients with gastric carcinoma undergoing a curative resection. Ann Surg Oncol 2005;12(5):347–53.
16. Mezhir JJ, Shah MA, Jacks LM, et al. Positive peritoneal cytology in patients with gastric cancer: natural history and outcome of 291 patients. Ann Surg Oncol 2010;17(12):3173–80.

17. Cunningham D, Allum WH, Stenning SP, et al. Perioperative chemotherapy versus surgery alone for resectable gastroesophageal cancer. N Engl J Med 2006; 355(1):11–20.

18. Al-Batran SE, Homann N, Pauligk C, et al. Perioperative chemotherapy with fluorouracil plus leucovorin, oxaliplatin, and docetaxel versus fluorouracil or capecitabine plus cisplatin and epirubicin for locally advanced, resectable gastric or gastro-oesophageal junction adenocarcinoma (FLOT4): a randomised, phase 2/3 trial. Lancet 2019;393(10184):1948–57.

19. Postlewait LM, Maithel SK. The importance of surgical margins in gastric cancer. J Surg Oncol 2016;113(3):277–82.

20. Japanese Gastric Cancer Association. Japanese gastric cancer treatment guidelines 2014 (ver. 4). Gastric Cancer 2017;20(1):1–19.

21. Bozzetti F, Marubini E, Bonfanti G, et al. Subtotal versus total gastrectomy for gastric cancer: five-year survival rates in a multicenter randomized Italian trial. Italian Gastrointestinal Tumor Study Group. Ann Surg 1999;230(2):170–8.

22. Mita K, Ito H, Fukumoto M, et al. Surgical outcomes and survival after extended multiorgan resection for T4 gastric cancer. Am J Surg 2012;203(1):107–11.

23. Brar SS, Seevaratnam R, Cardoso R, et al. Multivisceral resection for gastric cancer: a systematic review. Gastric Cancer 2012;15(Suppl 1):S100–7.

24. Macdonald JS, Smalley SR, Benedetti J, et al. Chemoradiotherapy after surgery compared with surgery alone for adenocarcinoma of the stomach or gastroesophageal junction. N Engl J Med 2001;345(10):725–30.

25. Schwarz RE, Smith DD. Clinical impact of lymphadenectomy extent in resectable gastric cancer of advanced stage. Ann Surg Oncol 2007;14(2):317–28.

26. Biondi A, D'Ugo D, Cananzi FC, et al. Does a minimum number of 16 retrieved nodes affect survival in curatively resected gastric cancer? Eur J Surg Oncol 2015;41(6):779–86.

27. Hoshi H. Standard D2 and modified nodal dissection for gastric adenocarcinoma. Surg Oncol Clin N Am 2012;21(1):57–70.

28. Songun I, Putter H, Kranenbarg EM, et al. Surgical treatment of gastric cancer: 15-year follow-up results of the randomised nationwide Dutch D1D2 trial. Lancet Oncol 2010;11(5):439–49.

29. Sano T, Sasako M, Mizusawa J, et al. Randomized controlled trial to evaluate splenectomy in total gastrectomy for proximal gastric carcinoma. Ann Surg 2017;265(2):277–83.

30. Degiuli M, Sasako M, Ponti A. Morbidity and mortality in the Italian Gastric Cancer Study Group randomized clinical trial of D1 versus D2 resection for gastric cancer. Br J Surg 2010;97(5):643–9.

31. Degiuli M, Sasako M, Ponti A, et al. Randomized clinical trial comparing survival after D1 or D2 gastrectomy for gastric cancer. Br J Surg 2014;101(2):23–31.

32. Cuschieri A, Weeden S, Fielding J, et al. Patient survival after D1 and D2 resections for gastric cancer: long-term results of the MRC randomized surgical trial. Surgical Co-operative Group. Br J Cancer 1999;79(9–10):1522–30.

33. Bonenkamp JJ, Hermans J, Sasako M, et al. Extended lymph-node dissection for gastric cancer. N Engl J Med 1999;340(12):908–14.

34. Bonenkamp JJ, Hermans J, Sasako M, et al. Quality control of lymph node dissection in the Dutch randomized trial of D1 and D2 lymph node dissection for gastric cancer. Gastric Cancer 1998;1(2):152–9.

35. Lee JH, Ryu KW, Lee JH, et al. Learning curve for total gastrectomy with D2 lymph node dissection: cumulative sum analysis for qualified surgery. Ann Surg Oncol 2006;13(9):1175–81.

36. Parikh D, Johnson M, Chagla L, et al. D2 gastrectomy: lessons from a prospective audit of the learning curve. Br J Surg 1996;83(11):1595–9.

37. Tsujinaka T, Sasako M, Yamamoto S, et al. Influence of overweight on surgical complications for gastric cancer: results from a randomized control trial comparing D2 and extended para-aortic D3 lymphadenectomy (JCOG9501). Ann Surg Oncol 2007;14(2):355–61.

38. Cats A, Jansen EPM, van Grieken NCT, et al. Chemotherapy versus chemoradiotherapy after surgery and preoperative chemotherapy for resectable gastric cancer (CRITICS): an international, open-label, randomised phase 3 trial. Lancet Oncol 2018;19(5):616–28.

39. Park SH, Sohn TS, Lee J, et al. Phase III trial to compare adjuvant chemotherapy with capecitabine and cisplatin versus concurrent chemoradiotherapy in gastric cancer: final report of the adjuvant chemoradiotherapy in stomach tumors trial, including survival and subset analyses. J Clin Oncol 2015;33(28):3130–6.

40. Leong T, Smithers BM, Michael M, et al. TOPGEAR: a randomised phase III trial of perioperative ECF chemotherapy versus preoperative chemoradiation plus perioperative ECF chemotherapy for resectable gastric cancer (an international, intergroup trial of the AGITG/TROG/EORTC/NCIC CTG). BMC Cancer 2015; 15:532.

41. Leong T, Smithers BM, Haustermans K, et al. TOPGEAR: a randomized, phase III trial of perioperative ECF chemotherapy with or without preoperative chemoradiation for resectable gastric cancer: interim results from an international, intergroup trial of the AGITG, TROG, EORTC and CCTG. Ann Surg Oncol 2017;24(8): 2252–8.

42. Slagter AE, Jansen EPM, van Laarhoven HW, et al. CRITICS-II: a multicentre randomised phase II trial of neo-adjuvant chemotherapy followed by surgery versus neo-adjuvant chemotherapy and subsequent chemoradiotherapy followed by surgery versus neo-adjuvant chemoradiotherapy followed by surgery in resectable gastric cancer. BMC Cancer 2018;18(1):877.

43. Davis JL, Selby LV, Chou JF, et al. Patterns and predictors of weight loss after gastrectomy for cancer. Ann Surg Oncol 2016;23(5):1639–45.

44. Aoyama T, Yoshikawa T, Shirai J, et al. Body weight loss after surgery is an independent risk factor for continuation of S-1 adjuvant chemotherapy for gastric cancer. Ann Surg Oncol 2013;20(6):2000–6.

Primary Liver Cancers

Intrahepatic Cholangiocarcinoma and Hepatocellular Carcinoma

Juan C. Mejia, MD*, Jennifer Pasko, MD

KEYWORDS

- Intrahepatic cholangiocarcinoma • Hepatocellular carcinoma • Primary liver cancers
- Liver resection • Cholangiocarcinoma • Cirrhosis

KEY POINTS

- Educate about primary liver cancers, specifically hepatocellular carcinoma and intrahepatic cholangiocarcinoma.
- Inform the general surgeon of important factors in the workup and diagnosis of hepatocellular carcinoma and intrahepatic cholangiocarcinoma.
- Discuss relevant treatment options for hepatocellular carcinoma and intrahepatic cholangiocarcinoma.
- Highlight relevant multidisciplinary approaches to patients with primary liver cancers.

INTRAHEPATIC CHOLANGIOCARCINOMA
Background

Intrahepatic cholangiocarcinoma (iCCA) is the second most common primary liver tumor after hepatocellular carcinoma (HCC). Studies suggest that iCCA makes up 10% to 15% of primary liver cancers.[1] Over the last several decades there has been a marked increase in the incidence of iCCA and a concomitant increase in mortality worldwide.[2] The incidence of iCCA in the United States is lower than in Eastern countries, with an incidence rate of 1.67 per 100,000.[3] However, it is projected that by 2030 primary liver cancers will be the second leading cause of cancer death in the United States.[4]

Types of Cholangiocarcinoma

Cholangiocarcinoma is a broad category of disease that is classified into distinct entities based on the origin of tumor. The 3 types of cholangiocarcinoma are iCCA, perihilar cholangiocarcinoma (pCCA), and distal cholangiocarcinoma (dCCA). The most

Providence Sacred Heart Medical Center, 101 West 8th Avenue, Suite 7050, Spokane, WA 99204, USA
* Corresponding author.
E-mail address: Juan.Mejia@providence.org

Surg Clin N Am 100 (2020) 535–549
https://doi.org/10.1016/j.suc.2020.02.013
0039-6109/20/© 2020 Elsevier Inc. All rights reserved.

common type of cholangiocarcinoma is pCCA constituting 50% of cases, compared with iCCA consisting of 10% of cases and dCCA accounting for 40%.[5,6] Perihilar disease, often referred to as a Klatskin tumor, is defined as any lesion above the cystic duct up to second biliary radicals within the liver.[5,6]

Presentation

Unfortunately, patients with iCCA are often found incidentally. Patients may not have symptoms at all, unlike other types of cholangiocarcinoma that often present with jaundice. As a result, patients with iCCA can present with locally advanced or metastatic disease at presentation. Patients can have vague abdominal symptoms, right upper quadrant pain, or weight loss, which may prompt imaging studies.

Imaging Characteristics of Intrahepatic Cholangiocarcinoma

Recommended imaging studies for a patient with iCCA is a triple-phase computed tomography (CT) scan of the liver or MRI (**Fig. 1**). A multiphase CT scan allows for an arterial and venous phase to be evaluated and can be helpful for surgical planning. Typical CT appearance for iCCA is a hypodense, irregular lesion in the unenhanced phase, peripheral rim enhancement in the arterial phase, and progressive hyperattenuation in the venous phase.[7] MRI of the liver can also be a helpful tool because iCCA appears hypodense on T1-weighted images and hyperintense on T2-weighted images.[8] The use of MRI with cholangiopancreatography can add additional information to help better understand the involvement of the biliary system and extent of tumor invasion.

Preoperative Workup for Intrahepatic Cholangiocarcinoma

Preoperative workup for any patient with iCCA is essential. With only 15% of patients presenting with resectable disease, it is imperative to have a thorough workup to rule out metastatic disease (**Box 1**).[9] Although most patients present with some imaging at their initial visit, there should be a recently obtained dedicated CT multiphase or MRI liver images. In addition it is recommended that a CT of the chest without contrast is obtained to rule out metastatic disease to the lungs. A full set of blood work is also recommended. With chronic liver disease and cirrhosis being a risk factor for developing iCCA, the blood work can be helpful to determining intrinsic liver function.

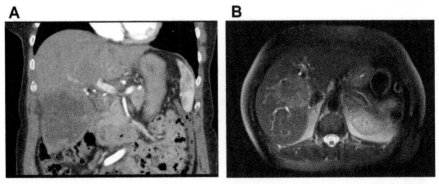

Fig. 1. (*A*) A large hypodense intrahepatic cholangiocarcinoma arising from the right liver on CT scan. (*B*) A central intrahepatic cholangiocarcinoma on MRI (T2), which is hyperintense.

Box 1
Preoperative workup for intrahepatic cholangiocarcinoma

Necessary Workup for Intrahepatic Cholangiocarcinoma
- Multiphase liver CT or liver MRI
- Chest CT without contrast
- Complete metabolic panel including liver enzymes, complete blood count, international normalized ratio, CA19-9, AFP, CEA

Considerations
- Biopsy of mass
- PET scan

Lastly, the use of fluorodeoxyglucose PET for iCCA is controversial and is not a standard part of the workup.

Tumor Markers of Intrahepatic Cholangiocarcinoma

Tumor markers are also considered a necessary portion of the workup. Carbohydrate antigen 19-9 (CA19-9) is the most sensitive at 50% and specific at 75% to 90% based on a level >100 U/mL.[10] It can also be a useful tool in surveillance postoperatively. However, as previously indicated CA19-9 is not always elevated preoperatively, obtaining α-fetoprotein (AFP) and carcinoembryonic antigen (CEA) levels is warranted.[11] A rare subgroup of primary liver tumors (HCC/cholangiocarcinoma) makes up a small proportion (approximately 0.4% to 4.7%) of all tumors, and AFP can be elevated in this group.[12]

To Biopsy or Not to Biopsy?

The role of biopsy in iCCA before surgery is debatable. An expert consensus statement in 2015 focused on its necessity and concluded that biopsy was not necessary in iCCA if the surgeon planned a resection with curative intent.[13] However, if patients have locally advanced nonresectable metastatic disease or are considering neoadjuvant treatment, there is usefulness in obtaining a biopsy to confirm diagnosis. If a biopsy is indeterminate it is necessary to rule out occult primary tumor with colonoscopy, mammography, and/or esophagogastroduodenoscopy.

Surgical Treatment of Intrahepatic Cholangiocarcinoma

Resection of iCCA is the only chance for a cure and is currently the standard of care for treatment. iCCA often presents at late stages, which can result in larger more advanced tumors that involve vascular and biliary pedicles. Patients should be seen by a surgical specialist, such as an HPB/surgical oncologist, because they often require a complex surgical operation. It is important to rule out multifocal disease or metastatic disease because these are contraindications to resection and are associated with worse overall survival (OS).[14,15] The goal of a surgical resection is to remove the tumor with an R0 resection and still leave the liver with adequate drainage and future liver remnant (FLR). These operations usually require a major hepatectomy with or without biliary reconstruction. Portal vein embolization may need to be performed to ensure adequate FLR.

Role of Lymphadenectomy in Intrahepatic Cholangiocarcinoma

In addition to resection, a lymphadenectomy of the regional lymph nodes should be performed. There has been controversy regarding the benefit of lymphadenectomy, but recent studies suggest that it not only helps to adequately stage the patient but also serves as a prognosticator for survival.[13,15,16] When a lymphadenectomy is performed, approximately one-third of nodes are positive. A lymphadenectomy for iCCA includes the regional nodal drainage basin; in particular the nodes of the hepatoduodenal ligament and hepatic artery, periduodenal nodes, and hilar nodes are considered N1 nodes.[17] Nodes in the celiac axis or para-aortic area are considered N2 and represent metastatic disease.[17] The most recent American Joint Committee on Cancer (AJCC) guidelines recommend at least 6 nodes at lymphadenectomy.[17]

Diagnostic Laparoscopy

Staging laparoscopy has become important in ruling out occult metastatic disease in patients with resectable iCCA. Two prospective trials showed that laparoscopy precluded resection in 25% to 36% of patients originally deemed resectable,[18,19] thus supporting the argument for routine use of laparoscopy in patients undergoing resection for iCCA, especially those deemed high risk.

Current Staging Guidelines

The staging guidelines for iCCA are published in the 8th edition of the AJCC/International Union Against Cancer staging manual (**Box 2**). In the 7th edition, iCCA was not classified as its own entity but was merged with HCC.[13] The most recent guidelines have been updated to reflect the importance of tumor size.[20] In addition, lymph node involvement previously was considered stage IVa disease but in the newest edition has been downstaged to stage IIIb.[20]

Surgical Factors Affecting Outcome

Patients who undergo resection have the best chance of long-term survival, with 5-year survival between 20% and 40%.[21–24] A recent meta-analysis performed by

---

Box 2
Staging for intrahepatic cholangiocarcinoma

T category
  T1a: solitary tumor $\leq$5 cm without vascular invasion
  T1b: solitary tumor >5 cm without vascular invasion
  T2: solitary tumor with intrahepatic vascular invasion or multiple tumors without or without vascular invasion
  T3: tumor perforating the visceral peritoneum
  T4: tumor involving local extrahepatic structures by direct invasion

N category
  N0: no regional lymph node metastasis
  N1: regional lymph node metastasis present

TNM Staging
  IA: T1aN0M0
  IB: T1bN0M0
  II: T1N0M0
  IIIA: T3N0M0
  IIIB: T4 and/or NI, M0
  IV: any T, any N, M1

Adapted from Lafaro KJ, Cosgrove D, Geschwind, JF et al. Multidisciplinary Care of Patients with Intrahepatic Cholangiocarcinoma: Updates in Management. Gastroenterol Res Pract. 2015.

Mavros and colleagues[23] evaluated the tumor characteristics associated with increased survival after surgical resection. Characteristics that were predictors of survival included larger tumors, presence of multiple tumors, lymph node metastasis, vascular invasion, and poor tumor differentiation.[24] Studies have demonstrated that lymph node metastasis is the most important indicator of survival.[13,25] However, patients who undergo a curative-intent resection have a high likelihood of recurrence. Most studies suggest that the risk of recurrence is greater than 50%, with most recurrences in the liver.[26]

Chemotherapy and Adjuvant Chemotherapy

The recent BILCAP trial was the first prospective trial to publish an OS benefit in patients who have undergone resection with adjuvant capecitabine in comparison with observation alone.[27] It is noteworthy that because of the rare nature of the disease, other biliary tract cancers were included in the study and iCCA made up only 8% of the study group.

Valle and colleagues[27] established the standard of care for nonresectable and metastatic iCCA with a randomized controlled trial evaluating patients with metastatic biliary cancer who received cisplatin/gemcitabine in comparison with patients who received gemcitabine alone. The results showed that patients who received gemcitabine and cisplatin had an overall and progression-free survival benefit.[28] This continues to be standard of care for metastatic disease to date.

Treatment Options for Metastatic and Unresectable Disease

Unfortunately, most patients present with metastatic or unresectable disease. The average survival for these patients is 6 to 12 months without treatment. The current practice for metastatic or unresectable disease is palliative chemotherapy. Although radiation therapy can be considered to decrease tumor burden,[29,30] no prospective randomized trials exist that show benefit in patients with iCCA.

There have been promising data regarding locoregional therapy. Studies using transarterial chemoembolization (TACE), drug-eluting beads, and yttrium-labeled selective internal radiation therapy have shown evidence for extended OS and are considered safe and effective in stabilizing disease.[31–34] However, unlike HCC there have been no randomized trials establishing the role of locoregional therapies in iCCA treatment.

The use of radiofrequency or microwaves can be considered for iCCA. This therapy is best used in small tumors ranging from 3 to 5 cm and has been shown to be effective in treating iCCA.[35] However, owing to the aggressive nature and usually advanced stage of tumor at presentation, the true value of ablation is unclear.

Promising results for metastatic iCCA have been seen in patients with hepatic arterial infusion (HAI) pumps. Initially used in patients with unresectable colorectal metastases, the use of HAI was expanded to include patients with iCCA. Initial results from Memorial Sloan Kettering have shown that patients with iCCA who received HAI and systemic chemotherapy had a statistically significant OS compared with those who received systemic chemotherapy alone.[36] To date, however, no prospective or large multi-institutional studies have been published.

HEPATOCELLULAR CARCINOMA
Epidemiology

Hepatocellular carcinoma (HCC) is the most common type of primary liver cancer.

In 2019 there will be an estimated 42,030 new cases of HCC and 31,780 estimated cancer-related deaths in the United States.[37] HCC arises against a background of cirrhosis in more than 80% of individuals.[38]

The major causes of cirrhosis in the United States are hepatitis C virus (HCV), alcohol, and nonalcoholic fatty liver disease (NAFLD). Less prevalent conditions of cirrhosis in the United States such as hepatitis B virus (HBV), hereditary hemochromatosis, and primary biliary cholangitis are also associated with HCC.[38]

Historically, HCV has been the leading cause of cirrhosis and liver transplantation in the United Sates. However, over the last decade with the advent of highly effective antiviral therapies and because of the obesity epidemic, alcoholic liver disease (ALD) and NAFLD are surpassing HCV as the leading causes of cirrhosis and, hence, HCC.

A recent study using the SEER (Surveillance Epidemiology End Results) data of the National Cancer Institute projects that the incidence of HCC will continue to increase until 2030.[39]

Clinical Presentation

Most patients with HCC are asymptomatic until intermediate-stage or advanced-stage cancer develops, defined by the Barcelona Clinic Liver Cancer (BCLC) staging system as stage B, C, or D (**Fig. 2**). Patients undergoing routine HCC screening are usually diagnosed at earlier stages (BCLC stages 0 and A); hence, they tend to be asymptomatic from the liver tumor standpoint.

Signs and symptoms related to HCC can include abdominal pain, anorexia, weight loss, palpable mass on examination of the abdomen, and hepatic decompensation manifested as variceal bleeding, new-onset or worsening ascites, coagulopathy, jaundice, and encephalopathy. HCC can also present with intratumoral and/or capsular rupture resulting in bleeding, which can lead to acute-onset abdominal pain and hemorrhagic shock. Less common symptoms include jaundice secondary to central biliary tree compression and fever from tumor necrosis.

Approximately 10% of patients will have metastasis at the time of diagnosis.[40] The most common sites of metastasis are lung, intra-abdominal lymph nodes, bone, and adrenal gland.

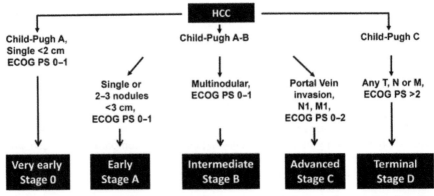

Fig. 2. Barcelona Clinic Liver Cancer staging system. ECOG, Eastern Cooperative Oncology Group; PS, performance status. (*From* Llovet JM, Bru C, Bruix J. Prognosis of hepatocellular carcinoma: the BCLC staging classification. Semin Liver Dis. 1999;19(3):329-338; with permission.)

Screening

The annual risk of developing HCC varies depending on the cause of chronic liver disease. The annual estimated risk is 1% to 8% for HCV, 1% to 15% for HBV, 1% for ALD, and 2.6% for NAFLD.[41]

The risk of HCC for patients with HCV-related cirrhosis who develop a sustained virological response after direct-acting antiviral therapy is lowered, with recent studies showing a 71% reduction in HCC risk. However, the risk is not completely eliminated and it is recommended that routine surveillance of this population is continued.[42]

The NAFLD/nonalcoholic steatohepatitis population represents a particular challenge for surveillance given that recent studies have reported the absence of cirrhosis in up to 50% of patients who have subsequently developed HCC.[43,44] The lack of clinical or radiographic findings indicating the presence of cirrhosis suggests that most of these patients are not enrolled in a surveillance program, and emerging data suggest that these patients are presenting with later-stage disease.[43,45] The American Association for the Study of Liver Diseases (AASLD) recently released practice guidelines for the management of NAFLD that do not recommend routine screening of HCC for patients with NAFLD.[46] However, the AASLD does recommend further assessment of patients incidentally found to have hepatic steatosis. Further assessment of hepatic steatosis with the goal of identifying patients with advanced fibrosis can be accomplished with noninvasive tools such as the NAFLD Fibrosis Score[47] and transient elastography. Patients with fibrosis stage 3 or higher should be started on a routine HCC surveillance program.

Any known cirrhotic patient or patient with a risk factor for chronic liver disease should be considered for surveillance. Current guidelines for HCC surveillance in adults include ultrasonography, with or without AFP, every 6 months. HCC surveillance is not recommended for patients with cirrhosis with Child-Pugh class C unless they are on the transplant waiting list, given their low anticipated survival. The current guidelines do not support HCC screening for patients with HCV or NAFLD without advanced fibrosis or cirrhosis.[42]

Although current guidelines do not support screening at a higher cadence or with other imaging modalities such as CT or MRI, it is recognized that there will be a small subset of patients that will fail current screening protocols. Screening failures are generally defined as patients who are diagnosed with HCC at an advanced stage whereby goals of therapy would usually be considered palliative.[48]

Diagnosis

Laboratory data

AFP is the most frequently used tumor marker for HCC. AFP is considered positive at a level of greater than 20 ng/mL and can be part of a surveillance program; however, in the absence of a concerning lesion it is not considered diagnostic.[49] AFP can be negative in up to 40% of patients with HCC.[50] When elevated, as with other tumors it is often used to assess response to treatment and to detect tumor recurrence after treatment, in conjunction with imaging such as CT or MRI.

Imaging

Diagnosis of HCC can usually be made with a good-quality 3- or 4-phase multidetector CT scanner, abdominal MRI with intravenous contrast, or contrast-enhanced ultrasonography in patients with risk factors for HCC.

The American College of Radiology created the Liver Imaging Reporting and Data System (LI-RADS) as a comprehensive system to standardize terminology, interpretation, and reporting of liver imaging.[51] LI-RADS reporting is applicable to patients with cirrhosis, chronic hepatitis B, and current or prior HCC.

There are 8 LI-RADS diagnostic categories (**Table 1**), which estimate the relative likelihood of HCC and malignancy based on the specific imaging features and when specific imaging features are present. LI-RADS represent a valuable tool for the radiographic diagnosis of HCC.

On CT or MRI, HCC (LI-RADS 5) would have the following features:

- Nonrim arterial-phase hyperenhancement, 10–19 mm in size, and have 2 additional major features, or
- Nonrim arterial-phase hyperenhancement, >20 mm in size, with one or more major additional features:
  o Enhancing capsule, nonperipheral washout, or threshold growth. Threshold growth is defined as ≥50% size increase of a mass in ≤6 months.

Pathology

The unique angiogenetic features of HCC that lead to specific diagnostic radiologic features, the low but not negligible risk of complications from a liver biopsy such as bleeding and track seeding, and the potential for sampling errors have significantly downplayed the role of liver biopsies as a diagnostic tool for HCC. Nonetheless, based on national guidelines such as the AASLD and National Comprehensive Cancer Network, there are still a few clinical scenarios in which a liver biopsy should be considered[42,52]:

- The lesion is probably HCC (LI-RADS 4) or highly concerning for malignancy (LI-RADS M), and a definitive tissue diagnosis would change next steps in management
- The lesion meets imaging criteria for HCC, but:
  o Patient does not have risk factors for HCC (ie, no history of cirrhosis or chronic hepatitis B)
  o Patient has cardiac cirrhosis, congenital hepatic fibrosis, or cirrhosis caused by a vascular disorder such a Budd-Chiari syndrome, hereditary hemorrhagic telangiectasis, or nodular regenerative hyperplasia
- Histologic confirmation of metastatic disease would change clinical decision making
- Histologic grading or molecular characterization is desired for potential molecular targeted therapies (within the context of a clinical trial)

Table 1 LI-RADS	
LR-NC	Not categorizable
LR-1	Definitely benign
LR-2	Probably benign
LR-3	Intermediate probability of malignancy
LR-4	Probably HCC
LR-5	Definitely HCC
LR-M	Probably or definitely malignant, not necessarily HCC
LR-TIV	Tumor in vein

Abbreviation: LR/LI-RADS, Liver Reporting and Data System.

Available at: https://www.acr.org/Clinical-Resources/Reporting-and-Data-Systems/LI-RADS. Accessed on August 30, 2019.

- Repeat biopsies can be considered when a previous biopsy was nondiagnostic or discordant with the clinical history, imaging, and biomarkers

Management of lesions concerning for malignancy should take place in a multidisciplinary fashion, including the decision to proceed with a liver biopsy.

Clinical implications of histologic grading of HCC are currently limited by the known intratumoral heterogeneity.[53,54] In patients with advanced-stage HCC, molecular profiling to determine eligibility for clinical trials of potential molecular targeted agents is an increasing area of interest and may be the future direction for liver biopsies.

Treatment

Treatments for HCC can be broadly divided into therapies with curative intent (liver transplant, resection and ablation) and noncurative therapies (locoregional therapies and systemic therapies).

Resection

Assessing resectability of a hepatocellular carcinoma(s) requires taking into consideration the degree of underlying liver disease, the tumor characteristics, the patient's performance status and overall health, and FLR.

In general, ideal candidates for resection are patients without cirrhosis. However, this accounts only for about 10% of HCC cases in Western countries. In patients with cirrhosis and HCC, resection is indicated in the setting of favorably located lesions with an expected adequate FLR, patients with Child-Pugh score A, and those with no portal hypertension. However, resection can also be considered in highly selected patients with Child-Pugh B score or minimal portal hypertension in the setting of HCC that can be managed with a limited resection.

Resection is considered a curative therapy for HCC, with results of large retrospective studies showing that in appropriately selected patients 5-year survival rates are approximately 70%.[55,56]

There are no specific limitations on the size or number of tumors that are eligible for resection. A retrospective analysis looking at patients with a single tumor ≤5 cm or 3 or fewer tumors ≤3 cm who underwent resection reported an OS at 5 years of 81%.[57] However, multifocal disease and macrovascular invasion features are considered predictive of a high risk of recurrence.[58]

Liver transplant

Transplantation is the treatment of choice for patients with HCC and clinically significant portal hypertension and/or decompensated cirrhosis, with reported 4-year OS of 85% and recurrence-free survival of 92%[59] for appropriately selected patients.

The Model for End-Stage Liver Disease (MELD) score, adopted in 2002,[60] was created to prioritize allocation of organs. In addition, MELD score exception points were designed to give certain clinical conditions including HCC adequate priority on the transplant list. The exception points for HCC when initially implemented created an unintended overprioritization of HCC patients resulting in higher transplant rates and slightly inferior long-term outcomes compared with non-HCC patients.[61] Hence, the MELD score exception points for HCC have undergone various iterations since its inception.

Patients with HCC are eligible for exception points if they have a T2 lesion and an AFP level of less than or equal to 1000 ng/mL. A T2 lesion is defined by the Organ Procurement and Transplantation Network (OPTN) as[62]:

- One lesion greater than or equal to 2 cm and less than or equal to 5 cm in size

- Two or 3 lesions each greater than or equal to 1 cm and less than or equal to 3 cm in size

Locoregional therapies

These therapies, which include ablation, radiation, and arterially directed therapies, are frequently part of the treatment plan for patients who are not candidates for resection, patients listed for transplantation as a bridge therapy, or when the goal is to downstage to meet liver transplant criteria.

Locoregional therapies may be repeated or sequentially combined based on tumor response and the patient's overall health. There is no strong evidence to support locoregional therapies in patients with Child's C cirrhosis, and the use of these therapies needs to be carefully considered.

- *Ablation*. In current practice, radiofrequency ablation (RFA) and microwave ablation (MWA) are the more commonly used modalities. A comparison of these 2 modalities using a propensity score analysis found that RFA was inferior to MWA for treating T2 lesions but had efficacy comparable to that of MWA for a solitary HCC $\leq$3 cm.[63] Ablative techniques are usually considered for patients who are not candidates for resection with lesions under 3 cm and not near major vascular or biliary structures. When considering a resection versus an ablation, size, location of the lesion, patient's performance status, and background liver disease need to be considered.
- *Arterially directed therapies*. These therapies are usually considered for patients with BCLC stage B HCC. Among these therapies, TACE has been the therapy with the longest track record of evidential support in treating HCC[64]; however, over the past decade transarterial radioembolization has been emerging as a solid alternative to TACE, with similar rates of local control and progression-free survival.[65]
- *Radiation therapy*. Options for patients with HCC who are not candidates for resection include external beam radiation therapy and stereotactic body radiation therapy (SBRT). SBRT is a technique that is able to deliver high ablative doses of radiation. Small single-center studies have compared SBRT with TACE[66] and ablation[67] and have shown similar local control rates. However, prospective comparative randomized studies are still needed to better define the role of SBRT. At the moment, expert panels consider SBRT as an alternative to ablation and/or embolization techniques or when these therapies have failed or are contraindicated for patients mainly within the T2 OPTN definition.[52]

Systemic therapies

Systemic therapies are recommended in patients with good performance status (ie, less than 2), Child-Pugh A cirrhosis, or highly selected Child-Pugh B cirrhosis in the setting of advanced HCC with macrovascular invasion and/or metastatic disease. Studies to date have shown no benefit of systemic therapies in the adjuvant setting, and they are currently not recommended. In patients with Child-Pugh C cirrhosis or poor performance status with advanced HCC, no therapy may be the best option.[42]

There are currently 2 approved first-line agents (sorafenib and lenvatinib) for HCC and 6 subsequent-line therapies if disease progresses on first-line therapy. Sorafenib, which was the first approved first-line therapy for those with advanced HCC (defined as patients not eligible for transplant or those who had disease progression after surgical or locoregional therapies), was based on the results of the SHARP trial, showing a median OS in the sorafenib arm of 10.7 months versus 7.9 months in the placebo group.[68] Lenvatinib, the other available first-line option, was approved in 2018 based on the results of the REFLECT trial showing noninferiority compared with sorafenib, with OS of 13.6 months in the lenvatinib arm and 12.3 months in the sorafenib arm.[69]

SUMMARY

The incidence of primary liver cancers is expected to continue to increase over the next few decades, and OS from primary liver cancers has not changed significantly in the last decade. Although there are potential curative therapies such as liver transplantation and surgical resection, only a small number of patients are eligible for these therapies. Ongoing efforts, as for many other cancers, revolve around emphasizing the importance of a multidisciplinary approach, early diagnosis, and improving systemic therapy options.

DISCLOSURE

No disclosures.

REFERENCES

1. Aljiffry M, Abudelah A, Walsh M, et al. Evidence-based approach to cholangiocarcinoma: a systemic review of current literature. J Am Coll Surg 2009;208: 134–47.
2. Patel T. Increasing incidence and mortality of primary intrahepatic cholangiocarcinoma in the United States. Hepatology 2001;33(6):1353–7.
3. Bridgewater J, Galle P, Khan S, et al. Guidelines for diagnosis and management of intrahepatic cholangiocarcinoma. J Hepatol 2014;60(6):1268–89.
4. Rahib L, Smith BD, Alizenberg R, et al. Projecting cancer incidence and deaths to 2030: the unexpected burden of thyroid, liver, and pancreas cancers in the United States. Cancer Res 2014;74(11):2913–21.
5. DeOliveira ML, Cunningham SC, Cameron JL, et al. Cholangiocarcinoma: thirty-one year experience with 564 patients at a s single institution. Ann Surg 2007; 245:755–62.
6. Blechacz B, Komuta M, Roskams T, et al. Clinical diagnosis and staging of cholangiocarcinoma. Nat Rev Gastroenterol Hepatol 2011;(8):512–22.
7. Valls C, Guma A, Puig I, et al. Intrahepatic peripheral cholangiocarcinoma: CT evaluation. Abdom Imaging 2000;25:490–6.
8. Murakami T, Nakamura H, Tsuda k, et al. Contrast enhanced MR imaging of intrahepatic cholangiocarcinoma: pathologic correlation study. J Magn Reson Imaging 1995;5:165–70.
9. Buettner S, Vugt J, Ijzermans J, et al. Intrahepatic cholangiocarcinoma: current perspectives. Onco Targets Ther 2017;(10):1131–42.
10. LaRusso NF, Gores GJ. The utility of CA 19-9 in the diagnosis of cholangiocarcinoma in patients with primary sclerosing cholangitis. Am J Gastroenterol 2000;95: 204–7.
11. Lubezky N, Facciuto M, Harimoto N, et al. Surgical Treatment of intrahepatic cholangiocarcinoma in the USA. J Hepatobiliary Pancreat Sci 2014;22(2):124–30.
12. Maximin S, Ganeshan D, Shanbhogue A, et al. Current update on combined hepatocellular-cholangiocarcinoma. Eur J Radiol Open 2014;1:40–8.
13. Weber S, Ribero D, O'Reilly E, et al. Intrahepatic cholangiocarcinoma: expert consensus statement. HPB (Oxford) 2015;17(8):669–80.

14. Ribero D, Pinna A, Guglielmi A, et al. Surgical approach for long term survival of patients with intrahepatic cholangiocarcinoma a multi-institutional analysis of 434 patients. Arch Surg 2012;147(12):1107–13.

15. Ek Rassie ZE, Partensky C, Scoazec JY, et al. Peripheral cholangiocarcinoma: presentation, diagnosis, pathology, and management. Eur J Surg Oncol 1999; 25:375–80.

16. Endo I, Gonen M, Yopp AC, et al. Intrahepatic cholangiocarcinoma: rising frequency, improved survival and determinants of outcome after resection. Ann Surg 2008;243:84–96.

17. Lee A, Chun Y. Intrahepatic cholangiocarcinoma the AJCC/UICC 8th edition updates. Chin Clin Oncol 2018;7(5):1–5.

18. Goere D, Waghoilkar GD, Pessaux P, et al. Utility of staging laparoscopy in subsets of biliary cancers: laparoscopy is a powerful diagnostic tool in patients with intrahepatic and gallbladder carcinoma. Surg Enodsc 2006;20:721–5.

19. D'Angelica M, Fong Y, Weber S, et al. The role of staging laparoscopy in hepatobiliary malignancy: prospective analysis of 401 cases. Ann Surg Oncol 2003;10: 183–9.

20. Kim Y, Moris DP, Zhang XF, et al. Evaluation of the 8th edition American Joint Commission on Cancer (AJCC) staging system for patients with intrahepatic cholangiocarcinoma: a surveillance, epidemiology, and end results (SEER) analysis. J Surg Oncol 2017;116:643–50.

21. Mechteld de Jong, Nathan H, Sotiropoulos G, et al. Intrahepatic cholangiocarcinoma: an international multi-institutional analysis of prognostic factors and lymph node assessment. J Clin Oncol 2011;29(23):3140–5.

22. Nathan H, Pawlik TM, Wolfgang C, et al. Trends in survival after surgery for cholangiocarcinoma: a 30 year population based SEER database analysis. J Gastrointest Surg 2007;11(11):1488–97.

23. Mavros M, Economopoulos K, Alexio V. Treatment and prognosis for patients with intrahepatic cholangiocarcinoma: systematic review and meta analysis. JAMA Surg 2014;149(5):565–74.

24. De Jong MC, Nathan M, Sotiropoulos GC. Intrahepatic cholangiocarcinoma: an international multi-institution analysis of prognostic factors and lymph node assessment. J Clin Oncol 2001;29:3140–5.

25. Choi SB, Kim KS, Choi JY, et al. The prognosis and survival outcome of intrahepatic cholangiocarcinoma following surgical resection: association of lymph node metastasis and lymph node dissection on survival. Ann Surg Oncol 2009;16: 3048–56.

26. Primrose J, Fox RP, Palmer DH, et al. Capecitabine compared with observation in resected biliary tract cancer(BILCAP): a randomized, controlled, multicenter, phase 3 study. Lancet Oncol 2019;20:663–73.

27. Valle J, Wasan H, Palmer DH. Cisplatin plus gemcitabine versus gemcitabine for biliary tract cancer. N Engl J Med 2010;362(14):1273–81.

28. Chen YX, Zent ZC, Tang ZY, et al. Determining the role of external beam radiotherapy in unresectable intrahepatic cholangiocarcinoma: a retrospective analysis of 84 patients. BMC Cancer 2010;10:492.

29. Barney BM, Olivier KR, Miller RC, et al. Clinical outcome toxicity using stereotactic body radiotherapy (SBRT) for advanced cholangiocarcinoma. Radiat Oncol 2012;7:67.

30. Park SY, Kim JH, Yoon HJ, et al. Transarterial chemoembolization versus supportive therapy in palliative treatment of resectable intrahepatic cholangiocarcinoma. Clin Radiol 2011;66(4):322–8.

31. Kulhman JB, Euringer W, Spangenberg HC, et al. Treatment of unresectable chol-angiocarcinoma: conventional transarterial chemoembolization compared with drug eluting bead-transarterial chemoembolization and systemic chemotherapy. Eur J Gastroenterol Hepatol 2012;24:437–43.
32. Ibrahim SM, Mulcahy MF, Lewandoswki RJ, et al. Treatment of unresectable chol-angiocarcinoma using yttrium-90 microspheres: results from a pilot study. Cancer 2008;113:2119–28.
33. Maithel S, Gamblin TC, Kamel I, et al. Multidisciplinary approaches to intrahe-patic cholangiocarcinoma. Cancer 2013;119(22):3929–42.
34. Kim JH, Won HJ, Shin YM, et al. Radiofrequency ablation for the treatment of pri-mary intrahepatic cholangiocarcinoma. AJR AM J Roentgenol 2011;196:W205–9.
35. Konstantinidis IT, Koerkamp BG, Do RG, et al. Unresectable intrahepatic cholan-giocarcinoma: systemic plus hepatic arterial infusion chemotherapy is associated with longer survival compared to systemic chemotherapy alone. Cancer 2016; 122(5):758–65.
36. Pellino A, Loupakis F, Cadamuro M, et al. Precision medicine in cholangiocarci-noma. Transl Gastroenterol Hepatol 2018;3:40.
37. Siegel RL, Miller KD, Jemal A. Cancer statistics, 2019. Cancer J Clin 2019; 69:7–34.
38. Bruix J, Sherman M, American Association for the Study of Liver Diseases. Man-agement of hepatocellular carcinoma: an update. Hepatology 2011;53:1020–2.
39. Petrick JL, Kelly SP, Altekruse SF, et al. Futures of hepatocellular carcinoma inci-dence in the United States forecast through 2030. J Clin Oncol 2016;34:1787–94.
40. Uka K, Aikata H, Shirakawa H, et al. Clinical features and prognosis of patients with extrahepatic metastases from hepatocellular carcinoma. World J Gastroen-terol 2007;13(3):414–20.
41. Sanyal AJ, Yoon SK, Lencioni R. The etiology of hepatocellular carcinoma and consequences for treatment. Oncologist 2010;15(4):14–22.
42. Marrero J, Kulik L, Sirlin C, et al. Diagnosis, staging, and management of hepa-tocellular carcinoma: 2018 practice guidance by the American Association for the Study of Liver Diseases. Hepatology 2018;68:723–50.
43. Piscaglia F, Svegliati-Baroni G, Barchetti A, et al. Clinical patterns of hepatocellu-lar carcinoma in nonalcoholic fatty liver disease: a multicenter prospective study. Hepatology 2016;63(3):827–38.
44. Reddy SK, Steel JL, Chen HW, et al. Outcomes of curative treatment for hepato-cellular cancer in nonalcoholic steatohepatitis versus hepatitis C and alcoholic liver disease. Hepatology 2012;55:1809–19.
45. Aby E, Phan J, Truong E, et al. Inadequate hepatocellular carcinoma screening in patients with nonalcoholic steatohepatitis cirrhosis. J Clin Gastroenterol 2019; 53(2):142–6.
46. Chalasani N, Younossi Z, Lavine J, et al. The diagnosis and management of nonalcoholic fatty liver disease: practice guidance from the American Association for the Study of Liver Diseases. Hepatology 2017;67(1):328–57.
47. Angulo P, Hui J, Marchensi G, et al. The NAFLD fibrosis score: a noninvasive sys-tem that identifies liver fibrosis in patients with NAFLD. Hepatology 2007;45(4): 846–54.
48. Mancebo A, Varela M, Rodriguez M. Incidence and risk factors associated with hepatocellular carcinoma surveillance failure. J Gastroenterol Hepatol 2018; 33(8):1524–9.

49. Gupta S, Bent SK. Test characteristics of alpha-fetoprotein for detecting hepatocellular carcinoma in patients with hepatitis C. A systematic review and critical analysis. Ann Intern Med 2003;139(1):46–50.

50. Chen DS, Sung JL, Sheu JC, et al. Serum alpha-fetoprotein in the early stage of human hepatocellular carcinoma. Gastroenterology 1984;86(4):1404.

51. Van der Pol C, Lim C, McGrath T, et al. Accuracy of the liver imaging reporting and data system in computed tomography and magnetic resonance image analysis of hepatocellular carcinoma or overall malignancy—a systematic review. Gastroenterology 2019;159(4).

52. Benson, D'Angelica, Abbott, et al. NCCN. 2019. Available at: https://www.nccn.org/. Accessed July 16, 2019..

53. Pawlik T, Gleisner AL, Anders RA, et al. Preoperative assessment of hepatocellular carcinoma tumor grade using needle biopsy: implications for transplant eligibility. Ann Surg 2007;245:435–42.

54. Friemel J, Rechsteiner M, Frick L, et al. Intratumor heterogeneity in hepatocellular carcinoma. Clin Cancer Res 2015;21:1951–61.

55. Kianmanesh R, Regimbeau J, Belghiti J. Selective approach to major hepatic resection for hepatocellular carcinoma in chronic liver disease. Surg Oncol Clin N Am 2003;12:51–63.

56. Llovet J, Fuster J, Bruix J. Intention to treat analysis of surgical treatment for early hepatocellular carcinoma: resection versus transplantation. Hepatology 1999;30:1434–40.

57. Yamakado K, Nakatsuka A, Takaki H. Early-stage hepatocellular carcinoma: radiofrequency ablation combined with chemoembolization versus hepatectomy. Radiology 2008;247:260–6.

58. Truty M, Vauthey J. Surgical resection of high-risk hepatocellular carcinoma; patient selection, preoperative considerations, and operative technique. Ann Surg Oncol 2010;17:1219–25.

59. Mazzaferro V, Regalia E, Doci R. Liver transplantation for the treatment of small hepatocellular carcinomas in patient with cirrhosis. N Engl J Med 1996;334:693.

60. Kmath P, Wiesner R, Malinchoc M, et al. A model to predict survival in patients with end stage liver disease. Hepatology 2001;33:464.

61. Washburn K, Edwards E, Harper A. Hepatocellular carcinoma patients are advantaged in the current liver transplant allocation system. Am J Transplant 2010;10:1643–8.

62. Organ Procurement and Transplantation Network (OPTN). Allocation of liver and liver-intestines. Available at: https://optn.transplant.hrsa.gov/media/1200/optn_policies.pdf. Accessed April 6, 2020.

63. Liu W, He W, Zous R, et al. Microwave vs radiofrequency ablation for hepatocellular carcinoma within the Milan criteria: a propensity score analysis. Aliment Pharmacol Ther 2018;48(6):671–81.

64. Llovet J, Real M, Motana X, et al. Arterial embolisation or chemoembolisation versus symptomatic treatment in patients with unresectable hepatocellular carcinoma: a randomized controlled trial. Lancet 2002;359:1734.

65. Facciorusso A, Serviddio G, Mscatiello N. Transarterial radioembolization vs chemoembolization for hepatocarcinoma patients: a systematic review and meta-analysis. World J Hepatol 2016;8:770–8.

66. Bush d, Smith J, Cheng J. Randomized clinical trial comparing proton beam radiation therapy with transarterial chemoembolization for hepatocellular carcinoma: results of an interim analysis. Int J Radiat Oncol Biol Phys 2016;95:477.

67. Wahl D, Stenmark M, Tao Y, et al. Outcomes after stereotactic body radiotherapy or radiofrequency ablation for hepatocellular carcinoma. J Clin Oncol 2016; 452:34.
68. Llovet J, Ricc S, Mazzaferro V. Sorafenib in advanced hepatocellular carcinoma. N Engl J Med 2008;359:378–90.
69. Kudo M, Finn RQ. Lenvatinib versus sorafenib in first-line treatment of patients with unresectable hepatocellular carcinoma; a randomized phase 3 non-inferiority trial. Lancet 2018;391:1163.

Cancers Metastatic to the Liver

Nikdokht Rashidian, MD, FEBS[a], Adnan Alseidi, MD, EdM, FACS[b],*, Russell C. Kirks, MD[b]

KEYWORDS

- Liver metastases • Colorectal cancer • Hepatectomy • Metastasectomy
- Liver surgery

KEY POINTS

- A diagnosis of liver metastases often can be established based on thorough clinical assessment, laboratory tests, and appropriate imaging. Liver biopsy is indicated only when the clinical diagnosis remains in doubt after appropriate radiological work-up and if the biopsy result will alter the management strategy.
- The treatment plan for patients with liver metastases should be determined case-by-case in a multidisciplinary setting and in a center that performs liver resections.
- Current principles of liver resection in colorectal liver metastases are the anticipation of achieving a negative margin while preserving an adequate functional liver remnant.
- Surgical resection is the treatment of choice for resectable colorectal and neuroendocrine liver metastases.
- Long term survival outcome data following treatment of hepatic metastases of non-colorectal non-neuroendocrine tumors are less robust than metatases of colorectal and neuroendocrine origin.
- Depending on surgeon and center experience with management of liver tumors, transfer to a high-volume liver surgery center may be needed.

INTRODUCTION

The liver is a common site of metastatic cancer spread, second only to lymph nodes.[1] Although metastatic lesions account for approximately 70% of malignant liver tumors, colorectal liver metastases (CRLMs) probably are the most relevant to surgeons due to the well-documented potential for improved survival, or even cure, after surgical resection.[2] Surgery is the only potentially curative treatment of CRLMs and it is associated with overall 5-year survival of more than 55% after resection; furthermore, the combination of surgery with curative intent and systemic chemotherapy results in a

[a] Department of GI Surgery, Ghent University Hospital, C. Heymanslaan 10, 2K12C Route1275, UZ Gent, Ghent 9000, Belgium; [b] Division of Pancreas, Liver and Biliary Surgery, Virginia Mason Medical Center, Virginia Mason HPB Surgery, 1100 Ninth Avenue, MC GS C6, Seattle, WA 98101, USA
* Corresponding author.
E-mail address: adnan.alseidi@ucsf.edu

Surg Clin N Am 100 (2020) 551–563
https://doi.org/10.1016/j.suc.2020.02.005
0039-6109/20/© 2020 Elsevier Inc. All rights reserved.

10-year survival of approximately 30%.[3–5] Also, the liver is the most common site of distant metastasis for neuroendocrine tumors (NETs) (neuroendocrine liver metastases [NELMs]) arising from the gastrointestinal (GI) tract and pancreas.[6] Liver-directed therapies are recommended with curative intent in the absence of extrahepatic metastasis or for symptom control in functional NELM when the liver carries the major tumor burden.[7,8] Liver metastasis may develop from many other cancers, which often are categorized into the heterogeneous group of noncolorectal non-NELMs (nCRnNELMs), including upper GI system cancers, soft tissue sarcoma, melanoma, genitourinary malignancies, breast carcinomas, and so forth. Although the data of long-term survival after metastasectomy for these tumors are sparse, a careful patient selection for surgery via multidisciplinary tumor board discussions may improve the outcome.[9,10]

INCIDENTALLY DETECTED SOLID LIVER LESIONS

Incidental identification of single or multiple solid liver lesions is not an uncommon scenario in general surgery practice. Clinical presentations in these cases include patients whose evaluation for a complaint discovered an unexpected liver lesion or patients with a history of malignancy being followed by surveillance imaging. The sequence of diagnostic steps depends in part on when a surgeon sees the patient. In general, assessment of patients with a newly discovered hepatic lesion, suspected to metastasis, includes clinical assessment, laboratory tests, complete liver imaging, whole-body staging, and attempts to locate a primary tumor or recurrence of previously treated lesions.

Clinical Assessment

A thorough patient history and physical examination as well as an assessment of functional status are required. Although metastatic lesions occur more commonly than primary hepatobiliary tumors, if imaging suggests portal hypertensive changes in the abdomen, ascites, or a cirrhotic contour to the liver, medical and social-historical factors associated with chronic liver disease should be elicited; these include viral hepatitis diagnosis or exposure, previous trauma or blood product transfusion, tattoos, promiscuous sexual activity, illicit substance use, and chronic or heavy ethanol consumption. For patients presenting with symptoms of jaundice or pruritis, available imaging should be reviewed to exclude main bile duct obstruction and imaging findings suggestive of cirrhosis; in a nonobstructed biliary system, clinical jaundice may signal diffuse tumor infiltration or replacement of liver parenchyma. Heavy tumor burden in a diseased liver (chronic liver disease, steatohepatitis, multiple intrahepatic biliary obstructions, and so forth) may yield a similar effect. In conjunction with a detailed social history and review of symptoms, a procedural history should be elicited, taking note of the date of last colonoscopy as well as a history of upper endoscopy and, in female patients, mammography and previous breast biopsies. If possible, previous endoscopy records and pathology results should be reviewed.

Especially in patients without a history of cancer or in those without regular medical care, a thorough physical examination must be undertaken to examine the draining nodal basins of the head and neck, chest and axilla, periumbilical region, and inguinal regions bilaterally. In women, breast and pelvic examinations should be performed unless recently documented and without change by long-term care providers. An abdominal examination can identify not only areas of fullness, discomfort, and mass or organomegaly but also previous incisions, generalized distension, and hernias. A digital rectal examination is considered in patients with an unknown primary site as well as patients with symptoms or a history of anorectal malignancies.

Laboratory Work-up

In assessment of a liver mass, serum studies are performed to evaluate the hemoglobin level, renal function, and electrolyte abnormalities (complete blood cell count and basic metabolic profile), the liver's synthetic function including liver function tests (LFTs), prothrombin time (PT)/international normalized ratio (INR), and the presence of specific tumor markers, such as carcinoembryonic antigen (CEA), cancer antigen 19-9, α-fetoprotein, and so forth. For those with a known history of malignancy, knowing historical tumor marker values or if a patient has a history of a nonproducing tumor helps compare previous values to newly obtained laboratory tests. If a combination of imaging and patient historical factors raises suspicion for hepatocellular carcinoma (HCC), laboratory analysis for viral hepatitis serology should be obtained. Assessment of a patient with suspected cirrhosis should include Child-Turcotte-Pugh scoring as well as a calculation of sodium-corrected Model for End-Stage Liver disease (MELD) score. A growing body of literature demonstrates the perioperative prognostic value of the MELD score in both cirrhotic and noncirrhotic patients.[11–13]

Assessment of nutritional status by serologic markers (albumin and prealbumin) for those reporting dysphagia, muscle wasting, or weight loss of more than 5 kg may help determine the sequence of therapy events as well as allow surgeons and nutritionists to have an impact on patient outcomes positively. Severely deconditioned or malnourished patients may have findings of muscle wasting on examination or history of limited exercise tolerance or amount of time spent daily in bed or chair. In-office functional assessment with 6-minute walking distance or handgrip strength also can be obtained with appropriate equipment. Especially in patients who are planning to undergo neoadjuvant therapy before hepatectomy or combined surgical procedure, nutritional optimization exists as one of the few modifiable risk factors for adverse surgical outcomes.[14–16]

Imaging

For patients with a history of treated malignancy or in those undergoing a staging imaging as part of the evaluation for recently discovered cancer, identification of a solid liver lesion(s) with characteristic imaging certainly raises the suspicion for metachronous or synchronous hepatic metastasis. If the lesion of concern is identified unexpectedly on transabdominal ultrasound, ^{18}F-fluorodeoxyglucose (FDG) positron emission tomography (PET)/computed tomography (CT) scan or on single-phase abdominal CT, further details are required to describe a lesion and assess its surgical resectability accurately. Anatomic factors of the lesion's relationship and proximity to segmental or lobar portal pedicles, hepatic veins, the biliary system, the inferior vena cava, and surrounding organs (diaphragm, stomach, retroperitoneum, and so forth) are crucial in consideration of the treatment of multiple lesions. Reviewing the lesion with an experienced radiologist can identify tumor-specific imaging characteristics in the event of an unknown primary or a liver with chronic or equivocal findings. The chest also needs to be staged.

Cross-sectional imaging used to define hepatic anatomy and lesion characteristics further usually is either multiphase liver CT (CT abdomen and pelvis with thin cuts through the liver during the noncontrasted, hepatic artery, portal vein, and delayed phases) or magnetic resonance imaging (MRI) of the liver. If an MRI of the liver is chosen, CT of the abdomen and pelvis also may be required to stage the remainder of the abdominal cavity. Institutional, patient, and surgeon factors must be considered when selecting the cross-sectional imaging modality used to assess liver lesions. This may include patients' ability to tolerate the enclosed space of an MRI and their ability to lie flat for longer periods. Institutional familiarity with multiphase CT, as well as the strength of MRI magnets for improved resolution, should be considered. Finally, as a surgeon assesses anatomic resectability in the setting of a multidisciplinary plan of care, the surgeon's comfort with the different imaging modalities should be part of the decision process to characterize lesions as part of a surgical or interventional plan for liver-directed therapy.

Additional imaging modalities may be required in the evaluation of certain tumor types, the evaluation of indeterminate findings on staging imaging, or if a primary lesion is not readily identified. FDG-PET imaging currently is not supported for routine use in staging or surveilling colorectal cancer (CRC) but is used in staging or evaluating treatment response in other GI malignancies, such as esophageal and gastric cancers. PET also may be more commonly encountered in a routine practice centered on pulmonary malignancies as well as melanoma.[17,18] In the setting of GI malignancy, PET may be useful for evaluating the metabolic avidity of equivocal findings on staging imaging, such as indeterminate pulmonary nodules or omental or peritoneal thickening; evaluating for metabolic response of initially equivocal lesions after chemotherapy also may play a role in determining the aggressiveness of surgical resection, if previously indeterminate lesions respond to chemotherapy, confirming a more widespread disease pattern.

COLORECTAL LIVER METASTASES

CRC is the third most commonly diagnosed cancer worldwide. Despite clinical advances in treatment, it remains the second leading cause of cancer-related death.[19] The liver is the most common site of metastases in CRC, and more than half of the patients eventually develop liver metastasis during their disease course.[20] Surgical resection is the treatment of choice for CRLMs, but only 20% of patients are deemed to be eligible for surgery at the time of diagnosis.[21,22] It seems, however, that the incidence of resectability in CRLMs is underestimated because many cases are deemed unresectable by nonliver surgeons, and, therefore, it cannot be overemphasized that the decision to preclude surgery for CRLMs must be made as part of a multidisciplinary team that incorporates oncologic planning as well as the technical aspects of resection as determined by a surgeon with liver-specific training and experience.

Patient Selection

Advances in surgical technique and systemic therapies have expanded the resectability criteria for initially unresectable CRLMs dramatically, and many factors previously considered contraindications for surgery have been challenged.[23] Traditionally, only patients with fewer than 3 lesions, tumors smaller than 5 cm, unilobar metastases, and anticipated free margin of greater than 1 cm and without extrahepatic disease were considered eligible for liver resection.[24] Current principles for liver resection in CRLMs are the anticipation of achieving a negative margin while preserving a liver remnant of adequate size, vascular perfusion, and venous and biliary drainage.[25] To determine the adequate remnant liver size, several factors must be considered, including the body mass index; presence of fatty liver disease, fibrosis, or cirrhosis; and amount of chemotherapy that a patient may have received.[26] In cases of extrahepatic metastases, liver metastasectomy still may be indicated as part of a staged intervention if the extrahepatic disease is resectable or controllable with systemic therapies (eg, small lung metastases).[27] Observed disease biology or patient fitness, however, may preclude definitive hepatic resection even in cases that are deemed technically resectable. In order to weigh these considerations, optimize perioperative results, and improve oncologic outcomes, the treatment strategy for patients with CRLMs should be determined case-by-case in a multidisciplinary setting and in a center with experience in hepatic resections.[2,28]

Preoperative Evaluation

Preoperative considerations in CRLMs are to (1) evaluate the status of primary disease: staging and resectability assessment in synchronous metastases and evaluation of local recurrence or residual disease in metachronous metastases; (2) determine the extent of hepatic disease and predict the future remnant liver size and function; and (3) identify possible extrahepatic disease.[27,29] Surgical risk assessment is essential and involves the evaluation of a patient's general health, liver health, and tumor factors. Liver surgery often is associated with considerable physiologic stress to patients; therefore, a thorough assessment of comorbidities and preoperative medical optimization is mandatory. Estimation of sufficient future liver remnant also is crucial. The chosen method for volumetric analysis depends on availability of software and expertise. Most centers calculate the liver volumes directly from cross-sectional images, whereas others use standardized formulas adjusted for various parameters, such as body surface area, body mass index, and gender and age of patients. The generally accepted minimum values for liver remnant to proceed with safe hepatic resection are summarized in **Table 1**.[30–32] Preoperatively, a standard blood work-up, including LFTs, albumin, and PT/INR, is needed. Also, a baseline CEA level should be obtained because of its utility in predicting prognosis and recurrence of the disease in the follow-up.[33]

Multiphase contrast-enhanced imaging using CT or MRI frequently is used in the preoperative evaluation of patients with CRLM. The choice of imaging technique depends on local availability and expertise. A multiphase contrast-enhanced CT scan commonly is used to detect lung and liver metastases. MRI offers a higher sensitivity in detecting small metastases (≤ 1 cm), particularly in a fatty liver background associated with chemotherapy-induced changes.[27] In the assessment of CRLMs, gadoxetic acid-enhanced MRI is superior to multidetector contrast-enhanced CT scan, especially after chemotherapy, in subcapsular metastases and in peribiliary lesions.[34] According to National Comprehensive Cancer Network (NCCN) guidelines, a hepatic MRI with intravenous routine extracellular or hepatocyte-specific contrast is the modality of choice to assess number and distribution of metastatic foci before planning liver-directed therapies. FDG-PET/CT is useful to evaluate equivocal lesions and to diagnose extrahepatic metastases but it is less accurate for detection of small liver and

Table 1	
Minimum future liver remnant for safe hepatic resection	
FLR >20%	Normal liver function
	After short-duration chemotherapy
FLR >30%	Steatosis
	After long-duration (>12 wk) chemotherapy
FLR >40%	Well-compensated hepatic fibrosis or cirrhosis
	Cholestasis

Abbreviation: FLR, future liver remnant.

pulmonary nodules. NCCN guidelines recommend PET scan for patients with potentially surgically curable metastatic CRC.[17]

Biopsy

Liver biopsy is indicated when the clinical diagnosis is in doubt despite appropriate radiological work-up and when it is likely that the biopsy result will alter the management strategy. As such, histologic confirmation of resectable liver metastases may not be required before surgery if the clinical picture is compatible with metastases of a known primary tumor. For instance, liver biopsy is not indicated to confirm a diagnosis when rising in CEA levels leads to identifying a characteristic liver lesion during the surveillance of a patient with resected CRC. During surgery, if histologic confirmation of liver metastases is clinically indicated, a needle biopsy is recommended over incising tumors with scalpels or biopsy forceps to minimize the potential risk of peritoneal seeding. To retrieve a sufficient sample, using a cutting needle device of 16 gauge or larger is recommended. Biopsy of 1 accessible and representative lesion generally is sufficient in the setting of multifocal disease.[35,36]

Treatment

The approach to CRLMs depends mainly on when in the course of the disease patient encounter liver metastases. Neoadjuvant chemotherapy often is indicated before metastasectomy to evaluate the natural behavior of the disease and, in some cases, to improve the resectability of large or critically located tumors.

Although the surgical approach to the small-volume, oligometastatic metachronous CRLMs may be straightforward, considering optimization of the future liver remnant through hepatic molding strategies may be required in cases of large tumors or bilobar disease. Referring such patients to specialized hepatobiliary units for evaluating the possibility of radioembolization, portal vein embolization, staged resection, associating liver partition and portal vein ligation for staged hepatectomy surgery, or a hybrid resection-ablation procedure is recommended.[27]

Synchronously detected CRLM is considered to represent less favorable biology and portend worse survival than metachronous disease. The surgical approach to synchronous CRLM can be simultaneous resections of the primary tumor and liver metastasis or staged resection; the latter is either colorectal-first (classic approach) or liver-first (reverse approach). The treatment sequence should be tailored to each patient, and it largely depends on a patient's symptoms, the extent of primary and metastatic disease, and the expertise of the medical center. Patients with a symptomatic colorectal tumor, such as bleeding, obstruction, and perforation, benefit from the classic staged resection with the treatment of their symptomatic tumor first. In general, combined resection should be reserved for selected patients, when both lesions are uncomplicated and resectable, requiring limited surgical procedures. Liver-first approach may be beneficial for patients with extensive CRLMs when simultaneous resection is not feasible.[37,38]

Although minimally invasive liver surgery has been used steadily in the treatment of CRLMs and getting worldwide acceptance, the optimal extent of liver resection for CRLMs still is a matter of debate. Minimally invasive nonanatomic parenchymal preserving liver surgery, in high-volume hepatobiliary centers with extensive laparoscopic experience, is cost-effective and associated with significantly reduced postoperative complication rate and similar margin positivity rates compared with open hepatectomy.[39]

NEUROENDOCRINE LIVER METASTASES

NETs with metastatic spread to the liver can originate in many sites throughout the body, including the thyroid, lung, and sites within the GI tract. Focusing on abdominal NETs, pancreatic islet cell tumors (pancreatic NETs [pNETs]), and bowel neuroendocrine (carcinoid) tumors represent a spectrum of disease whose first likely site of metastasis is the liver. Although functional pNETs may present with characteristic endocrinopathies based on the cell type (insulinoma, glucagonoma, somatostatinoma, and so forth), functional manifestations of carcinoid tumors, termed *carcinoid syndrome* or *carcinoid crisis*, are vasomotor effects of hypotension and tachycardia with resulting flushing, anxiety, and potentially syncope. The GI effects of this symptom may include diarrhea. In nonfunctional neuroendocrine lesions, on the contrary, no significant hormonal or endocrine symptoms may be apparent. Symptoms of NELM also can arise from tumor size and burden, producing compression of nearby organs or biliary structures. Primary intestinal carcinoid tumors also can present with obstruction or bleeding and require surgical management.[40]

NETs typically present as arterial phase hyperenhancing solid lesions. A primary site within the pancreas or bowel may be visible on abdominal imaging; in the case of carcinoids, mesenteric lymphadenopathy may be visible to suggest the location of a primary lesion. When evaluating for symptomatology related to NELM, review of systems should include discussing common symptoms of functional NETs, such as refractory gastroesophageal reflux or peptic ulcer disease, jejunal ulcerative disease despite *Helicobacter pylori* eradication and acid-suppressing medication (gastrinoma); syncope or near-syncope associated with hypoglycemia and potentially mood changes or confusion (insulinoma); or the constellation of symptoms associated with carcinoid syndrome, listed previously. Especially in patients with pNETs, family history should be evaluated for other tumors reminiscent of multiple endocrine neoplasia type 1.

Serum studies to evaluate or follow NETs include the assessment of chromogranin A or specific hormones in functional tumors. For patients with NET, nuclear medicine whole-body imaging with somatostatin receptor scintigraphy (SRS), or Octreoscan, historically has been used to evaluate the location of a primary lesion as well as the extent of metastatic disease. Compared with traditional SRS, gallium-68-DOTATATE-PET/CT is a cross-sectional study using gallium-labeled radiotracer combining avidity for somatostatin receptors with CT format cross-sectional imaging. Although DOTATATE-PET has been found to change operative plans by identifying lesions occult on traditional CT and/or OctreoScan, both DOTATATE-PET and traditional SRS may have difficulty in characterizing lesions less than 1 cm in size. In cases of poorly differentiated or dedifferentiated NETs, somatostatin receptors may not be fully expressed, limiting the sensitivity of both SRS and DOTATATE-PET. FDG-labeled PET scan may be more useful with these lesions, but assessment of extent of intrahepatic disease could be limited by background hepatic metabolic activity.[41,42]

NELM typically represents an indolent disease course that can evolve over longer periods than those seen in GI adenocarcinoma liver metastases. Although surgical intervention provides the only chance for cure in the setting of NELM, outcomes from the surgical intervention are divided into the operative goal: complete clearance of disease, cytoreduction, and palliation. Curative resection traditionally has been limited to those with an unilobar disease with or without peripheral lesions elsewhere; the addition of surgical ablation lends more definitive treatment options to those with bilobar disease so that a resect/ablate strategy can be adopted based on disease location and extent. For patients with symptoms related to hormonally active tumors, a goal of 90% cytoreduction has been sought if curative resection is not possible based on performance status, liver remnant, or tumor location. Specific consider-ations are required in the preoperative and perioperative management of symptomatic carcinoid tumors. Echocardiography is obtained as a part of routine surveillance of these patients as advocated by NCCN guidelines for functional carcinoid tumors.[43] As relates to surgery, echocardiography assesses cardiac function, valvular disease, and resulting pulmonary hypertension, considering that central and hepatic venous hypertension can result in hemorrhage during hepatic resection. Given the vasoactive and compensatory cardiac effects of carcinoid crisis, preoperative and intraoperative somatostatin analog administration often is performed to mediate intraoperative carci-noid crisis physiology precipitated by tumor manipulation.[44]

In those unable to tolerate curative resection, medical therapy is centered on so-matostatin analog therapy to control symptoms. New advances in somatostatin receptor-targeted antibody therapy (peptide receptor radionuclide therapy) may lend additional treatment options to select patients.[45,46] Regional therapy in the form of transarterial chemoembolization or radioembolization also plays a role in those patients with disease who cannot be controlled with surgery or ablation alone, although no trial has compared regional therapy to surgical cytoreduction in a randomized fashion.[45,47] Combinations of surgery and interventional or tumor-directed systemic treatments also are described.[45,48,49] With the evolving landscape of NELM treatment, surgery and somatostatin analogs no longer are the only tools in the armamentarium of treatment. The modern selection of thera-pies and the often indolent disease course argue against burning bridges as related to local or regional options, again underscoring the need for optimal patient and treatment selection through a multidisciplinary, data-supported, and NCCN-supported approach involving medical oncology, interventional radiology, and sur-gical perspectives.

NONCOLORECTAL NON-NEUROENDOCRINE LIVER METASTASES

Although the surgical treatment of metachronous CRC is recognized as critical in obtaining long-term survival from metastatic disease, outcomes for the treatment of hepatic metastases of noncolorectal, non-NETs are less robust. This category is composed of a variety of tumor types, including breast, melanoma (cutaneous and ocular), soft tissue sarcomas, and tumors of genitourinary origin, among others, in sur-gical series. Fit patients with favorable disease biology, as evidenced by chemotherapy-responsive disease, limited hepatic tumor burden, and a longer post-resection interval from their primary lesion, may be candidates for local or regional therapy. Retrospective surgical series considering this problem does show the oppor-tunity for long-term survival after liver-directed therapy, with each study acknowl-edging the caveat of selection bias in terms of patients with favorable disease biology being those considered for hepatectomy with curative intent.[50–54] In these se-ries, GI adenocarcinomas (esophagus, gastric, and small bowel) typically have inferior survival compared with non-GI disease metastases, highlighting the natural history of both disease processes as well as the inherent limitations of assessing survival out-comes from a variety of tumors being treated.[53] In these settings, full-body FDG-PET, as well as staging specific to the known previous disease, is required to evaluate for other sites of distant or locally recurrent disease.

Surgical series evaluating outcomes after partial hepatectomy for nCRnNELM typi-cally consider limited, liver-only disease in patients fit to undergo hepatectomy or other local therapy, such as ablation. Although earlier surgical series argue for hepatectomy for tumor clearance,[53] modern reviews of surgical thermal ablation have identified that tumor size and histology may be independent factors for local recurrence and that patients treated with ablation typically benefit from lower surgical morbidity when ablations are performed in high-volume centers. In a multi-institutional retrospective

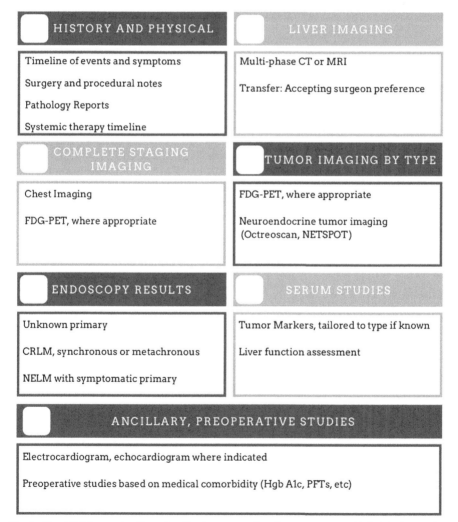

EVALUATION AND REFERRAL

Liver Metastases Checklist

HISTORY AND PHYSICAL

Timeline of events and symptoms

Surgery and procedural notes

Pathology Reports

Systemic therapy timeline

LIVER IMAGING

Multi-phase CT or MRI

Transfer: Accepting surgeon preference

COMPLETE STAGING IMAGING

Chest Imaging

FDG-PET, where appropriate

TUMOR IMAGING BY TYPE

FDG-PET, where appropriate

Neuroendocrine tumor imaging (Octreoscan, NETSPOT)

ENDOSCOPY RESULTS

Unknown primary

CRLM, synchronous or metachronous

NELM with symptomatic primary

SERUM STUDIES

Tumor Markers, tailored to type if known

Liver function assessment

ANCILLARY, PREOPERATIVE STUDIES

Electrocardiogram, echocardiogram where indicated

Preoperative studies based on medical comorbidity (Hgb A1c, PFTs, etc)

Fig. 1. Checklist for evaluation of patients suspected to liver metastases. Hgb A1c, hemoglobin A1c; PFT, pulmonary function test.

series comparing local recurrence and incomplete ablation between HCC, CRLM, NELM, and nCRnNELM, there was no statistical difference in recurrence when considering the histologies of CRLM, NELM, and nCRnNELM.[55] HCC, however, was noted to recur locally more frequently, a finding the authors attribute to the oncogenic liver milieu in the setting of cirrhosis.

Advances in interventional therapy for these lesions include stereotactic radiation as well as radioembolization as treatment of lesions based on size and location.[56,57] Given the heterogeneity of disease, patient selection bias, and the variety of options for treatment, the decision to intervene surgically on nCRnNELM requires a comprehensive patient evaluation in the form of a multidisciplinary tumor board to discuss the timing and role of systemic therapy, disease-targeted therapy, surgery, interventional regional therapy, and, ultimately, a patient's willingness and candidacy to undergo various treatment options.

WHEN TO REFER AND WHAT TO INCLUDE?

Depending on surgeon and center experience and comfort with the management of a liver lesion or diffuse lesions, transfer to a high-volume liver surgery center may be needed. These reasons could include the need for additional interventional or diagnostic evaluation, such as radioembolization or endoscopic ultrasound with biopsy, experience with thermal ablation techniques (interventional radiology or surgery), the magnitude of hepatectomy needed (extended resection, staged hepatectomy, liver molding intervention needed, and so forth), or if novel therapeutics or clinical trials are indicated. By reviewing this article, a condensed checklist can be formed to guide plans for appropriate, patient-individualized disease management, whether it be a primary center, a referring surgeon, or a combination (**Fig. 1**). Compiling a comprehensive cancer treatment history, current disease evaluation, and patient and liver assessment can expedite the formulation of a treatment plan as well as minimize redundant studies and charges to the patient and the health care system.

DISCLOSURE

The authors have nothing to disclose.

REFERENCES

1. Clark AM, Ma B, Taylor DL, et al. Liver metastases: microenvironments and ex-vivo models. Exp Biol Med 2016;241(15):1639–52.
2. Adam R, Kitano Y. Multidisciplinary approach of liver metastases from colorectal cancer. Ann Gastroenterol Surg 2019;3(1):50–6.
3. Tabchouri N, Gayet B, Okumura S, et al. Recurrence patterns after laparoscopic resection of colorectal liver metastases. Surg Endosc 2018;32(12):4788–97.
4. Creasy JM, Sadot E, Koerkamp BG, et al. Actual 10-year survival after hepatic resection of colorectal liver metastases: what factors preclude cure? Surgery 2018;163(6):1238–44.
5. Engstrand J, Nilsson H, Strömberg C, et al. Colorectal cancer liver metastases - a population-based study on incidence, management and survival. BMC Cancer 2018;18(1):78.
6. Saxena A, Chua TC, Perera M, et al. Surgical resection of hepatic metastases from neuroendocrine neoplasms: a systematic review. Surg Oncol 2012;21(3):e131–41.
7. Pavel M, Baudin E, Couvelard A, et al. ENETS consensus guidelines for the management of patients with liver and other distant metastases from neuroendocrine

neoplasms of foregut, midgut, hindgut, and unknown primary. Neuroendocrinology 2012;95(2):157–76.

8. Pavel M, O''Toole D, Costa F, et al. ENETS consensus guidelines update for the management of distant metastatic disease of intestinal, pancreatic, bronchial neuroendocrine neoplasms (NEN) and NEN of unknown primary site. Neuroendocrinology 2016;103(2):172–85.

9. Parisi A, Trastulli S, Ricci F, et al. Analysis of long-term results after liver surgery for metastases from colorectal and non-colorectal tumors: a retrospective cohort study. Int J Surg 2016;30:25–30.

10. Groeschl RT, Nachmany I, Steel JL, et al. Hepatectomy for noncolorectal non-neuroendocrine metastatic cancer: a multi-institutional analysis. J Am Coll Surg 2012;214(5):769–77.

11. Havens JM, Columbus AB, Olufajo OA, et al. Association of model for end-stage liver disease score with mortality in emergency general surgery patients. JAMA Surg 2016;151(7):e160789.

12. Godfrey EL, Kueht ML, Rana A, et al. MELD-Na (the new MELD) and perioperative outcomes in emergency surgery. Am J Surg 2018;216(3):407–13.

13. Fromer MW, Aloia TA, Gaughan JP, et al. The utility of the MELD score in predicting mortality following liver resection for metastasis. Eur J Surg Oncol 2016; 42(10):1568–75.

14. van Stijn MFM, Korkic-Halilovic I, Bakker MSM, et al. Preoperative nutrition status and postoperative outcome in elderly general surgery patients. JPEN J Parenter Enteral Nutr 2013;37(1):37–43.

15. Norman K, Stobäus N, Gonzalez MC, et al. Hand grip strength: outcome predictor and marker of nutritional status. Clin Nutr 2011;30(2):135–42.

16. Burden S, Todd C, Hill J, et al. Pre-operative nutrition support in patients undergoing gastrointestinal surgery. Cochrane Database Syst Rev 2012;(11):CD008879.

17. National Comprehensive Cancer Network (NCCN). NCCN Clinical practice guidelines in oncology. Available at: https://www.nccn.org/professionals/physician_gls/default.aspx. Accessed October 17, 2019.

18. Serrano PE, Gafni A, Gu C-S, et al. Positron Emission Tomography–Computed Tomography (PET-CT) versus no PET-CT in the management of potentially resectable colorectal cancer liver metastases: cost implications of a randomized controlled trial. J Oncol Pract 2016;12(7):e765–74.

19. Bray F, Ferlay J, Soerjomataram I, et al. Global cancer statistics 2018: GLOBOCAN estimates of incidence and mortality worldwide for 36 cancers in 185 countries. CA Cancer J Clin 2018;68(6):394–424.

20. Manfredi S, Lepage C, Hatem C, et al. Epidemiology and management of liver metastases from colorectal cancer. Ann Surg 2006;244(2):254–9.

21. Adam R, Wicherts DA, de Haas RJ, et al. Patients with initially unresectable colorectal liver metastases: is there a possibility of cure? J Clin Oncol 2009;27(11):1829–35.

22. Tomlinson JS, Jarnagin WR, DeMatteo RP, et al. Actual 10-year survival after resection of colorectal liver metastases defines cure. J Clin Oncol 2007;25(29):4575–80.

23. Imai K, Adam R, Baba H. How to increase the resectability of initially unresectable colorectal liver metastases: a surgical perspective. Ann Gastroenterol Surg 2019; 3(5):476–86.

24. Fong Y, Fortner J, Sun RL, et al. Clinical score for predicting recurrence after hepatic resection for metastatic colorectal cancer: analysis of 1001 consecutive cases. Ann Surg 1999;230(3):309–21.

25. van Dam RM, Lodewick TM, van den Broek MAJ, et al. Outcomes of extended versus limited indications for patients undergoing a liver resection for colorectal cancer liver metastases. HPB (Oxford) 2014;16(6):550–9.

26. Chapelle T, Op De Beeck B, Huyghe I, et al. Future remnant liver function estimated by combining liver volumetry on magnetic resonance imaging with total liver function on (99m)Tc-mebrofenin hepatobiliary scintigraphy: can this tool predict post-hepatectomy liver failure? HPB (Oxford) 2016;18(6):494–503.

27. Adams RB, Aloia TA, Loyer E, et al. Selection for hepatic resection of colorectal liver metastases: expert consensus statement. HPB (Oxford) 2013;15(2):91–103.

28. Chow FC-L, Chok KS-H. Colorectal liver metastases: An update on multidisciplinary approach. World J Hepatol 2019;11(2):150–72.

29. Charnsangavej C, Clary B, Fong Y, et al. Selection of patients for resection of hepatic colorectal metastases: expert consensus statement. Ann Surg Oncol 2006; 13(10):1261–8.

30. Shindoh J, Tzeng C-WD, Aloia TA, et al. Optimal future liver remnant in patients treated with extensive preoperative chemotherapy for colorectal liver metastases. Ann Surg Oncol 2013;20(8):2493–500.

31. Martel G, Cieslak KP, Huang R, et al. Comparison of techniques for volumetric analysis of the future liver remnant: implications for major hepatic resections. HPB (Oxford) 2015;17(12):1051–7.

32. Vauthey J-N, Dixon E, Abdalla EK, et al. Pretreatment assessment of hepatocellular carcinoma: expert consensus statement. HPB (Oxford) 2010;12(5):289–99.

33. Sasaki K, Margonis GA, Andreatos N, et al. Pre-hepatectomy carcinoembryonic antigen (CEA) levels among patients undergoing resection of colorectal liver metastases: do CEA levels still have prognostic implications? HPB (Oxford) 2016; 18(12):1000–9.

34. Granata V, Fusco R, de Lutio di Castelguidone E, et al. Diagnostic performance of gadoxetic acid–enhanced liver MRI versus multidetector CT in the assessment of colorectal liver metastases compared to hepatic resection. BMC Gastroenterol 2019;19(1):129.

35. Rockey DC, Caldwell SH, Goodman ZD, et al. Liver biopsy. Hepatology 2009; 49(3):1017–44.

36. Cresswell AB, Welsh FKS, Rees M. A diagnostic paradigm for resectable liver lesions: to biopsy or not to biopsy? HPB (Oxford) 2009;11(7):533–40.

37. Adam R, de Gramont A, Figueras J, et al. Managing synchronous liver metastases from colorectal cancer: a multidisciplinary international consensus. Cancer Treat Rev 2015;41(9):729–41.

38. Kardassis D, Ntinas A, Miliaras D, et al. Patients with multiple synchronous colonic cancer hepatic metastases benefit from enrolment in a "liver first" approach protocol. World J Hepatol 2014;6(7):513–9.

39. Fretland ÅA, Dagenborg VJ, Bjørnelv GMW, et al. Laparoscopic versus open resection for colorectal liver metastases: the OSLO-COMET randomized controlled trial. Ann Surg 2018;267(2):199–207.

40. Chakedis J, Beal EW, Lopez-Aguiar AG, et al. Surgery provides long-term survival in patients with metastatic neuroendocrine tumors undergoing resection for non-hormonal symptoms. J Gastrointest Surg 2019;23(1):122–34.

41. Hendifar AE, Ramirez RA, Anthony LB, et al. Current practices and novel techniques in the diagnosis and management of neuroendocrine tumors of unknown primary. Pancreas 2019;48(9):1111–8.

42. Babazadeh NT, Schlund DJ, Cornelius T, et al. Should 68Ga-DOTATATE PET/CT be performed routinely in patients with neuroendocrine tumors before surgical resection? World J Surg 2020;44(2):604–11.

43. Shah MH, Goldner WS, Halfdanarson TR, et al. NCCN Guidelines Insights: Neuroendocrine and Adrenal Tumors, Version 2.2018. J Natl Compr Canc Netw 2018; 16(6):693–702.

44. Sarmiento JM, Que FG. Hepatic surgery for metastases from neuroendocrine tumors. Surg Oncol Clin N Am 2003;12(1):231–42.

45. Ito T, Lee L, Jensen RT. Treatment of symptomatic neuroendocrine tumor syndromes: recent advances and controversies. Expert Opin Pharmacother 2016; 17(16):2191–205.

46. Pusceddu S, De Braud F, Festinese F, et al. Evolution in the treatment of gastroenteropancreatic-neuroendocrine neoplasms, focus on systemic therapeutic options: a systematic review. Future Oncol 2015;11(13):1947–59.

47. Osborne DA, Zervos EE, Strosberg J, et al. Improved outcome with cytoreduction versus embolization for symptomatic hepatic metastases of carcinoid and neuroendocrine tumors. Ann Surg Oncol 2006;13(4):572–81.

48. Maccauro M, Follacchio GA, Spreafico C, et al. Safety and efficacy of combined peptide receptor radionuclide therapy and liver selective internal radiation therapy in a patient with metastatic neuroendocrine tumor. Clin Nucl Med 2019; 44(4):e286–8.

49. Bertani E, Fazio N, Radice D, et al. Resection of the primary tumor followed by peptide receptor radionuclide therapy as upfront strategy for the treatment of G1–G2 pancreatic neuroendocrine tumors with unresectable liver metastases. Ann Surg Oncol 2016;23(5):981–9.

50. Tsang ME, Mahar AL, Martel G, et al. Assessing tools for management of noncolorectal nonneuroendocrine liver metastases: External validation of a prognostic model. J Surg Oncol 2018;118(6):1006–11.

51. Ercolani G, Ravaioli M, Grazi GL, et al. The role of liver resections for metastases from lung carcinoma. HPB (Oxford) 2006;8(2):114–5.

52. Reddy SK, Barbas AS, Marroquin CE, et al. Resection of noncolorectal nonneuroendocrine liver metastases: a comparative analysis. J Am Coll Surg 2007; 204(3):372–82.

53. Cordera F, Rea DJ, Rodriguez-Davalos M, et al. Hepatic resection for noncolorectal, nonneuroendocrine metastases. J Gastrointest Surg 2005;9(9):1361–70.

54. Kassahun WT. Controversies in defining prognostic relevant selection criteria that determine long-term effectiveness of liver resection for noncolorectal nonneuroendocrine liver metastasis. Int J Surg 2015;24:85–90.

55. Groeschl RT, Pilgrim CHC, Hanna EM, et al. Microwave ablation for hepatic malignancies: a multiinstitutional analysis. Ann Surg 2014;259(6):1195–200.

56. Robin TP, Raben D, Schefter TE. A contemporary update on the role of stereotactic body radiation therapy (SBRT) for liver metastases in the evolving landscape of oligometastatic disease management. Semin Radiat Oncol 2018;28(4):288–94.

57. Padia SA. Y90 clinical data update: cholangiocarcinoma, neuroendocrine tumor, melanoma, and breast cancer metastatic disease. Tech Vasc Interv Radiol 2019; 22(2):81–6.

Pancreas Solid Tumors

George Younan, MD, FACS[a,b,]*

KEYWORDS

• Pancreas • Neoplasm • Mass • Pancreatectomy • Adenocarcinoma

KEY POINTS

- Solid tumors of the pancreas include tumors of pancreatic cells of origin and tumors of extrapancreatic cells of origin.
- Pancreatic ductal adenocarcinoma is the most common pancreatic solid malignant tumor.
- Differential diagnosis includes exocrine tumors, neuroendocrine tumors, focal autoimmune pancreatitis, solid pseudopapillary tumors of the pancreas, primary pancreatic lymphoma, and metastatic tumors to the pancreas.

INTRODUCTION

Solid tumors of the pancreas encompass a variety of diagnoses, the vast majority are aggressive malignant tumors; however, some carry a lower malignant potential.[1] Pancreatic exocrine tumors, in all their subtypes, account for approximately 85% to 90% of all pancreatic solid tumors.[2] Despite advances in surgical and oncological care of pancreatic ductal adenocarcinoma, cure is exceedingly rare and long-term survival is less than 10%.[3] The need to differentiate pancreatic ductal adenocarcinoma from other pancreatic solid tumors is paramount, as treatments greatly differ.[4] Whereas surgical resection and perioperative systemic chemotherapy offer the best chance at long-term survival for patients with pancreatic ductal adenocarcinoma, approach to nonfunctioning small pancreatic neuroendocrine tumors can be based on observation alone.[5] Focal autoimmune pancreatitis lesions can present as hypodense pancreatic masses on contrast imaging studies, mimicking pancreatic ducal cancers; however, treatment can rely solely on corticosteroids and supportive care.[6,7]

We describe in this article the classification, epidemiology, screening, clinical presentation, diagnostic workup, and generalized treatment strategies for all varieties of pancreatic solid tumors. This article is intended to be an additional tool and a guideline for general surgeons when faced with a pancreatic mass diagnosis and allows them to direct their patients' care to improve outcomes.

---

[a] Department of Surgery, Inova Fair Oaks Hospital, Fairfax, VA, USA; [b] Division of Hepato-Pancreato-Biliary Surgery, Virginia Surgery Associates, 13135 Lee Jackson Memorial Highway, Suite #305, Fairfax, VA 22033, USA
* Division of Hepato-Pancreato-Biliary Surgery, Virginia Surgery Associates, 13135 Lee Jackson Memorial Highway, Suite #305, Fairfax, VA 22033.
E-mail address: grg.younan@gmail.com

Surg Clin N Am 100 (2020) 565–580
https://doi.org/10.1016/j.suc.2020.02.008
0039-6109/20/© 2020 Elsevier Inc. All rights reserved.

surgical.theclinics.com

CLASSIFICATION AND EPIDEMIOLOGY

Solid tumors of the pancreas can be broadly classified into 2 main categories based on their cell of origin. They can originate either from intrapancreatic cells, forming tumors that start in the pancreas gland; or extrapancreatic cells that are not pancreas-specific, however forming tumors inside the substance of the pancreas. The exocrine pancreatic system is the origin of the most common type of pancreatic tumors.[1,8] Pancreatic ductal adenocarcinomas arise from ductal cells, and comprise approximately 90% of pancreatic malignant tumors.[9] Patients are typically affected in their seventh decade of life, with most patients having metastatic, or surgically inoperable disease, and a 5-year overall survival of less than 10%.[10]

Acinar cell carcinomas are a rare variant of pancreatic exocrine cells of origin with acinar differentiation, comprising less than 1% of pancreatic malignant tumors.[9] They are morphologically and genetically different from ductal adenocarcinomas.[11] Age of onset is similar to patients with ductal adenocarcinoma. Pancreatoblastomas are also very rare pancreatic tumors with acinar differentiation, believed to arise from pancreatic exocrine stem cells, and are thought to be related to acinar cell carcinomas.[9] They are diagnosed in children approximately 5 years old and are associated with Beckwith-Wiedemann syndrome.[12]

Cells of the pancreatic endocrine system are the origin of pancreatic neuroendocrine tumors, also known as islet cell tumors.[1,13] These are overall rare and account for 1% to 2% of all pancreatic tumors, and approximately 5% of all pancreatic malignant tumors.[9,14] Their incidence rate is approximately 1 per 100,000 people, and patients affected are most commonly diagnosed in their fourth to sixth decades of life.[15] Most pancreatic neuroendocrine tumors are nonfunctioning and are not related to a hormone-secreting syndrome, whereas hormone-secreting tumors are the minority and are classified based on the hormone they secrete the most.[16–18] Examples of functioning pancreatic neuroendocrine tumors include insulinomas, gastrinomas, glucagonomas, somatostatinomas, and VIPomas.[19,20]

Pancreatic tumors of extrapancreatic cells of origin comprise metastatic tumors to the pancreas, solid pseudopapillary tumors of the pancreas, focal autoimmune pancreatitis, and primary pancreatic lymphoma. Metastatic tumors to the pancreas are a rare entity among pancreatic solid cancers; they include renal cell carcinomas, melanomas, breast carcinomas, colorectal carcinomas, and sarcomas.[21,22] These can be a sign of widespread metastatic disease or isolated and solitary metastases to the pancreas, amenable to surgical resection.[23]

Focal autoimmune pancreatitis is another disease that can present as a pancreatic solid tumor.[24] Another terminology of this disease is sclerosing pancreatitis.[25] Clinical presentations of autoimmune pancreatitis vary, and one of them is a pancreatic mass that can be suspicious for a malignancy.[24,26] This is specifically significant in the focal form of the disease.[27,28]

Solid pseudopapillary tumors of the pancreas are very rare tumors, first described by Franz in 1959 and thus called Franz tumors.[29] They comprise approximately 1% to 2% of all pancreatic tumors.[9] They are not believed to originate from pancreatic tissue lineage; however, their exact cell of origin is still unknown.[30,31] They occur predominantly in young women in their third or fourth decade of life and carry a 10% to 15% chance of malignancy.[32]

Primary pancreatic lymphomas originate from extrapancreatic cells and are a rare entity when they occur in the pancreas, accounting for fewer than 0.5% of pancreatic malignancies and 1% of extranodal lymphomas.[33,34] Because of the overlapping clinical picture, it is hard to distinguish a pancreatic lymphoma from a pancreatic adenocarcinoma.[35] Large B-cell lymphoma tends to be the most common variant occurring in the pancreas.[36]

Periampullary tumors can be misdiagnosed as pancreatic solid tumors, and sometimes even after surgical resection, differentiating them remains difficult. These include solid tumors of the ampulla, duodenum, or the biliary tree. The discussion of these is beyond the scope of this article.

SCREENING

Pancreatic solid tumors are diagnosed in 1 of 3 general scenarios. They are either symptomatic and found after a workup for those symptoms, or incidentally found during a workup for unrelated medical issues or found based on screening protocols in high-risk individuals.

Pancreatic ductal adenocarcinoma carries a poor prognosis, even when diagnosed and treated early.[2] It constitutes the fourth most common cause of cancer-related death in the United States and projected to be higher in the coming decades.[3] Screening protocols are being considered around the world; however, no one screening algorithm has been consolidated yet.[37,38] Screening is currently considered in individuals who have a high lifetime risk of getting the disease, and these include, in general, patients with a family history of pancreatic cancer with affected first-degree relatives, patients with Peutz-Jeghers syndrome, and patients carrying genetic mutations (BRCA2, p16, HNPCC, and PALB2 with affected first-degree relatives). National Comprehensive Cancer Network guidelines were updated in 2018 to recommend genetic testing to any patient with pancreatic cancer.[39] Patients with a positive family history for pancreatic cancer carry a high risk of getting the disease, and 10% of patients who are diagnosed with pancreatic cancer have a positive family history.[40] An effective screening method can ideally be a blood test to detect early disease; however, this is not available yet. Screening relies on axial imaging with pancreas-protocol computed tomography (CT) or MRI scans, in addition to more accurate tests to detect small pancreatic lesions through endoscopic ultrasound.[37,41,42]

Pancreatic neuroendocrine tumors are mostly sporadic but can be associated with familial syndromes, including multiple endocrine neoplasia type I, Von-Hippel-Lindau syndrome, tuberous sclerosis, and neurofibromatosis type I syndrome.[15] Familial types of the disease tend to be indolent, however necessitating treatment; thus, screening protocols have been suggested to this subtype of patients.[43] Lifetime risk of developing pancreatic neuroendocrine tumors is the highest in patients with MEN1 syndrome and lowest in patients with tuberous sclerosis.[44,45]

Solid pseudopapillary tumors of the pancreas have not been found to have any genetic associated syndromes or any other known risk factors.[32,46]

CLINICAL PRESENTATION

Pancreatic exocrine cancers are often diagnosed late in their development and most patients tend to have metastatic disease.[40] Their clinical presentation differs from that of neuroendocrine tumors, especially in recent decades when neuroendocrine tumors are diagnosed earlier.[47] Symptoms in general are related to either the local activity of the tumor and its relationship to surrounding structures, organs, nerves, blood vessels (eg, jaundice, pain, vomiting), or systemic effects, related to chemicals secreted by those tumors, creating a whole cascade of effects targeting the body universally (eg, cachexia, depression, weight loss).[40] Pancreatic exocrine tumors present most commonly with abdominal pain, jaundice, and weight loss. Some other symptoms include pancreatic insufficiency symptoms and deep vein thrombosis.[48,49] Most pancreatic exocrine tumors are located in the head and neck of the gland compared with the body and tail; this dictates the initial presentation of patients. Symptoms are usually insidious in onset and take a few weeks to be clinically significant. Pain and jaundice might take a few weeks and up to 2 months to be noticeable by patients before seeking medical advice. New-onset diabetes mellitus has been hypothesized to be an early finding associated with pancreatic cancers.[50]

Pancreatic neuroendocrine tumors, on the other hand, are a different breed when it comes to clinical presentation.[51] It is now known that most are nonfunctioning (up to 75%–80%) and only a minority of them are diagnosed based on their associated hormonal syndrome.[44,52]

Nonfunctioning tumors are either found incidentally or when they become symptomatic due to a locoregional tumor effect or when metastatic.[18,53] The most common symptom remains abdominal pain in up to 70% of patients, followed by weight loss.[13,18] Obstructive jaundice is a much less frequent sign when compared with exocrine tumors.[54] Other signs include a palpable intra-abdominal mass, whether primary or metastatic, the liver being the most common organ of metastasis from a pancreatic origin, in addition to less frequent signs like intra-abdominal bleeding.[55] Approximately 30% to 70% are found to be metastatic at diagnosis.[15]

The clinical presentation of metastatic tumors of the pancreas is a function of the primary disease.[22] Whereas most metastatic disease is found in a synchronous fashion, some patients present with recurrent metastatic disease on restaging or when symptomatic, hence the importance of tissue diagnosis.[21–23] Solitary or multifocal pancreatic lesions can be found in this subcategory. Solitary lesions are the most common; however, multifocal lesions are present up to 45% of the time.[56]

Focal lesions related to autoimmune pancreatitis tend to show up with pancreatitis type symptoms.[24,27] Patients tend to be younger with a history of other autoimmune diseases, and they usually have a history of chronic pancreatitis with a previous negative workup.[57] The abdominal pain is usually more chronic in nature and tends to be stable compared with progressing abdominal pain in real tumors of the pancreas.[27,28] Other locoregional signs and symptoms can be very similar to those of other pancreatic tumors.[6]

Solid pseudopapillary tumors of the pancreas are a disease of young women in their third or fourth decade of life.[32] Most patients present with symptoms, and abdominal pain is the most common finding in approximately 80% of patients, followed by nausea or vomiting in 20% of the cases.[30,58] An interesting finding is that, even when located in the head of the pancreas, fewer patients present with jaundice compared with patients with pancreatic ductal adenocarcinoma, and the rate of jaundice has been reported to be lower than 5%.[59] Fewer than 20% of patients are diagnosed with metastasis at the time of the diagnosis of the primary tumor, the liver and peritoneum being the most common sites of metastasis.[32]

Primary pancreatic lymphoma presents in a more systemic fashion rather than locoregional symptoms.[33,34] Constitutional symptoms, such as weight loss, fever, and night sweats, are common. They are typically large tumors with significant surrounding lymphadenopathy.[36,60] Obstructive jaundice tends to be rare in pancreatic lymphoma.[35,36]

DIAGNOSTIC TOOLS AND LOCALIZATION

The usual universal approach to patients with pancreatic solid tumors must be used by the general surgeon, including a comprehensive history and physical examination and a comprehensive personal and family cancer history, in addition to a history of risk factors.[48] General surgeons dealing with pancreatic solid tumors must be able to direct the care of these patients based on 2 general tests: serologic tests and radiological tests.

Laboratory Tests

A full laboratory panel must be obtained, including a comprehensive blood count, a full chemistry panel, including liver functional tests, amylase and lipase, nutritional status, and coagulation profiles.[40,48]

Tumor markers are useful in the evaluation of pancreatic tumors. These include carbohydrate antigen 19 to 9 (CA19–9), carcinoembryonic antigen, alpha-fetoprotein (AFP), chromogranin A, neuron-specific enolase, pancreatic polypeptide, and functional neuroendocrine tumor hormonal measurement.[61,62] CA19 to 9 remains the only biomarker that is routinely used in the workup of pancreatic ductal adenocarcinoma.[63] Although not used for diagnosis, it is routinely tested after diagnosis of pancreatic ductal adenocarcinoma and followed throughout treatment.[63] Normalization of CA19 to 9 carries important prognostic factors after neoadjuvant therapy for pancreatic cancer.[64] The Lewis blood group antigen must0 be expressed in individuals who are diagnosed with pancreatic cancer before this antigen can be tracked, 5% to 10% of the population does not express a Lewis antigen, and thus CA19 to 9 cannot be used in their cases. AFP has been found to be elevated in acinar cancers of the pancreas.[11] Work is under way to find new pancreatic cancer biomarkers to help in early detection and treatment of this lethal disease. Circulating tumor cells and tumor DNA have been well studied and carry a promising value.[65,66] Tumor marker measurement in the case of neuroendocrine tumors is a class 3 recommendation currently from the National Comprehensive Cancer Network recommendations due to lack of sensitivity and specificity.

Imaging and Endoscopic Tests

Once a pancreatic solid mass is detected, additional specific noninvasive imaging studies and invasive endoscopic procedures are used to help guide diagnosis and management, as pancreatic solid tumor treatments differ significantly.

IMAGING STUDIES
Ultrasound

Transabdominal ultrasounds are usually the first tests used because they are noninvasive, low cost, and have high availability. They tend to have a low sensitivity and specificity when scanning small tumors. Ultrasound sensitivity ranges from 50% to 90%.[67] Ultrasound is more useful in pancreatic head tumors compared with body and tail tumors.[68] Pancreatic ductal adenocarcinoma presents as an irregular hypoechoic mass on ultrasound with associated ductal dilation. Pancreatic neuroendocrine tumors are well circumscribed, with smooth margins on ultrasound, hypoechoic in nature, and can demonstrate a hypervascular enhancement with contrast.[69] Focal autoimmune pancreatitis is hypoechoic and nonspecific on ultrasound.[70] Pancreatic lymphomas appear as large, hypoechoic, bulky masses within the pancreatic parenchyma.[71] Solid pseudopapillary tumors are hypoechoic masses that can be solid, cystic, or a combination.[31] In general, ultrasound is an accepted first-line study in symptomatic patients; however, its use is very limited, as it cannot differentiate between different types of pancreatic solid tumors.

Computed Tomography

A triphasic pancreas-protocol CT scan is the best and the most common first imaging test used if a solid pancreatic lesion needs investigation.[40] CT scans allow radiological staging of the disease and assess resectability, in addition to searching for metastatic disease.[68,72] Sensitivity of a multidetector pancreas-protocol CT (MDCT) can reach up to 97% in all tumors and even 100% in tumors larger than 2 cm.[72] Typical findings of a pancreatic ductal adenocarcinoma on CT include a hypoattenuating (sometimes iso-attenuating) mass, irregular in shape, with upstream pancreatic duct dilation, and biliary duct dilation if the mass is in the head area of the pancreas, hence the term "double duct sign."[73] MDCT is the test of choice during restaging of pancreatic adenocarcinoma in conjunction to PET/CT, as a regular CT might not detect small metastatic lesions (Fig. 1).[74]

Acinar cell carcinomas tend to be similar in attenuation to ductal adenocarcinomas; however, they are much larger. They can contain calcifications and usually have a cystic component.[75] Whenever cystic, they show less hypervascularity than the cystic variant of neuroendocrine tumors (see Fig. 1).

Neuroendocrine tumors are hypervascular, well-circumscribed masses on early arterial phases of an abdominal CT, usually homogenous; however, they can be heterogeneous with a hyperattenuating rim due to a cystic degeneration and central necrosis of these tumors as they grow in size.[69] Metastatic neuroendocrine tumors to peripancreatic lymph nodes and distant organs tend to be hypervascular as well (see Fig. 1).

Focal autoimmune pancreatitis lesions appear as hypointense or iso-intense pancreatic head enlargement.[6,70] The striking difference compared with regular pancreatitis findings is the absence of peripancreatic fat stranding (see Fig. 1).[70]

Pancreatic lymphomas occur in 2 morphologic forms: a localized form, acting like a focal hypodense mass, and a diffuse infiltrating form, looking like inflammation of the pancreas.[71] If in the head of the pancreas, a lymphoma does not usually cause upstream pancreatic ductal dilation, in comparison with ductal adenocarcinomas, and if presenting as an infiltrating pattern through the whole gland, patients do not typically have the clinical presentation of acute pancreatitis.[71] Central necrosis or calcifications are virtually nonexistent in primary pancreatic lymphomas (see Fig. 1).[71]

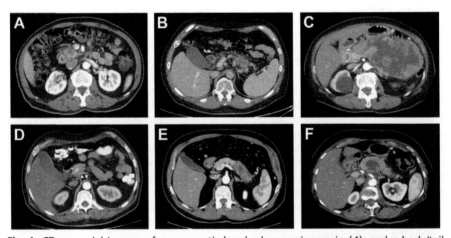

Fig. 1. CT scan axial images of a pancreatic head adenocarcinoma in (A), and a body/tail adenocarcinoma in (B). (C) Mixed solid/cystic acinar cell carcinoma. A typical hypervascular pancreatic head neuroendocrine tumor is shown in (D). An axial CT of a focal body/tail autoimmune pancreatitis lesions is shown in (E). A primary pancreatic head lymphoma is shown in (F). Blue arrows point to tumors.

Solid pseudopapillary tumors of the pancreas show a pattern of heterogeneity with a mixture of solid and cystic components.[31] They are well encapsulated with heterogenous attenuation.[76] Metastatic tumors to the pancreas usually show the enhancement pattern of their primary tumor, colon cancer metastases to the pancreas are hypoattenuating on a contrast study compared with the pancreas parenchyma, whereas renal cell carcinoma metastases to the pancreas are hyperattenuating.[56]

MRI

MRI/magnetic resonance cholangiopancreatography (MRCP) has been widely used in recent years in the workup of pancreatic tumors. It has many advantages over MDCT, especially in small tumors, iso-attenuating tumors, and pancreatic head hypertrophy, and is the state-of-art noninvasive method to replace endoscopic retrograde cholangiopancreatography (ERCP), in delineating pancreatic and biliary ductal anatomy.[77–80] On MRI, pancreatic adenocarcinomas appear hypointense on T1-weighted, and can be variable on T2-weighted images (**Fig. 2**).[81]

MRI is similar to CT in detecting pancreatic neuroendocrine tumors; they are round hypointense lesions on T1 and hyperintense compared with pancreas on T2-weighted images. Liver metastases show the same pattern of enhancement (see **Fig. 2**).[69]

Focal autoimmune pancreatitis lesions are usually found in the head of the pancreas, with mild upstream pancreatic ductal dilation.[6,70] The lesions of the focal form are hypointense on T1-weighted, and hyperintense on T2-weighted images. Focal lesions can show segmental nonvisualization of the main pancreatic duct and no significant upstream dilation, and this finding tends to be specific for focal autoimmune pancreatitis lesions on MRCP.[70] Secretin stimulation during MRCP has the potential to differentiate ductal adenocarcinoma from focal pancreatitis lesions.[82]

Pancreatic lymphomas show a pattern of low intensity compared with the gland on T1-weighted, and slightly increased signal on T2-weighted images, in cases of focal involvement (see **Fig. 2**).[71]

Solid pseudopapillary tumors present as masses with a hemorrhagic component with a high intensity on T1-weighted, and low intensity on T2-weighted images

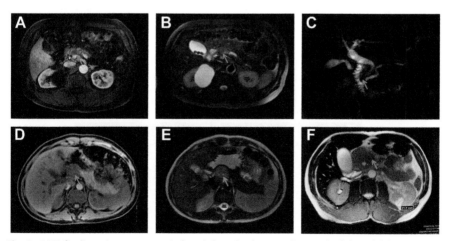

Fig. 2. MRI findings in a pancreatic head ductal adenocarcinoma in (*A*) and (*B*). An MRCP reconstruction of the biliary and pancreatic ductal dilation is delineated in (*C*). A large pancreatic neck gastrinoma on MRI is depicted in (*D*) and (*E*). A primary pancreatic neck lymphoma on MRI is shown in (*F*). Blue arrows point to tumors.

compared with the hemorrhagic area.[76] Other characteristics of these tumors are similar to CT, showing an encapsulated, well-circumscribed tumor, usually in the tail of the pancreas, with solid and cystic components and hemorrhage.[76]

Metastatic tumors to the pancreas are hypointense on T1-weighted, and hyperintense on T2-weighted images compared with pancreas parenchyma.[56] Rim enhancement can be seen, either homogeneously in small lesions or heterogeneously in larger lesions.[56] Upstream pancreatic duct dilation is not usual with metastatic tumors to the pancreas, and if multifocal, lesions tend to show the same pattern on imaging.[56]

Nuclear Imaging

The most common used radiotracer with PET/CT is 18-fluorodeoxyglucose, hence the term FDG-PET. It is the most commonly used test to assess metastatic disease and more sensitive than MDCT in treatment restaging and monitoring and to detect occult metastatic disease.[83,84] Focal autoimmune pancreatitis lesions tend to show avid uptake on FDG-PET imaging due to the inflammatory status of the mass (**Fig. 3**).[70]

Nuclear medicine studies are used in the localization of pancreatic neuroendocrine tumors. Somatostatin receptor scintigraphy takes advantage of somatostatin receptors on these tumors.[69] These imaging modalities not only localize neuroendocrine tumors, they also provide data on the somatostatin receptor status of these tumors for potential therapeutic interventions. Improvement on the initial octreotide analog scintigraphy came long when Gallium 68 dotatate PET scans were introduced. These, combined with CT, improved detection and sensitivity of nuclear imaging studies of neuroendocrine tumors.[85] Insulinomas remain the one subgroup of neuroendocrine tumors that are poorly localized with this study due to the low numbers of somatostatin receptor 2 in them; the same issue is present with poorly differentiated neuroendocrine tumors, as they have a low number of this receptor (see **Fig. 3**).[86]

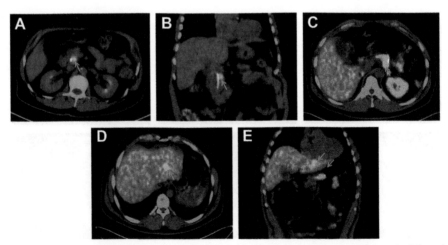

Fig. 3. FDG-PET/CT of a small pancreatic head ductal adenocarcinoma is shown in (A) and (B). Axial images of a Gallium-68 PET scan in a case of a nonfunctioning pancreatic body neuroendocrine tumor that has metastasized to the liver in (C) and (D); both lesions are depicted in the same coronal cut of the same scan in (E). Blue arrows point to tumors.

INVASIVE ENDOSCOPIC STUDIES
Endoscopic Retrograde Cholangiopancreatography

This is an invasive diagnostic and therapeutic endoscopic procedure found to be highly sensitive and specific in diagnosing pancreatic cancer.[87] Findings include malignant-looking pancreatic duct and distal bile duct strictures and upstream duct dilation.[88] ERCP is used to stent the biliary tree and treat obstruction-induced cholestasis and brush intraductal tumors for tissue diagnosis.[89] ERCP carries a risk of procedure-related pancreatitis that can be detrimental to the treatment of patients with pancreatic adenocarcinoma, delaying their surgeries or their systemic therapies and thus there has been questioning of the need of preoperative biliary stenting that was addressed by multiple studies.[90,91] The general consensus points toward surgical resection and drainage versus biliary stenting; however, if biliary stenting is needed, as in the setting of neoadjuvant therapy, then biliary stenting with self-expanding metallic stents is preferred (**Fig. 4**).[90]

Endoscopic Ultrasound

The use of endoscopic ultrasound (EUS) in pancreatic solid lesions encompasses diagnosis, staging and treatment. The accuracy of EUS for staging has been debated and is highly variable and is operator dependent.[92] As for diagnosis of tumors, EUS is used to obtain a fine needle aspirate or a core biopsy, from a primary pancreatic mass, a peripancreatic lymph node, or a metastatic liver or peritoneal nodule, with all the subsequent treatment implications. There is still controversy on the use of neoadjuvant therapy in cases of resectable pancreatic ductal adenocarcinoma, thus there has been questions about the need for an EUS-guided biopsy in cases of tumors that will be primarily resected. The importance of EUS in these cases lies in the diagnosis of tumors that mimic adenocarcinoma and that might not require surgical

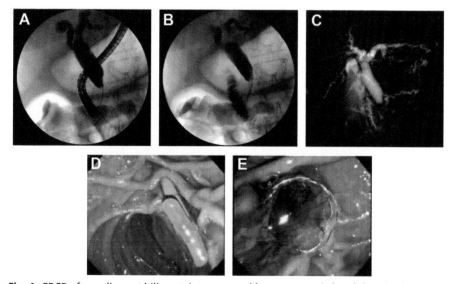

Fig. 4. ERCP of a malignant biliary stricture caused by a pancreatic head ductal adenocarcinoma, typical findings of a distal malignant-looking stricture with upstream dilation are shown in (*A*), deployment of a metallic wallstent is shown in (*B*), with the corresponding MRCP shown in (*C*). A plastic (*D*) and metallic (*E*) stents are depicted on endoscopic imaging.

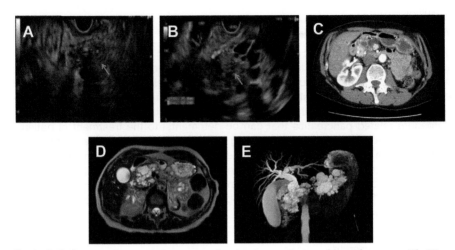

Fig. 5. EUS-diagnosed pancreatic neuroendocrine tumor that could not be seen with CT or MRI in a patient with Von Hippel-Lindau syndrome. (*A*) and (*B*) show 2 cuts of the tumor on endoscopy. Respective CT, MRI, and MRCP of the same area are shown in (*C*), (*D*), and (*E*), failing to identify any tumors other than the cysts. Blue arrows point to tumors.

resection, such as focal autoimmune pancreatitis or primary pancreatic lymphoma.[26,27,68] This controversy does not exist in cases of borderline resectable or locally advanced disease, or non-surgical candidates, where patients will require systemic chemotherapy, thus needing a histologic confirmation.[93] EUS aspiration or biopsy has been shown to be very sensitive in acquiring a definitive cytologic diagnosis, with a sensitivity reaching up to 95%.[94,95] It is best if EUS is used before a biliary stent is inserted in obstructing tumors as this will affect accuracy and yield (**Fig. 5**).

EUS can be additionally used for assisting in celiac plexus neurolysis, a procedure that is widely used for cancer-related pain, although its benefit has been questioned.[96] EUS also has been used in multiple studies for endoscopic ablation of pancreatic lesions and drainage of the biliary tree independently from ERCP.

SUMMARY

The scope of this article was to be a guide for general surgeons when being consulted on a patient with a solid pancreatic mass. We describe the classification, epidemiology, screening, clinical presentation, and the diagnostic workup from a surgical oncology standpoint. The treatment for this differential of diagnoses is a whole different subject and is not meant to be part of this article; however, we opted to include some generalized referral and treatment strategies. Referral patterns concerning pancreatic surgery have been changing over the past decade and pancreatic surgery outcomes have been widely studied; definitions and guidelines have been widely published. High-volume surgeons and high-volume institutions have improved outcomes after pancreatic surgery.[97] These trends advocated for centralization of complex abdominal surgeries to high-volume tertiary care centers, nationally and internationally.[98,99] Obstacles to centralization include feasibility of access to cancer care, disparity between patient groups, commercial insurance variability, and changing government health policies.[100,101]

Multidisciplinary approach to tumors of the pancreas is key, especially when dealing with lesions that mimic pancreatic adenocarcinoma.[102] Emphasis must be stressed on the use of clinical trials in the treatment of pancreatic disease as new treatments are being discovered, in addition to the early diagnosis and quick initiation of treatment in hopes of obtaining long-term survival in patients with a lethal disease.

CONFLICTS OF INTEREST

None.

REFERENCES

1. Wood LD, Hruban RH. Pathology and molecular genetics of pancreatic neoplasms. Cancer J 2012;18(6):492–501.
2. Winter JM, Brennan MF, Tang LH, et al. Survival after resection of pancreatic adenocarcinoma: results from a single institution over three decades. Ann Surg Oncol 2012;19(1):169–75.
3. Allen PJ, Kuk D, Castillo CF, et al. Multi-institutional validation study of the American Joint Commission on Cancer (8th Edition) changes for T and N staging in patients with pancreatic adenocarcinoma. Ann Surg 2017;265(1):185–91.
4. Yadav S, Sharma P, Zakalik D. Comparison of demographics, tumor characteristics, and survival between pancreatic adenocarcinomas and pancreatic neuroendocrine tumors: a population-based study. Am J Clin Oncol 2018; 41(5):485–91.
5. Klimstra DS. Nonductal neoplasms of the pancreas. Mod Pathol 2007;20(Suppl 1):S94–112.
6. Finkelberg DL, Sahani D, Deshpande V, et al. Autoimmune pancreatitis. N Engl J Med 2006;355(25):2670–6.
7. Sahani DV, Kalva SP, Farrell J, et al. Autoimmune pancreatitis: imaging features. Radiology 2004;233(2):345–52.
8. Kloppel G, Luttges J. WHO-classification 2000: exocrine pancreatic tumors. Verh Dtsch Ges Pathol 2001;85:219–28.
9. Hackeng WM, Hruban RH, Offerhaus GJ, et al. Surgical and molecular pathology of pancreatic neoplasms. Diagn Pathol 2016;11(1):47.
10. Siegel RL, Miller KD, Jemal A. Cancer statistics, 2018. CA Cancer J Clin 2018; 68(1):7–30.
11. Abraham SC, Wu TT, Hruban RH, et al. Genetic and immunohistochemical analysis of pancreatic acinar cell carcinoma: frequent allelic loss on chromosome 11p and alterations in the APC/beta-catenin pathway. Am J Pathol 2002; 160(3):953–62.
12. Chisholm KM, Hsu CH, Kim MJ, et al. Congenital pancreatoblastoma: report of an atypical case and review of the literature. J Pediatr Hematol Oncol 2012; 34(4):310–5.
13. Kulke MH, Shah MH, Benson AB 3rd, et al. Neuroendocrine tumors, version 1.2015. J Natl Compr Canc Netw 2015;13(1):78–108.
14. Hallet J, Law CH, Cukier M, et al. Exploring the rising incidence of neuroendocrine tumors: a population-based analysis of epidemiology, metastatic presentation, and outcomes. Cancer 2015;121(4):589–97.
15. Dasari A, Shen C, Halperin D, et al. Trends in the incidence, prevalence, and survival outcomes in patients with neuroendocrine tumors in the United States. JAMA Oncol 2017;3(10):1335–42.

16. Rindi G, Klimstra DS, Abedi-Ardekani B, et al. A common classification frame-work for neuroendocrine neoplasms: an International Agency for Research on Cancer (IARC) and World Health Organization (WHO) expert consensus pro-posal. Mod Pathol 2018;31(12):1770–86.

17. Kloppel G. Neuroendocrine neoplasms: dichotomy, origin and classifications. Visc Med 2017;33(5):324–30.

18. Kuo JH, Lee JA, Chabot JA. Nonfunctional pancreatic neuroendocrine tumors. Surg Clin North Am 2014;94(3):689–708.

19. Clancy TE. Surgical management of pancreatic neuroendocrine tumors. Hema-tol Oncol Clin North Am 2016;30(1):103–18.

20. Falconi M, Eriksson B, Kaltsas G, et al. ENETS consensus guidelines update for the management of patients with functional pancreatic neuroendocrine tumors and non-functional pancreatic neuroendocrine tumors. Neuroendocrinology 2016;103(2):153–71.

21. Cheng SK, Chuah KL. Metastatic renal cell carcinoma to the pancreas: a review. Arch Pathol Lab Med 2016;140(6):598–602.

22. Sperti C, Pozza G, Brazzale AR, et al. Metastatic tumors to the pancreas: a sys-tematic review and meta-analysis. Minerva Chir 2016;71(5):337–44.

23. Maeda A, Uesaka K, Matsunaga K, et al. Metastatic tumors of the pancreas. Pancreas 2008;37(2):234–6.

24. Tabata M, Kitayama J, Kanemoto H, et al. Autoimmune pancreatitis presenting as a mass in the head of the pancreas: a diagnosis to differentiate from cancer. Am Surg 2003;69(5):363–6.

25. DiMagno EP. Autoimmune chronic pancreatitis: a plea for simplification and con-sistency. Clin Gastroenterol Hepatol 2003;1(6):421–2.

26. Horiuchi A, Kaneko T, Yamamura N, et al. Autoimmune chronic pancreatitis simulating pancreatic lymphoma. Am J Gastroenterol 1996;91(12):2607–9.

27. Buscarini E, Frulloni L, De Lisi S, et al. Autoimmune pancreatitis: a challenging diagnostic puzzle for clinicians. Dig Liver Dis 2010;42(2):92–8.

28. Frulloni L, Scattolini C, Falconi M, et al. Autoimmune pancreatitis: differences between the focal and diffuse forms in 87 patients. Am J Gastroenterol 2009; 104(9):2288–94.

29. Reddy S, Cameron JL, Scudiere J, et al. Surgical management of solid-pseudopapillary neoplasms of the pancreas (Franz or Hamoudi tumors): a large single-institutional series. J Am Coll Surg 2009;208(5):950–7 [discussion: 957–9].

30. Wright MJ, Javed AA, Saunders T, et al. Surgical resection of 78 pancreatic solid pseudopapillary tumors: a 30-year single institutional experience. J Gastrointest Surg 2019. [Epub ahead of print].

31. Antoniou EA, Damaskos C, Garmpis N, et al. Solid pseudopapillary tumor of the pancreas: a single-center experience and review of the literature. In Vivo 2017; 31(4):501–10.

32. Reddy S, Wolfgang CL. Solid pseudopapillary neoplasms of the pancreas. Adv Surg 2009;43:269–82.

33. Mishra MV, Keith SW, Shen X, et al. Primary pancreatic lymphoma: a population-based analysis using the SEER program. Am J Clin Oncol 2013;36(1):38–43.

34. Ramesh J, Hebert-Magee S, Kim H, et al. Frequency of occurrence and charac-teristics of primary pancreatic lymphoma during endoscopic ultrasound guided fine needle aspiration: a retrospective study. Dig Liver Dis 2014;46(5):470–3.

35. Rock J, Bloomston M, Lozanski G, et al. The spectrum of hematologic malignancies involving the pancreas: potential clinical mimics of pancreatic adenocarcinoma. Am J Clin Pathol 2012;137(3):414–22.

36. Alexander RE, Nakeeb A, Sandrasegaran K, et al. Primary pancreatic follicle center-derived lymphoma masquerading as carcinoma. Gastroenterol Hepatol (N Y) 2011;7(12):834–8.

37. Canto MI, Harinck F, Hruban RH, et al. International Cancer of the Pancreas Screening (CAPS) Consortium summit on the management of patients with increased risk for familial pancreatic cancer. Gut 2013;62(3):339–47.

38. Lennon AM, Hruban RH, Klein AP. Screening for pancreatic cancer—is there hope? JAMA Intern Med 2019;179(10):1313–5.

39. Syngal S, Furniss CS. Germline genetic testing for pancreatic ductal adenocarcinoma at time of diagnosis. JAMA 2018;319(23):2383–5.

40. Vincent A, Herman J, Schulick R, et al. Pancreatic cancer. Lancet 2011; 378(9791):607–20.

41. Ngamruengphong S, Canto MI. Screening for pancreatic cancer. Surg Clin North Am 2016;96(6):1223–33.

42. Canto MI, Goggins M, Yeo CJ, et al. Screening for pancreatic neoplasia in high-risk individuals: an EUS-based approach. Clin Gastroenterol Hepatol 2004;2(7): 606–21.

43. Pea A, Hruban RH, Wood LD. Genetics of pancreatic neuroendocrine tumors: implications for the clinic. Expert Rev Gastroenterol Hepatol 2015;9(11): 1407–19.

44. Metz DC, Jensen RT. Gastrointestinal neuroendocrine tumors: pancreatic endocrine tumors. Gastroenterology 2008;135(5):1469–92.

45. Leoncini E, Carioli G, La Vecchia C, et al. Risk factors for neuroendocrine neoplasms: a systematic review and meta-analysis. Ann Oncol 2016;27(1):68–81.

46. Law JK, Ahmed A, Singh VK, et al. A systematic review of solid-pseudopapillary neoplasms: are these rare lesions? Pancreas 2014;43(3):331–7.

47. Leoncini E, Boffetta P, Shafir M, et al. Increased incidence trend of low-grade and high-grade neuroendocrine neoplasms. Endocrine 2017;58(2):368–79.

48. McGuigan A, Kelly P, Turkington RC, et al. Pancreatic cancer: a review of clinical diagnosis, epidemiology, treatment and outcomes. World J Gastroenterol 2018; 24(43):4846–61.

49. Ansari D, Ansari D, Andersson R, et al. Pancreatic cancer and thromboembolic disease, 150 years after Trousseau. Hepatobiliary Surg Nutr 2015;4(5):325–35.

50. Pannala R, Basu A, Petersen GM, et al. New-onset diabetes: a potential clue to the early diagnosis of pancreatic cancer. Lancet Oncol 2009;10(1):88–95.

51. Turaga KK, Kvols LK. Recent progress in the understanding, diagnosis, and treatment of gastroenteropancreatic neuroendocrine tumors. CA Cancer J Clin 2011;61(2):113–32.

52. Kasumova GG, Tabatabaie O, Eskander MF, et al. National rise of primary pancreatic carcinoid tumors: comparison to functional and nonfunctional pancreatic neuroendocrine tumors. J Am Coll Surg 2017;224(6):1057–64.

53. Singh S, Dey C, Kennecke H, et al. Consensus recommendations for the diagnosis and management of pancreatic neuroendocrine tumors: guidelines from a Canadian National Expert Group. Ann Surg Oncol 2015;22(8):2685–99.

54. Milan SA, Yeo CJ. Neuroendocrine tumors of the pancreas. Curr Opin Oncol 2012;24(1):46–55.

55. Zerbi A, Falconi M, Rindi G, et al. Clinicopathological features of pancreatic endocrine tumors: a prospective multicenter study in Italy of 297 sporadic cases. Am J Gastroenterol 2010;105(6):1421–9.
56. Triantopoulou C, Kolliakou E, Karoumpalis I, et al. Metastatic disease to the pancreas: an imaging challenge. Insights Imaging 2012;3(2):165–72.
57. Takuma K, Kamisawa T, Gopalakrishna R, et al. Strategy to differentiate autoimmune pancreatitis from pancreas cancer. World J Gastroenterol 2012;18(10):1015–20.
58. Salvia R, Bassi C, Festa L, et al. Clinical and biological behavior of pancreatic solid pseudopapillary tumors: report on 31 consecutive patients. J Surg Oncol 2007;95(4):304–10.
59. Papavramidis T, Papavramidis S. Solid pseudopapillary tumors of the pancreas: review of 718 patients reported in English literature. J Am Coll Surg 2005;200(6):965–72.
60. Saif MW. Primary pancreatic lymphomas. JOP 2006;7(3):262–73.
61. Reiter MJ, Costello JE, Schwope RB, et al. Review of commonly used serum tumor markers and their relevance for image interpretation. J Comput Assist Tomogr 2015;39(6):825–34.
62. Oberg K, Modlin IM, De Herder W, et al. Consensus on biomarkers for neuroendocrine tumour disease. Lancet Oncol 2015;16(9):e435–46.
63. Ansari D, Gustafsson A, Andersson R. Update on the management of pancreatic cancer: surgery is not enough. World J Gastroenterol 2015;21(11):3157–65.
64. Tsai S, George B, Wittmann D, et al. Importance of normalization of CA19-9 levels following neoadjuvant therapy in patients with localized pancreatic cancer. Ann Surg 2020;271(4):740–7.
65. Allenson K, Castillo J, San Lucas FA, et al. High prevalence of mutant KRAS in circulating exosome-derived DNA from early-stage pancreatic cancer patients. Ann Oncol 2017;28(4):741–7.
66. Riva F, Dronov OI, Khomenko DI, et al. Clinical applications of circulating tumor DNA and circulating tumor cells in pancreatic cancer. Mol Oncol 2016;10(3):481–93.
67. Miura F, Takada T, Amano H, et al. Diagnosis of pancreatic cancer. HPB (Oxford) 2006;8(5):337–42.
68. Conrad C, Fernandez-Del Castillo C. Preoperative evaluation and management of the pancreatic head mass. J Surg Oncol 2013;107(1):23–32.
69. Lewis RB, Lattin GE Jr, Paal E. Pancreatic endocrine tumors: radiologic-clinicopathologic correlation. Radiographics 2010;30(6):1445–64.
70. Crosara S, D'Onofrio M, De Robertis R, et al. Autoimmune pancreatitis: multimodality non-invasive imaging diagnosis. World J Gastroenterol 2014;20(45):16881–90.
71. Merkle EM, Bender GN, Brambs HJ. Imaging findings in pancreatic lymphoma: differential aspects. AJR Am J Roentgenol 2000;174(3):671–5.
72. Brennan DD, Zamboni GA, Raptopoulos VD, et al. Comprehensive preoperative assessment of pancreatic adenocarcinoma with 64-section volumetric CT. Radiographics 2007;27(6):1653–66.
73. Zamboni GA, Kruskal JB, Vollmer CM, et al. Pancreatic adenocarcinoma: value of multidetector CT angiography in preoperative evaluation. Radiology 2007;245(3):770–8.
74. Sahani DV, Bonaffini PA, Catalano OA, et al. State-of-the-art PET/CT of the pancreas: current role and emerging indications. Radiographics 2012;32(4):1133–58 [discussion: 1158–60].

75. Tatli S, Mortele KJ, Levy AD, et al. CT and MRI features of pure acinar cell carcinoma of the pancreas in adults. AJR Am J Roentgenol 2005;184(2):511–9.

76. Rai S, Prabhu S, Rai S, et al. Image findings of solid pseudopapillary neoplasms of the pancreas on multiphasic multidetector CT scan-a single institute experience from Southern India. J Clin Diagn Res 2017;11(9):TC01–5.

77. Maccioni F, Martinelli M, Al Ansari N, et al. Magnetic resonance cholangiography: past, present and future: a review. Eur Rev Med Pharmacol Sci 2010; 14(8):721–5.

78. Raman SP, Horton KM, Fishman EK. Multimodality imaging of pancreatic cancer-computed tomography, magnetic resonance imaging, and positron emission tomography. Cancer J 2012;18(6):511–22.

79. Sandrasegaran K, Lin C, Akisik FM, et al. State-of-the-art pancreatic MRI. AJR Am J Roentgenol 2010;195(1):42–53.

80. Sandrasegaran K, Nutakki K, Tahir B, et al. Use of diffusion-weighted MRI to differentiate chronic pancreatitis from pancreatic cancer. AJR Am J Roentgenol 2013;201(5):1002–8.

81. Tamm EP, Bhosale PR, Vikram R, et al. Imaging of pancreatic ductal adenocarcinoma: State of the art. World J Radiol 2013;5(3):98–105.

82. Carbognin G, Girardi V, Biasiutti C, et al. Autoimmune pancreatitis: imaging findings on contrast-enhanced MR, MRCP and dynamic secretin-enhanced MRCP. Radiol Med 2009;114(8):1214–31.

83. Dibble EH, Karantanis D, Mercier G, et al. PET/CT of cancer patients: part 1, pancreatic neoplasms. AJR Am J Roentgenol 2012;199(5):952–67.

84. Yeh R, Dercle L, Garg I, et al. The role of 18F-FDG PET/CT and PET/MRI in pancreatic ductal adenocarcinoma. Abdom Radiol (N Y) 2018;43(2):415–34.

85. Sadowski SM, Neychev V, Millo C, et al. Prospective study of 68Ga-DOTATATE positron emission tomography/computed tomography for detecting gastro-entero-pancreatic neuroendocrine tumors and unknown primary sites. J Clin Oncol 2016;34(6):588–96.

86. Ludvigsen E, Stridsberg M, Janson ET, et al. Expression of somatostatin receptor subtypes 1-5 in pancreatic islets of normoglycaemic and diabetic NOD mice. Eur J Endocrinol 2005;153(3):445–54.

87. Hanada K, Minami T, Shimizu A, et al. Roles of ERCP in the early diagnosis of pancreatic cancer. Diagnostics (Basel) 2019;9(1) [pii:E30].

88. Ohtsuka T, Tamura K, Ideno N, et al. Role of ERCP in the era of EUS-FNA for preoperative cytological confirmation of resectable pancreatic ductal adenocarcinoma. Surg Today 2014;44(10):1887–92.

89. Jinkins LJ, Parmar AD, Han Y, et al. Current trends in preoperative biliary stenting in patients with pancreatic cancer. Surgery 2013;154(2):179–89.

90. Tol JA, van Hooft JE, Timmer R, et al. Metal or plastic stents for preoperative biliary drainage in resectable pancreatic cancer. Gut 2016;65(12):1981–7.

91. Scheufele F, Schorn S, Demir IE, et al. Preoperative biliary stenting versus operation first in jaundiced patients due to malignant lesions in the pancreatic head: a meta-analysis of current literature. Surgery 2017;161(4):939–50.

92. Tamburrino D, Riviere D, Yaghoobi M, et al. Diagnostic accuracy of different imaging modalities following computed tomography (CT) scanning for assessing the resectability with curative intent in pancreatic and periampullary cancer. Cochrane Database Syst Rev 2016;(9):CD011515.

93. Luz LP, Al-Haddad MA, Sey MS, et al. Applications of endoscopic ultrasound in pancreatic cancer. World J Gastroenterol 2014;20(24):7808–18.

94. Eloubeidi MA, Chen VK, Eltoum IA, et al. Endoscopic ultrasound-guided fine needle aspiration biopsy of patients with suspected pancreatic cancer: diagnostic accuracy and acute and 30-day complications. Am J Gastroenterol 2003;98(12):2663–8.

95. Eloubeidi MA, Jhala D, Chhieng DC, et al. Yield of endoscopic ultrasound-guided fine-needle aspiration biopsy in patients with suspected pancreatic carcinoma. Cancer 2003;99(5):285–92.

96. Chak A. What is the evidence for EUS-guided celiac plexus block/neurolysis? Gastrointest Endosc 2009;69(2 Suppl):S172–3.

97. Pugalenthi A, Protic M, Gonen M, et al. Postoperative complications and overall survival after pancreaticoduodenectomy for pancreatic ductal adenocarcinoma. J Surg Oncol 2016;113(2):188–93.

98. Fong Y, Gonen M, Rubin D, et al. Long-term survival is superior after resection for cancer in high-volume centers. Ann Surg 2005;242(4):540–4 [discussion: 544–7].

99. Swan RZ, Niemeyer DJ, Seshadri RM, et al. The impact of regionalization of pancreaticoduodenectomy for pancreatic cancer in North Carolina since 2004. Am Surg 2014;80(6):561–6.

100. Murphy MM, Simons JP, Ng SC, et al. Racial differences in cancer specialist consultation, treatment, and outcomes for locoregional pancreatic adenocarcinoma. Ann Surg Oncol 2009;16(11):2968–77.

101. Stitzenberg KB, Sigurdson ER, Egleston BL, et al. Centralization of cancer surgery: implications for patient access to optimal care. J Clin Oncol 2009;27(28):4671–8.

102. Fogel EL, Shahda S, Sandrasegaran K, et al. A multidisciplinary approach to pancreas cancer in 2016: a review. Am J Gastroenterol 2017;112(4):537–54.

Pancreas Cystic Lesions

Houssam Osman, MD[a,b], Dhiresh Rohan Jeyarajah, MD[a],*

KEYWORDS

- Pancreatic cysts • Cystic neoplasm • Pancreas

KEY POINTS

- The majority of pancreatic cystic neoplasms are discovered incidentally.
- Mucinous cystic neoplasms (MCN) are predominantly found in female. In general, all MCN need be evaluated for surgical resection.
- MD-IPMN carries the highest risk of malignant transformation among pancreatic cystic neoplasm. All MD-IPMN should be considered for surgical resection.
- SB-IPMN carries significantly less chance of malignant transformation. Observation should be considered especially in smaller, asymptomatic lesions, and with no worrisome features.
- The diagnosis of pancreatic cystic neoplasm should be considered when a mature cyst is seen early in the course of 1st pancreatitis attack.

CYSTIC NEOPLASMS

With the ease of cross-sectional imaging, cystic lesions of the pancreas have become more commonly identified. Therefore, it is highly likely that every general surgeon will be asked for an opinion regarding a patient with a cyst in their pancreas. It is important that the general surgeon has a working knowledge of the types of cystic lesions of the pancreas and, more important, when these need to be observed and when they need to be resected. The purpose of this article is to outline the basic pathway of management of cystic lesions of the pancreas.

SEROUS CYSTIC LESIONS

Serous cystic lesions of the pancreas are benign lesions and can be observed safely. Apart from one report from Hopkins,[1] where a few patients with serous lesions presented with metastatic lesions to the liver, there have been no reports of malignant potential in these tumors. Therefore, it is imperative that the diagnosis is made accurately.

[a] Department of Surgery, Methodist Richardson Medical Center, 2805 East President George Bush Highway, Richardson, TX 75082, USA; [b] Trinity Surgical Consultants, 2805 East President George Bush Highway, Richardson, TX 75082, USA
* Corresponding author. 2805 East President George Bush Highway, Richardson, TX 75082.
E-mail address: rohanjeyarajah@gmail.com

Surg Clin N Am 100 (2020) 581–588
https://doi.org/10.1016/j.suc.2020.02.006
0039-6109/20/© 2020 Elsevier Inc. All rights reserved.
surgical.theclinics.com

Serous lesions have the appearance of tiny cystic structures best seen on T2-weighted MRI imaging. These spaces are filled with thin fluid that does not contain any mucin. Imaging alone is sufficient for the diagnosis, as long as it is clearly the case. The authors are proponents of liberal use of endoscopic ultrasound (EUS) examination in cases where MRI imaging is not clear cut. In the case of EUS, the endosonographer can make a diagnosis by the EUS characteristics of the lesions; in fact, a fine needle aspiration (FNA) biopsy is rarely needed in these cases. If fluid is aspirated, the amylase and carcinoembryonic antigen (CEA) will be low, this will show that the lesion is not mucinous (low CEA <192 ng/mL)[2] and has no connection to the pancreatic duct (low amylase).

In some cases, serous lesions can cause symptoms related to mass effect. This effect can be from obstruction of the main pancreatic duct leading to pain and pancreatitis. Alternatively, large lesions can cause a local mass effect on the stomach or duodenum, resulting in symptoms of gastric outlet obstruction and pain. In these cases, surgical resection can be warranted for symptom control. As with any surgery that is performed for symptoms, it is important that the surgeon and the patient have a clear understanding regarding the expectations for the surgery. With the routine use of minimally invasive techniques, surgical resection of the left pancreas can be a relatively straightforward procedure. However, just because an minimally invasive surgical technique can be used should not alter the indications for surgery: Serous lesions do not need to be resected unless they are clearly symptomatic.

If resection is warranted, a spleen preserving approach can be considered for left-sided lesions. The authors are not advocates of spleen preservation; however, patients with serous lesions requiring resections can be candidates for spleen preservation.

Enucleation of serous lesions has been described.[3] However, the authors favor standard resection for those rare patients who require resection.

The pathology of serous lesions shows bland strands of tissue with clear fluid in between these septae.

MUCINOUS CYSTIC NEOPLASM

Mucinous cystic neoplasms (MCNs) are lesions that have a female predominance and affect patients in their middle age.[4] The main pathologic finding in resected MCN is a dense ovarian stroma, making it interesting that this is almost an exclusively female disease. MCNs tend to occur in the center of the pancreas and do not result in main pancreatic ductal dilation, a surprising finding considering that these lesions can be somewhat large. They tend to be located in the center of the gland and are

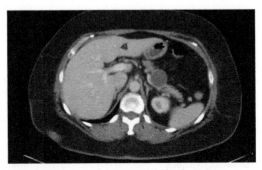

Fig. 1. Contrast-enhanced CT image of a pancreatic body MCN.

not excentric in location, like side branch intraductal papillary mucinous neoplasms (SB-IPMN) (described elsewhere in this article). This finding makes MCN recognizable to the trained eye.

With a good MRI, the main differential diagnosis for MCN is an IPMN. It is important to make this distinction, because all MCNs should be resected whereas there is room for observation in specific cases of side branch IPMN (described elsewhere in this article). The finding of a centrally located cystic lesion without main pancreatic duct dilation in a middle-aged woman should raise the question of MCN (**Fig. 1**).

Based on the Fukuoka guidelines,[5] all MCN should be resected owing to their risk for malignancy. Therefore, making an accurate diagnosis is critical. The authors use EUS examination in these patients to help make the diagnosis of MCN. The endosonographer will see that there is a cystic lesion that is not connected to the pancreatic duct. FNA will show mucinous epithelium. Sampling of fluid will show an elevated CEA (>192 ng/mL)[2] and a low amylase level, demonstrating that this is a mucinous lesion (elevated CEA) that does not communicate with the pancreatic duct. This combination of fluid studies is not 100% accurate but is a good framework to use in working up patients with cystic lesions.

Once there is suspicion for an MCN, surgery is recommended. Anatomic surgical resection is the preferred approach—a left-sided pancreatectomy or Whipple procedure. In select cases, a central pancreatectomy can be performed. The authors are reticent to perform this surgery because there are 2 places for potential pancreatic leak: the proximal transection and the anastomosis to the distal pancreas. All of these surgeries can be performed using a minimally invasive surgical technique. In fact, patients with MCN are excellent candidates for a minimally invasive pancreatectomy because they are often young and have relatively normal glands.

INTRADUCTAL PAPILLARY MUCINOUS NEOPLASM

IPMN is a relatively new entity, only being described in the late 1990s by the Japanese.[5] Before this, surgeons who saw patients with dilated pancreatic ducts assumed that the patients had alcohol-related chronic pancreatitis. In fact, many patients were accused of misrepresenting their alcohol intake and were treated as substance abusers when they had main duct IPMN (MD-IPMN).

IPMN can affect the main pancreatic duct (MD-IPMN) or the side branches (SB-IPMN). It is critical that the general surgeon be able to identify the differences between these 2 entities, because their management is very different. Missing an MD-IPMN can have serious consequences because these lesions have a high risk of malignant transformation.

Main Pancreatic Duct Intraductal Papillary Mucinous Neoplasm

MD-IPMN form when the lining of the main pancreatic duct transforms to a papillary type of epithelium that produces mucin. This transformation causes the duct to dilate and become obstructed. This process can lead to pancreatitis, the main manner in which these patients present for care. Typically, the patient with an MD-IPMN is diabetic and, if there is progression to malignancy, they have pain that is unrelenting. It is highly likely that a patient with an MD-IPMN will present to the emergency department of every general surgeon with the diagnosis of acute pancreatitis.

The finding of dilation of the main pancreatic duct without any calcifications on imaging to suggest a chronic pancreatitis history should be the main tip off to the diagnosis. If this finding is seen on presentation, the general surgeon should have a low threshold to consider MD-IPMN and begin a workup for this entity. If needed, referral to hepatic–pancreatic–biliary surgery should be initiated, because the imaging in itself can be enough to warrant intervention with major pancreatic resection.

If further verification of MD-IPMN is warranted, the use of endoscopic retrograde cholangiopancreatography, EUS examination, and pancreatoscopy can be undertaken. Endoscopic retrograde cholangiopancreatography can be helpful in that visualization of the ampulla with a side-viewing endoscope shows mucin extruding from the ampulla. The ampulla will have the classic fisheye appearance that is pathognomonic for MD-IPMN. This entity is the most common endoscopic retrograde cholangiopancreatography finding; MD-IPMN tend to occur more commonly in the head of the pancreas. EUS examination can be used to assess the extent of involvement of the main pancreatic duct. The endosonographer will see papillary projections and mucin involving the main pancreatic duct and will be able to assess where the transition occurs to normal duct. Pancreatoscopy is performed by placing a spy-scope into the dilated main pancreatic duct. This way is the best to biopsy and assess the extent of involvement with IPMN.

Together, these measures aid the surgeon in assessing or the extent of resection. The most common surgical intervention is the Whipple procedure. Assessing for associated malignancy and extent of involvement of the main pancreatic duct is a topic of much debate. It is the authors' practice to perform as limited a resection as possible and only chase the transected pancreatic neck margin if there is invasive cancer. The use of total pancreatectomy is avoided at all costs. The authors only consider total pancreatectomy in those patients who are already brittle diabetic and in pain.

An important point is that all patients with MD-IPMN should be considered for surgical intervention.

Side Branch Intraductal Papillary Mucinous Neoplasm

SB-IPMN occurs owing to transformation of the lining of the side branch ducts off the main pancreatic duct. This transformation leads to mucin production and dilation of these side branches. This phenomenon is seen on cross-sectional imaging as a classic cluster of grapes hanging off a branch. The imaging characteristics alone are enough to make the diagnosis if viewed by experienced eyes. SB-IPMN tend to eccentrically located cystic lesions, as opposed to MCN that is more centrally located. SB-IPMN are most commonly identified on an imaging study that is obtained for other reasons, for example in a patient with prostate cancer who is undergoing surveillance imaging.

Most asymptomatic SB-IPMN can be observed and not resected. This statement is bold, but is important to understand. In fact, the Fukuoko guidelines really leave room for observation in this entity. The older guidelines focused on size, but the more updated guidelines look at other factors in deciding whether to resect SB-IPMN.

It is important to know that if the SB-IPMN causes clear symptoms, usually unexplained acute pancreatitis, resection should be strongly considered. It is only in those patients who are asymptomatic that observation can be entertained. To consider observation, the cystic lesions must:

i. Not be associated with main pancreatic ductal dilation (6–8 mm being worrisome and >8 mm being considered high risk)
ii. Have no enhancing solid nodules
iii. No symptoms, including bile duct dilation

Consideration for surgery can be made if the lesion is larger than 3 cm and the patient does not want close observation. Lesions that do not have any of these features can be observed.

The authors use EUS examination liberally in these patients, especially to clinch the diagnosis of SB-IPMN and to ensure that there are no solid areas by EUS criteria. As noted elsewhere in this article, FNA will yield mucinous cells, which in itself is not cause for alarm. If there is associated dysplasia or malignancy, the lesion should be resected. The fluid analysis will reveal a high CEA (>192 ng/mL) and a high amylase, demonstrating communication with the pancreatic duct. The use of cytology to assess for dysplasia or cancer and the use of EUS imaging to look for solid areas is helping in the decision process of who can be followed and who needs resection.

If the patient has an SB-IPMN that does meet any of the worrisome features mentioned, serial imaging with magnetic resonance cholangiopancreatography and contrast-enhanced abdominal MRI is used to follow the patient. There is much debate about frequency of imaging. It is the authors' practice to obtain imaging at 6 months after presentation. As long as the patient does not show any high-risk features, imaging is then obtained in 1 year. The issue of what to do with a perfectly asymptomatic lesion that is growing and has reached a of size greater than 3 cm is a difficult topic. In general, the authors present observation versus resection to the patient. In these cases, the left-sided lesions present an easier pathway, because distal pancreatectomy is so much better tolerated and of lower morbidity and mortality than pancreaticoduodenectomy. In those with pancreatic head lesions, the authors have to be convinced that the morbidity and mortality of the surgery is less than that of the disease itself. This decision is tough and the authors are very conservative in patients with asymptomatic SB-IPMN. The presence of symptoms makes the decision much easier and the authors are very aggressive with offering resection to these patients.

PANCREATITIS-RELATED FLUID COLLECTIONS
Definition and Terminology

The 2012 revised Atlanta classification identified 2 types of pancreatitis: interstitial edematous pancreatitis and necrotizing pancreatitis.[6] The classification has also defined 4 types of pancreatic and peripancreatic fluid collection.

1. Acute peripancreatic fluid collections occur in the first 1 to 3 weeks of interstitial acute pancreatitis. They are characterized by the lack of well-defined wall.
2. Pancreatic pseudocysts are matured acute peripancreatic fluid collections beyond 4 weeks. They are characterized by the presence of s well-defined wall.
3. Acute necrotic collections happen during the first few weeks of necrotizing pancreatitis and contain variable amount of fluid and necrotic materials
4. Walled-off pancreatic collections (WOPN) occur when acute necrotic collection persists beyond 4 weeks. They are encapsulated fluid and necrotic materials

As we can see form this definition, true pancreatic pseudocysts are actually rare and most symptomatic pancreatic collections beyond 4 weeks are WOPN.

Clinical Presentation and Diagnosis

The diagnosis of acute pancreatitis requires the presence of 2 out of 3 criteria, namely, classic acute upper abdominal pain radiating to the back, amylase or lipase serum levels of greater than 3 times the upper limit, and a computed tomography (CT) scan consistent with acute pancreatitis.[6] A CT scan is not usually needed on presentation unless the diagnosis is questionable or to rule out other pathology.

There are 2 phases identified in the course of acute pancreatitis.

1. Phase 1 takes place in the first 1 to 4 weeks. The pathophysiology in this stage is related to cytokines release and true infection is rare. Most pancreatitis resolve spontaneously in this phase.
2. Phase 2 occurs after 4 weeks, in which local complication and infection take place. More than 90% pf pancreatitis attacks are mild and self-limiting. A CT scan is usually required in the first phase of pancreatitis when patients present with severe pancreatitis or shows lack of improvement. The role of the CT scan at presentation is controversial and is usually used to make the diagnosis of acute pancreatitis and ensure that there is not a perforated viscous masquerading as acute pancreatitis. Contrast-enhanced CT scanning is the modality of choice to evaluate the extent of pancreatitis in the early stage of the disease. In patients with a severe contrast allergy or those with renal failure, noncontrast CT scans or MRI can be used.

The distinction between acute pancreatic collection and acute necrotic collection can be difficult in the first 24 to 48 hours of pancreatitis. After 1 week from the onset of pancreatitis, acute necrotic collections appear heterogeneous and pancreatic necrosis can be better identified on contrast-enhanced CT scans.

Pancreatic pseudocysts, which occur 4 weeks from pancreatitis, appear as well-circumscribed thin-walled peripancreatic collection on contrast-enhanced CT scans. These collection are hyperintense on T2-weighted MRI. WOPN in contrast appear as a walled-off heterogeneous collection on CT scans, and MRI usually better delineate the solid component within the collection (**Fig. 2**).

The diagnosis of a pancreatitis-related cyst should be questioned when a mature cyst is seen on imaging obtained early in the course of first episode of pancreatitis and the possibility of cystic neoplasm should be considered. In the scenario where there is a cystic lesion seen at presentation of acute pancreatitis, one must consider the possibility that the cyst is causative rather than the result of the pancreatitis. This finding would suggest an IPMN is the diagnosis causing pancreatitis attack. This diagnosis would be an indication for resection.

EUS examination is usually not needed to make the diagnosis of pancreatitis related collections. In the instance that EUS examination is used to differentiate between cystic neoplasms and pseudocyst, the cystic fluid analysis typically reveals high amylase and low CEA level in pancreatitis related collections. EUS examination has more therapeutic value when dealing with pancreatitis-related collections.

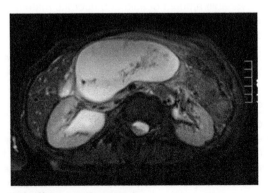

Fig. 2. MRI of a walled off pancreatic necrosis.

Management

The old dictum for intervention of pancreatitis-related fluid collections with surgery is no longer practiced.[7] The main indication for intervention are symptoms or infection. Preemptive drainage for the fear of rupture or bleeding is no longer performed.

There are generally 3 indications to intervene for pancreatic collection.

1. Infection
2. Persistent systemic inflammatory response syndrome and lack of improvement
3. Symptomatic pseudocyst and WOPN

Acute peripancreatic and necrotic collection occur in the first phase of pancreatitis and the treatment of these collection is the management of acute pancreatitis rather than addressing the local process and local intervention in the early phase should be avoided if possible.

The diagnosis of infection pancreatic collections is made when air is seen on imaging or when there is ongoing sepsis like picture. The use of FNA in making the diagnosis of infection has declined in recent years owing to the risk of secondary infection and bleeding.[8] The treatment of infected pancreatic collections in the early phase of pancreatitis is mostly percutaneous drainage and surgical intervention is generally avoided. Infected pseudocyst or WOPN can be addressed percutaneously, endoscopically, or surgically. The role of the Step Up approach has been popularized after the Dutch trial.[9] In this trial, patients with infected necrosis were treated with percutaneous drainage that was upsized aggressively to achieve adequate drainage of fluid collections. In the circumstance that this goal could not be achieved with a percutaneous approach, surgical minimally invasive debridement was used. This has been our approach in our patients with infected pancreatic fluid collections and we have been able to avoid surgery in most of these patients.

Symptomatic mature pseudocyst or WOPN are generally treated with endoscopic or surgical drainage procedures. The theory here is that the distal pancreas drains into the fluid collection via a disconnected duct; this fluid then drain into the viscous that is anastomosed to the cyst. In a certain percentage of patients, the distal gland duct stenosis or is inadequately drained. This circumstance results in repeated bouts of acute pancreatitis and pain that will need interval distal pancreatic resection. Surgical resection should be considered if the diagnosis of pancreatitis-related collection is uncertain and a cystic neoplastic lesion is a possibility.

DISCLOSURE

No conflicts of interest; no disclaimers.

REFERENCES

1. Cameron JL, Riall TS, Coleman J, et al. One thousand consecutive pancreaticoduodenectomies. Ann Surg 2006;244(1):10–5.

2. Linder JD, Geenen JE, Catalano MF. Cyst fluid analysis obtained by EUS-guided FNA in the evaluation of discrete cystic neoplasms of the pancreas: a prospective single-center experience. Gastrointest Endosc 2006;64(5):697–702.

3. Madura JA, Yum MN, Lehman GA, et al. Mucin secreting cystic lesions of the pancreas: treatment by enucleation. Am Surg 2004;70(2):106–12 [discussion: 113].

4. Scourtas A, Dudley JC, Brugge WR, et al. Preoperative characteristics and cyto-logical features of 136 histologically confirmed pancreatic mucinous cystic neo-plasms. Cancer Cytopathol 2017;125(3):169–77.
5. Kaimakliotis P, Riff B, Pourmand K, et al. Sendai and Fukuoka consensus guide-lines identify advanced neoplasia in patients with suspected mucinous cystic neo-plasms of the pancreas. Clin Gastroenterol Hepatol 2015;13(10):1808–15.
6. Bradley EL. A clinically based classification system for acute pancreatitis. Sum-mary of the International Symposium on Acute Pancreatitis, Atlanta, Ga, September 11 through 13, 1992. Arch Surg 1993;128(5):586–90. Available at: http://www.ncbi.nlm.nih.gov/pubmed/8489394. Accessed May 11, 2014.
7. Jeyarajah DR, Osman HG, Patel S. Advances in management of pancreatic necro-sis. Curr Probl Surg 2014;51(9):374–408.
8. Sarr MG, Banks PA, Bollen TL, et al. The new revised classification of acute pancreatitis 2012. Surg Clin North Am 2013;93(3):549–62.

FURTHER READING

Horvath K, Freeny P, Escallon J, et al. Safety and efficacy of video-assisted retroper-itoneal debridement for infected pancreatic collections: a multicenter, prospective, single-arm phase 2 study. Arch Surg 2010;145(9):817–25.
Fong Z, Ferrone CR, Lillemoe KD, et al. Intraductal papillary mucinous neoplasm of the pancreas: current state of the art and ongoing controversies. Ann Surg 2016; 263(5):908–17.
Pergolini I, Sahora K, Ferrone CR, et al. Long-term risk of pancreatic malignancy in patients with branch duct intraductal papillary mucinous neoplasm in a referral cen-ter. Gastroenterology 2017;153(5):1284–94.e1.
Mukewar S, de Pretis N, Aryal-Khanal A, et al. Fukuoka criteria accurately predict risk for adverse outcomes during follow-up of pancreatic cysts presumed to be intra-ductal papillary mucinous neoplasms. Gut 2017;66(10):1811–7.
Tamura K, Ohtsuka T, Ideno N, et al. Treatment strategy for main duct intraductal papillary mucinous neoplasms of the pancreas based on the assessment of recur-rence in the remnant pancreas after resection: a retrospective review. Ann Surg 2014;259(2):360–8.
Zaheer A, Singh VK, Qureshi RO, et al. The revised Atlanta classification for acute pancreatitis: updates in imaging terminology and guidelines. Abdom Imaging 2013;38(1):125–36.
Sheu Y, Furlan A, Almusa O, et al. The revised Atlanta classification for acute pancre-atitis: a CT imaging guide for radiologists. Emerg Radiol 2012;19(3):237–43.
Pelaez-Luna M, Vege SS, Petersen BT, et al. Disconnected pancreatic duct syndrome in severe acute pancreatitis: clinical and imaging characteristics and outcomes in a cohort of 31 cases. Gastrointest Endosc 2008;68:91–7.
Albashir S, Stevens T. Endoscopic ultrasonography to evaluate pancreatitis. Cleve Clin J Med 2012;79:202–6.

Peritoneal Cancers and Hyperthermic Intraperitoneal Chemotherapy

Eric Pletcher, MD, MS[a], Elizabeth Gleeson, MD, MPH[b],
Daniel Labow, MD[c],*

KEYWORDS

- Peritoneal metastasis • Hyperthermic intraperitoneal chemotherapy
- Cytoreductive surgery • Colorectal • Peritoneal mesothelioma
- Pseudomyxoma peritonei • Ovarian cancer • Peritoneal carcinoma index

KEY POINTS

- Peritoneal carcinomatosis can be primary disease due to peritoneal mesothelioma, peritoneal carcinoma, or desmoplastic small round cell tumor, or secondary disease as a site of metastasis such as colorectal, appendiceal, ovarian, or pseudomyxoma peritonei.
- Treatment of local regional disease with cytoreductive surgery and hyperthermic intraperitoneal chemotherapy can increase overall survival and is predicated on patient selection, peritoneal cancer index, and completeness of cytoreduction score.
- Patients may present with synchronous or metachronous peritoneal metastasis with no symptoms or vague abdominal pain, decreased appetite, and increased abdominal girth secondary to disease progression in the abdomen and pelvis.
- Workup begins with a computed tomography (CT) of the chest, abdomen, and pelvis to quantify peritoneal carcinoma index or identify extra-abdominal disease, but can be supplemented with MRI, PET-CT, or diagnostic laparoscopy.

INTRODUCTION: PERITONEAL MALIGNANCIES: MESOTHELIOMA, APPENDICEAL, COLORECTAL, PSEUDOMYXOMA PERITONEI, AND OVARIAN CANCER

Peritoneal carcinomatosis refers to the metastatic spread of cancer to the peritoneal lining of the abdomen. Primary tumors can originate both inside and, more rarely, outside the abdomen, and disseminate to the peritoneal surface via lymphatics, blood, peritoneal cavity, or direct invasion. The origin of peritoneal carcinomatosis can be

[a] Surgery Department, Mount Sinai West and Morningside, 425 West 59th Street, 7th Floor, New York, NY 10019, USA; [b] Division of Surgical Oncology, Mount Sinai Hospital, 19 East 98th Street, Suite 7A, New York, NY 10029, USA; [c] Surgery Department, Mount Sinai Hospital, Mount Sinai West and Morningside, 425 West 59th Street, 7th Floor, New York, NY 10019, USA
* Corresponding author.
E-mail address: daniel.labow@mountsinai.org

Surg Clin N Am 100 (2020) 589–613
https://doi.org/10.1016/j.suc.2020.02.009
0039-6109/20/© 2020 Elsevier Inc. All rights reserved.
surgical.theclinics.com

primary, derived from the peritoneal lining itself, such as in primary peritoneal meso-thelioma, primary peritoneal carcinoma, or desmoplastic small round cell tumor. It also can be due to a secondary cause, from another primary organ, such as carcinoma of the gastrointestinal or Müllerian tracts, resulting in locoregional disease. Peritoneal carcinomatosis previously represented terminal disease; however, today each primary cancer is considered as its own unique disease process, and treated accordingly.

Peritoneal carcinomatosis was first described in 1908 by Miller and Wynn[1] in a 32-year-old man with peritoneal mesothelioma who was found to have endothelioma with diffuse deposits and mucinous ascites that were not resected. In 1980, Dr Robert Fernandez and Dr John Daly[2] published a case series from MD Anderson that described various treatment regimens, including surgical resection and adjuvant chemoradio-therapy with fluorouracil or melphalan. This approach was supported by Antman and colleagues[3] in 1983, who reiterated mesothelioma as its own disease process and argued for operative resection, abdominal radiation, and adjuvant chemotherapy. The modern-day approach of cytoreductive surgery (CRS) and intraperitoneal chemo-therapy bloomed from Dedrick[4] in 1985 and was followed up by Sugarbaker[5] in 1995, demonstrating the efficacy of peritoneal stripping on long-term survival and curative intent of the procedure. In this article, primary peritoneal mesothelioma and colorectal, appendiceal, ovarian, and pseudomyxoma peritonei are discussed in detail.

As mentioned before, primary peritoneal malignancies include peritoneal mesothe-lioma, primary peritoneal carcinoma, and desmoplastic small round cell tumors, which develop from the serosal lining of the peritoneal cavity. Peritoneal spread represents the second most common site for mesothelioma following the pleura, making up 7% to 18% of reported cases with an incidence of 1 case per 100,000 people.[6,7] In the United States, men have a greater propensity for the development of mesothelioma, which may be secondary to work-related exposure to asbestos, the most well-known cause.[8] Currently, there is no American Joint Committee on Cancer (AJCC) tumor-node-metastasis (TNM) staging system for malignant peritoneal mesothelioma. The disease process usually involves diffusely distributed tumor nodules and associ-ated ascites, resulting in mass effect on intra-abdominal organs. Alexander and col-leagues[9] demonstrated increased median overall survival of 38.4 months following complete or near-complete resection and heated intraperitoneal chemotherapy treat-ment with cisplatin, versus 6 months median survival with systemic chemotherapy alone.[10]

Pseudomyxoma peritonei, like peritoneal mesothelioma, develops peritoneal im-plants and ascites, but in contrast, is typically secondary to a perforated mucinous appendiceal tumor. It can include both the omental caking and ovarian involvement.[11] In addition to the appendix as the primary source, the colon, ovaries, pancreas, and urachus can all provide the mucinous primary tumor, which can lead to peritoneal dissemination. This tends to collect within the pelvis, paracolic gutters, omentum, and liver capsule. Based on the results of the Peritoneal Surface Oncology Group In-ternational Modified Delphi Process, language classifying noncarcinoid epithelial neo-plasms based on architecture and cytology differentiated the primary tumors responsible for pseudomyxoma peritonei into 6 categories. Low-grade appendiceal mucinous neoplasm has low-grade cytology and no invasive architectural features, whereas high-grade appendiceal mucinous neoplasm has similar architecture and high-grade cytology. The remaining 4 categories have invasive architecture, but differ in the presence and abundance of signet ring cells with mucinous adenocarcinoma: poorly differentiated mucinous adenocarcinoma with signet ring cells (less than 50%), mucinous signet ring cell carcinoma (more than 50%), and adenocarcinoma (nonmucinous and no signet ring). Chua and colleagues[12] reported a multi-institutional study on Pseudomyxoma peritonei secondary to appendiceal neoplasm, and found a median overall survival of 16.3 years following CRS and intraperitoneal chemotherapy, depending on the completeness of resection.

Traditionally, resection of colonic primary with limited metastatic disease has been attempted with curative intent, and is the standard of care. This practice has been applied to the locoregional metastatic spread of appendiceal and colorectal adenocarcinoma associated with peritoneal carcinomatosis, although mixed evidence exists regarding the benefits of CRS and hyperthermic intraperitoneal chemotherapy (HIPEC). Elias and colleagues[13] demonstrated, in a retrospective cohort study, a 30% 5-year survival rate with 3% postoperative mortality and 23% morbidity. Two randomized trials have demonstrated that cytoreduction and HIPEC increased overall survival when compared with systemic chemotherapy alone.[14,15] This contrasts the preliminary results of the PRODIGE 7 trial, which found no difference in median overall survival, 5-year survival, or relapse-free survival for patients undergoing HIPEC and CRS.[16]

Approximately 87% of patients with ovarian cancer present with stage III disease secondary to metastasis outside the pelvis per AJCC and FIGO (International Federation of Gynecology and Obstetrics) staging guidelines.[17] In contrast to patients with peritoneal metastasis secondary to gastrointestinal malignancy, the treatment algorithm per National Comprehensive Cancer Network (NCCN) guidelines involves platinum-based systemic chemotherapy and evaluation for possible CRS depending on response. The major ovarian neoplasm subtypes include malignant germ cell cancer, sex-cord stromal cell tumors, and epithelial ovarian cancer, with the latter representing 90% of cases, and being the fifth most common cause of cancer mortality in women. A Phase 3 trial investigating the addition of HIPEC to CRS for ovarian cancer has been conducted and demonstrated an increase in recurrence-free survival from 11 to 14 months and median overall survival from 34 to 46 months.[18] Despite these drastic findings, practice guidelines have changed minimally with the addition of HIPEC for consideration at the time of interval debulking surgery for Stage III disease per NCCN guidelines. There are more than 40 clinical trials investigating the use of HIPEC for treatment of ovarian cancer at the time of publication.

RELEVANT ANATOMY/PATHOPHYSIOLOGY

The peritoneal cavity is contained by the peritoneum, a serous layer of simple squamous epithelium that lines the visceral and parietal surfaces covering approximately 1 to 2 m^2 of surface area.[19,20] It is bordered posteriorly by the retroperitoneum covering the anterior portions of the duodenum, left and right colon, pancreas, kidneys, and adrenal glands. Peritoneal fluid serves as lubrication between the organ spaces freely flowing throughout the 9 interconnected subdivisions within the peritoneal cavity. This free flow of fluid can subsequently provide transport for peritoneal metastasis passing by or attaching to the following ligaments or mesentery: coronary, gastrohepatic, hepatoduodenal, falciform, gastrocolic, duodenocolic, gastrosplenic, splenorenal, and phrenicocolic ligaments; transverse mesocolon; and small bowel mesentery. This is dependent on the movement of the diaphragm. It also can continue into 1 or more of the subdivisions into the left or right subphrenic spaces, which communicate with the left and right paracolic gutters, respectively, the supramesenteric or inframesenteric space divided by the transverse mesocolon, subhepatic space, pelvis, or lesser space via the Foramen of Winslow. Gravity-dependent regions also exist and include the paracolic gutters and pelvis.

The semipermeable nature of the peritoneum is responsible for passage of some cell types, molecules, and fluid, as well as production of peritoneal fluid.

The blood supply to the peritoneum is divided between the splanchnic vessels for the visceral peritoneum and the iliac, lumbar, and intercostal vessels for the parietal peritoneum. The arterial and venous supply are paralleled by a rich lymphatic network, providing means for lymphatic or hematogenous spread of cancer to the peritoneum.[21]

As stated previously, there are 2 categories of peritoneal cancer: tumors that have spread from other organs and tumors that originate from the peritoneal lining. Any cancer can spread to the peritoneum in the advanced stage; however, the most common cancers to spread to the peritoneum originate from organs that reside in the peritoneum. These include but are not limited to gastric, colorectal, appendiceal, and ovarian cancer. Some tumors that originate from the peritoneal lining include peritoneal mesothelioma, primary peritoneal carcinoma, and desmoplastic small round cell tumors.

For tumors originating in the peritoneal cavity, spread takes place via cancer cells shed from T4 tumors where tumors invade beyond the serosal layer.[22] Malignant cells are also thought to seed the abdominal cavity after malignant perforation, such as a perforating colon cancer. Another proposed mechanism of spread includes surgical contamination of the peritoneal cavity, when tumors are incompletely excised with positive margins, spread at port sites during the removal of surgical cancer specimen, or rupture of the specimen during handling. The peritoneal lining is well vascularized with cytokines and growth factors, and serves as an ideal place for seeding of tumor cells.[23]

CLINICAL PRESENTATION

Patients may have synchronous and metachronous presentation of peritoneal carcinomatosis. In a study following the natural history of patients with nongynecologic peritoneal carcinomatosis, 57% of the patients had synchronous peritoneal carcinomatosis in which ascites (34%) and bowel obstruction (19%) were the main symptoms.[24] With low cancer burden, patients may present with no symptoms at all. With synchronous presentation, patients may present with symptoms of the primary tumor. Further staging may lead to identification for peritoneal metastases. If not seen on imaging, peritoneal disease is often diagnosed at the time of surgery. Retrospectively, patients may report that they have noticed weight gain (particularly if they have mucinous ascites secondary to pseudomyxoma peritonei or ovarian cancer), weight loss, vague abdominal pain, or ascites. In advanced cases and high tumor burden, patients may present with symptoms of bowel obstruction. These patients often have a history of one of the known cancers that spread to the peritoneum, such as colorectal, appendiceal, or ovarian cancer. This is often the case for metachronous presentation, although these patients are usually enrolled in a surveillance program with the oncology team.

Most patients presenting with ovarian cancer have metastatic disease to their peritoneum and are Stage III. Tumor burden associated with disease progression leads to compressive forces within the pelvis, peritoneum, and retroperitoneum causing urinary, abdominal, and back discomfort. **Table 1** lists percentages of patients presenting with the respective symptoms. In contrast to ovarian cancer, only 7% of patients presenting with a new diagnosis will have synchronous metastasis to the peritoneum. Patients with peritoneal metastasis from a colorectal primary, if symptomatic, originally present with constitutional symptoms, including cachexia and fatigue, in addition to abdominal discomfort.[25]

As mentioned before, most pseudomyxoma peritonei are secondary to a mucinous tumor originating from the appendix. A mucocele at the base appendicitis can result in

Table 1	
Symptoms associated with presentation of ovarian cancer	
Abdominal bloating, fullness or increased girth	27%–71%
Pain (low back, abdominal)	22%–58%
Urinary symptoms	16%–34%
Constitutional symptoms (fatigue)	34%–50%

Data from Goff BA, Mandel LS, Melancon CH, et al. Frequency of symptoms of ovarian cancer in women presenting to primary care clinics. JAMA. 2004;291(22):2705; and Olson SH, Mignone L, Nakraseive C, et al. Symptoms of ovarian cancer.Obstet Gynecol. 2001;98(2):212.

a presentation consistent with acute appendicitis, which is present in up to 27% of cases. This is discussed in further detail in the "Diagnostic procedures" section. In women specifically, an ovarian neoplasm also can be the source of mucin, and ovarian mass represents 39% of the cases for female presentation. Increasing abdominal girth (23% of patients) followed by new onset of a hernia (14% of women) are 2 other common presentations in both men and women.[26]

Thirty percent to 50% of patients presenting with peritoneal mesothelioma report abdominal pain and distension, which can vary in its onset depending on subtype.[27,28] Decreased appetite and subsequent weight loss and hernia development are both byproducts of the increased abdominal pressure secondary to disease progression.[29–31]

DIAGNOSTIC PROCEDURES

Diagnostic imaging of primary and secondary peritoneal disease is paramount for management of potential CRS and HIPEC candidates and is used for the following:

- Identification of extraperitoneal disease
- Quantification of preoperative peritoneal carcinoma index (PCI)
- Localization of tumor deposits that would make the patient not a candidate for CRS
- Surveillance of possible recurrence

Computed tomography (CT), MRI, and PET-CT are all used during preoperative workup and range in their ability to localize and characterize disease. Identification of metastatic lesions can be limited by decreased tumor size, seen in miliary disease and plaquelike shape. These tumor characteristics coupled with location within the mesentery, porta hepatis, peritoneal reflection, diaphragmatic recess, and small bowel serosal make localization even more difficult.

The Peritoneal Surface Oncology Group International Consensus recommends initiating diagnostic imaging with a CT of the chest, abdomen, and pelvis, and supplementing with MRI, PET, or diagnostic laparoscopy for indeterminate findings.[32] A major role of preoperative imaging is to estimate the PCI. PCI is a measure of peritoneal disease within the abdomen and pelvis, where location and size of tumor implants are used to generate a summative value. **Fig. 1** identifies Sugarbaker's 13 regions[5] and corresponding lesion sizes used to generate PCI.

High-resolution CT requires differences in tissue density to discriminate between adjacent structures. Sheetlike deposits are often missed, as are lesions implanted in the small bowel serosal and mesentery where CT sensitivity ranges from 21% to 25%[33,34] Tumor deposits smaller than 0.5 cm are identified on CT with a sensitivity

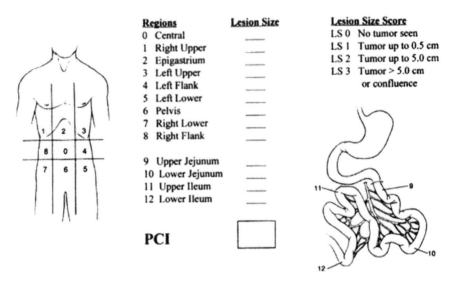

Regions	Lesion Size	Lesion Size Score
0 Central	_____	LS 0 No tumor seen
1 Right Upper	_____	LS 1 Tumor up to 0.5 cm
2 Epigastrium	_____	LS 2 Tumor up to 5.0 cm
3 Left Upper	_____	LS 3 Tumor > 5.0 cm
4 Left Flank	_____	or confluence
5 Left Lower	_____	
6 Pelvis	_____	
7 Right Lower	_____	
8 Right Flank	_____	
9 Upper Jejunum	_____	
10 Lower Jejunum	_____	
11 Upper Ileum	_____	
12 Lower Ileum	_____	

PCI

Fig. 1. Peritoneal carcinoma index (PCI). (*From* Jacquet P, Sugarbaker PH. Clinical research methodologies in diagnosis and staging of patients with peritoneal carcinomatosis. In: Sugarbaker PH, ed. Peritoneal carcinomatosis: principles of management. 1st ed. Norwell, MA: Kluwer Academic Publishers; 1996:359–74; with permission.)

ranging from 11% to 28%.[35,36] As a result, retrospective studies have found CT ultimately underestimates PCI in 33% of cases, with one-third of these cases actually having a PCI greater than 20.[37] Numerous mesenteric deposits and PCI greater than 20 are 2 intraoperative findings that can classify a patient as inoperable. Knowledge of surgical history and comparison of previous cross-sectional imaging are necessary steps. Scar from previous surgeries can be misinterpreted at disease. Listed in **Table 2** is an organ approach to identifying metastatic disease and key radiologic features to note. Despite these limitations, CT is often the imaging modality of choice for diagnosis and preoperative assessment because it is readily available and has high spatial resolution. **Table 3** depicts concerning findings seen on cross-sectional imaging associated with incomplete cytoreduction.

Oral and intravenous contrast are recommended to enhance evaluation of small bowel serosal involvement where CT is often limited.[38] CT can be supplemented with additional imaging, such as PET and MRI, to improve its sensitivity, as well as diagnostic laparoscopy. Retrospective studies comparing the accuracy of MRI and CT have demonstrated MRI as having superior 95% sensitivity for tumor sites, 70% specificity, and 88% accuracy in contrast to the site sensitivity of CT of 55%, a specificity of 86%, and accuracy of 63%.[39] When CT and MRI are combined in the preoperative setting, sensitivity increased to more than 80%.[40]

The sensitivity of PET-CT is predicated on tumor metabolism and can be predicted by tumor histology. Therefore, PET-CT provides the least value in identification of mucinous disease, which varies in its degree of cellularity. Metabolic activity of tumor deposits can corroborate suspicion for peritoneal metastasis in patients who had indeterminate MRI or CT when supplemented with PET. In addition, identification of extraperitoneal disease would preclude a patient from being a surgical candidate for HIPEC and CRS.[41]

Biopsy represents the gold standard of diagnosis and can be obtained percutaneously or via diagnostic laparoscopy. Diagnostic laparoscopy is a safe and sensitive

Table 2
Organ-specific computed tomography findings

Organ	Radiologic Finding
Diaphragm	Plaquelike thickening in the diaphragmatic/subdiaphragmatic region, nodularity, or stranding
Liver	Perihepatic nodularity or stranding
Gallbladder fossa	Nodularity or stranding, perihepatic and/or subcapsular and/or parenchyma hepatic metastatic disease
Porta hepatis/ Gastrohepatic ligament	Implants or nodes (noting size, heterogeneity, and borders)
Lesser sac	Nodularity or stranding
Pancreas	Any abnormality
Stomach	Nodular or stranding vs invasion
Spleen	Indeterminate perisplenic nodularity or stranding perisplenic and/or subcapsular and/or parenchyma splenic metastatic disease, with attention to ligament and hilum
Omentum	Deposit vs nodularity or caking
Root of SMA	Deposit vs nodularity or stranding
Small bowel mesentery	Deposit vs nodularity or stranding
Small bowel	No involvement vs indeterminate nodularity vs tumor abutting colon with no wall thickening or invasion vs tethering or angulation suggestive of mesenteric infiltration
Colon (note if above or below the peritoneal reflection)	No involvement vs indeterminate nodularity vs tumor abutting colon with no wall thickening or invasion vs diffuse or segmental wall thickening
Appendix	Implants or primary tumor
Peritoneal lining	Thickening/nodularity
Abdominal wall	Masses/nodularity
Uterus/ovaries/pelvic ligaments	Masses/nodularity
Bladder	Masses/nodularity
Peritoneal ascites	Absent vs small/moderate/large volume
Retroperitoneal lymph nodes	With respect (above or below) renal hilum, number and size of largest nodes
Lung and pleura	Pulmonary metastasis, pleural effusion, metastasis, or indeterminate nodularity/thickening
Cardiophrenic lymph nodes/ retrocrural lymph nodes	Number and size of largest nodes

Data from Bartlett DJ, Thacker PG, Sheedy SP. HIPEC and Peritoneal Carcinomatosis: Evolving Role of Imaging in Defining Treatment. SMA, superior mesenteric artery. Available at: https://cdn.ymaws.com/www.abdominalradiology.org/resource/collection/92FAB4A5-3BFE-44A1-9E66-271B8B1C744D/2018.95_Bartlett.pdf.

measure for not only obtaining tissue but also estimating PCI, and thus has become invaluable in guiding future management. Historically, diagnostic laparoscopy was not recommended secondary to feared complications associated with gaining access to a hostile abdomen, although morbidity is low (0.4%) and success rate is close to 93%.[42,43] In addition, this procedure has the advantage of providing direct

Table 3 Computed tomography findings associated with incomplete cytoreduction	
Organ/Area	**Radiologic Finding**
Small bowel/mesentery	Bowel obstruction or partial obstruction at more than 1 site, mesentery drawn together by tumor, tumor infiltrating between leaves of small bowel mesentery, tumor 5 cm in diameter in jejunal regions Peritoneal carcinoma index >20 (excluding pseudomyxoma peritonei, cystic mesothelioma, or low malignant potential ovarian tumors)
Retroperitoneum	Mesenteric or para-aortic lymphadenopathy, hydroureter, psoas muscle invasion
Pelvis	Pelvic sidewall invasion, seminal vesicle invasion
Gastrohepatic or hepatoduodenal ligaments	Porta hepatis infiltration and/or bile duct obstruction tumor 5 cm in diameter in gastrohepatic ligament or subpyloric space, gastric outlet obstruction
Ascites	Hemorrhagic ascites in any patient, serous ascites in setting of gastrointestinal malignancy

Adapted from Sugarbaker PH, Sardi A, Brown G, et al. Concerning CT features used to select patients for treatment of peritoneal metastases, a pictorial essay. Int J Hyperthermia. 2017;33(5):497-504; with permission.

visualization of the mesentery and porta hepatis, and identifying patients who are not resectable. This spares patients the morbidity associated with laparotomy and can hasten timing to adjuvant chemotherapy.[44] Finally, second-look laparoscopy, or the use of laparoscopy to identify locoregional spread following resection of primary or peritoneal disease, is being offered with the hope of identifying patients with limited peritoneal disease who would benefit most from CRS and HIPEC. This strategy has been used for high-risk primary tumors, including T4 colorectal cancers,[45] late-stage ovarian cancer, and gastric cancer.[46,47] In addition, this intervention is recommended by our institution for histologically proven peritoneal carcinomatosis of colorectal cancer and/or high-grade appendiceal origin during the first 6 to 13 months following HIPEC and CRS.

CT may illustrate an appendiceal mucocele, which is defined by the intraluminal distension with mucinous fluid. This finding can represent both neoplastic and benign processes, with the latter representing close to 20% of cases and being due to cysts and mucosal hyperplasia.[48] Any adjacent mucin identified in the peritoneum before resection likely represents pseudomyxoma peritonei secondary to a mucinous appendiceal neoplasm.

Specifically for pseudomyxoma, differentiation between tumor deposits and mucinous fluid or ascites can be a challenge using CT. Diffusion-weighted imaging added to routine MRI improves both the sensitivity and specificity for detection of these deposits. Peritoneal metastasis shows restricted diffusion on diffusion-weighted imaging, whereas ascites will show a low signal intensity. These differences improve discernibility between these 2 entities.[49]

PATIENT SELECTION

Every patient encounter begins with a thorough history and physical investigating comorbidities and functional status. Knowledge of individual risk factors associated with increased morbidity and mortality can help guide the interview process. In addition, patient selection is also dependent on certain criteria specific to the individual disease processes. Integrative care is necessary during preoperative workup, and all patients should be evaluated by a multidisciplinary board. Age older than 60 and malnutrition represented by an albumin less than 3 are both independent risk factors associated with increased morbidity.[50,51] Investigation into recent weight loss is mandatory and any symptoms consistent with a history of partial or complete small bowel obstruction could be a sign of unresectability. Overall functional status, which can be quantified with an Eastern Cooperative Oncology Group (ECOG) performance status, is also predictive of morbidity and has been associated with increased complications as patients regress from being fully active (ECOG 0) to restricted from strenuous or work activities (ECOG 1 and 2, respectively).[52]

Patients being evaluated for peritoneal carcinomatosis secondary to metasynchronous or synchronous colorectal or appendiceal adenocarcinoma should have an initial or repeat colonoscopy to assess for primary tumor or recurrence at the anastomosis. K-ras status for the previous or new pathology also should be evaluated to determine if the patient is a candidate for cetuximab. Blood work should be sent including complete blood count with differential, hepatic function panel, and carcinoembryonic antigen (CEA) to evaluate any underlying anemia, elevated bilirubin, or alkaline phosphatase, which could suggest an obstructive pattern, and CEA to establish a baseline before any type of therapy. CT of the chest, abdomen, and pelvis if not already obtained is necessary to evaluate for extra-abdominal metastasis. PCI greater than 20 is typically trialed with systemic chemotherapy before attempted CRS and HIPEC. Evidence of liver metastasis, which can be superficial or parenchymal, is not an absolute contraindication to HIPEC and CRS. Recent evidence suggests that patients with concurrent peritoneal and liver metastasis have improved survival after CRS and HIPEC with liver resection compared with systemic chemotherapy.[53–55] Number, size, and laterality of liver metastases, vascular or biliary tree invasion, and disease within the gastrohepatic ligament are all factors considered when trying to determine if resection is possible. **Fig. 2** depicts a management algorithm applied to patients with colorectal cancer. PCI greater than 20, gross invasion of the porta hepatis or root of the mesentary and unresectable liver lesions all represent contraindications to proceed with cytoreductive surgery.

For pseudomyxoma peritonei and peritoneal mesothelioma, there is no established PCI threshold in which CRS and HIPEC are contraindicated. With the exception of PCI, the selection process mirrors that of colorectal cancer. Algorithms detailing the management of low-grade mucinous neoplasms and primary peritoneal mesothelioma can been seen in **Figs. 3** and **4**, respectively.

PREOPERATIVE PLANNING/OPERATIVE TECHNIQUE
Preparation and Patient Positioning

The patient is positioned supine on the operating room table. If there is a known rectosigmoid mass and plans to perform a low anterior resection, then the patient will need to be placed in stirrups. Arms are left out, untucked.

We start by prepping the skin with ChloraPrep. In the presence of an ostomy or open wound, we use betadine. We prepare the area from the nipple line down to the mid-thigh and from table to table.

Diagnostic Laparoscopy

The procedure always begins with a diagnostic laparoscopy. We do this to estimate the extent of peritoneal disease before committing the patient to a midline laparotomy.

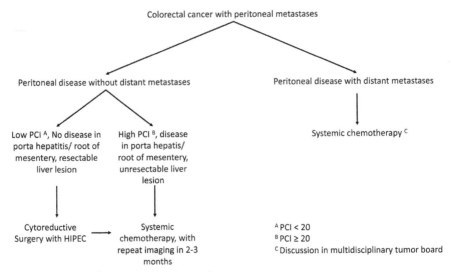

Fig. 2. Algorithm for treatment colorectal cancer.

Exploratory Laparotomy

Then, we make an incision for open HIPEC from xiphoid to pubic bone to access all quadrants of the peritoneum. Care is taken to ensure hemostasis. Once we have entered the abdomen, we begin to inspect the peritoneal cavity in a systematic fashion. The parietal peritoneum is inspected first in a clockwise fashion throughout the peritoneum. Nodules larger than a millimeter are removed. Those smaller than 1 mm can be ablated with the electrocautery. The visceral peritoneum is then inspected, examining each organ meticulously in all quadrants of the abdomen. The hilum of the liver cannot be missed. The lesser sac must be opened to see posteriorly to the stomach and at the foramen of Winslow. The omentum is resected in every case and is sent to pathology permanently. The paracolic gutters are inspected in great detail. In the pelvis, the reproductive organs should be fully examined. The pouch of Douglas must be inspected and the insertion sites of the ureters into the bladder.

Once the quadrants have been inspected, the bowel is run from the ligament of Treitz to the peritoneal reflection in the pelvis. The ligament of Treitz is often a place that can harbor a nodule. The bowel should be examined on both sides and with attention paid to the mesentery. When removing nodules from the mesentery, a leaf of mesentery is taken with the nodule to avoid injuring any vessels deep within the mesentery. The bowel is run at a minimum of 3 times. If the serosa appears compromised after resection of tumors, Lembert sutures are placed. Full-thickness tumors of the bowel are removed with bowel resection. Anastomoses are avoided until after infusion of heated chemotherapy.

Hyperthermic Intraperitoneal Chemotherapy

Once the CRS part is completed, the perfusion cannulas are placed into the peritoneum. We usually use a Y-shaped or wishbone cannula for the infusion side placing the limbs of the "Y" in each paracolic gutter. This is secured in the superior aspect of the incision. We use a lasso cannula placed over the liver for the output or drainage catheter and this is secured in the inferior aspect of the incision. These catheters are

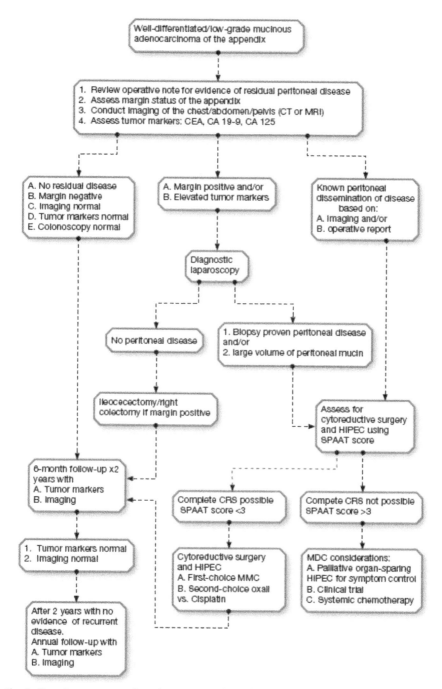

Fig. 3. Pseudomyxoma peritonei treatment algorithm. (*From* Grotz TE, Fournier KF, Mann GN. Peritoneal malignancies. MMC, mitomycin; SPAAT, simplified preoperative assessment for appendix tumor. In: Feig BW, Ching CD, eds. *The MD Anderson surgical oncology handbook*. 6th ed. Philadelphia, PA: Wolters Kluwer; 2019:281-303; with permission.)

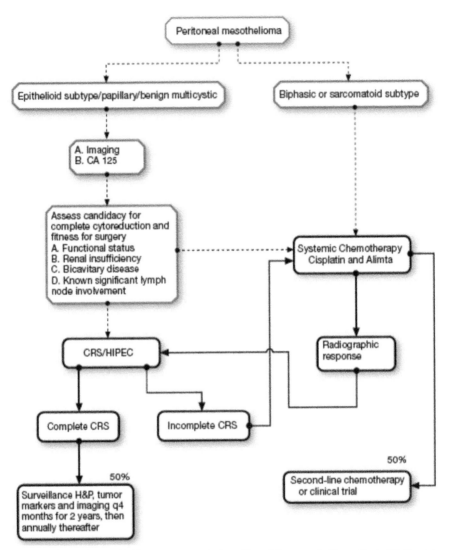

Fig. 4. Peritoneal mesothelioma treatment algorithm. Q4, every 4. (*From* Grotz TE, Fournier KF, Mann GN. Peritoneal malignancies. H&P, history and physical. In: Feig BW, Ching CD, eds. *The MD Anderson surgical oncology handbook.* 6th ed. Philadelphia, PA: Wolters Kluwer; 2019:281-303; with permission.)

secured in a water-tight fashion with a running locking 3 to 0 nylon suture. The catheters are connected to circuit tubing, which drains into a reservoir and contains the perfusate. A heat source and heat exchanger are a part of the roller pump with a suction system for circulation of perfusate. Temperature probes are connected to the inflow and outflow tubing. The peritoneum is first infused with 3 L of isotonic dialysis fluid until it reaches the goal outflow temperature of 42° Celsius. At this point, the mitomycin is instilled into the pump a dose of 17.5 mg/m², followed by 8.8 mg/m² every 30 minutes. We use mitomycin for pseudomyxoma peritonei, peritoneal mesothelioma, colorectal cancer, and appendical cancer per the regimen described by Verwaal et al.[56] The total dose was limited to 70 mg maximum per the regimen described by Verwaal et al.[56]. We have a surgeon scrubbed and monitoring the patient. For ovarian cancer, we use Cisplatnin with Sodium Thiosulfate for renal protection. Cisplatin is instilled at 100 mg/m2 with a flow rate of 1 L/minute (50% of the dose) for 30 minutes. At this time, we initiate an intravenous bolus of sodiumm thiosulphate at 9 g/m2 in 200 ml, followed by a continuous infusion of 12 g/m2 in 1000 ml for 6 hours. 25% of the cisplatin is instillations at the 30 minutes and 60 minutes time-points.[18] Occasional shaking of the peritoneal cavity can shift air bubbles out of the system. After 90 minutes, all the fluid is drained from the peritoneal cavity.

Anastomoses, Drains, Abdominal Closure

The bowel is run once more to ensure no serosal injuries are present. Anastomoses are now performed so that the bowel continuity is restored. A drain is left and the abdominal fascia and skin are closed.

PERIOPERATIVE MANAGEMENT

Recent evidence has emerged revealing the relatively low mortality and morbidity associated with HIPEC and CRS when compared with other high-risk surgical oncology procedures. This is likely secondary to improved perioperative and oncologic outcomes due to institutional experience.[13,57,58] Perioperative management represents a major challenge not only for the surgical team, but also anesthesia and intensivists. Although the intervention is meant for treatment of locoregional disease, the effects are widespread.

Thus, preoperative screening must be multifactorial, as well. Malnutrition is the most common cause of immunodeficiency in the general surgery population and is associated with decreased overall survival, infectious complications, and increased length of stay in patients undergoing HIPEC and CRS.[59,60] Because of this, preoperative and postoperative evaluation for malnutrition is necessary, and preoperative carbohydrate and protein supplementation has become incorporated into HIPEC enhanced recovery after surgery (ERAS) programs.[61,62]

Because the nature of this procedure, patients will experience numerous physiologic changes intraoperatively affecting the cardiovascular, respiratory, gastrointestinal, genitourinary, metabolic, and hematologic systems.

Hemodynamic stability is predicated on adequate fluid resuscitation. Operative time required for cytoreduction and thermal energy secondary to the HIPEC increase the capillary permeability of the peritoneum and are associated with vast fluid shifts. Patients can lose 12 mL/kg per hour intraoperatively and an estimated 4 L per day following the procedure.[63] To combat intravascular depletion, patients were historically over resuscitated, with some retrospective studies finding more than 60% of patients receiving 10 L of fluid and up to 5 units of packed red blood cells intraoperatively.[64] Implementation of a fluid-restricted or goal-directed protocols are currently being investigated and have shown to decrease complications and length of stay.[65–67] Changes to intraoperative monitoring have also been tested with the use of FloTrac/Vigileo, but no difference in the amount of fluid administered or perioperative outcomes were found following this addition.[68] Our institution favors goal-directed resuscitation perioperatively and recommends a preoperative discussion with the anesthesia team regarding threshold for transfusions, resuscitation, and blood products.

Despite measures taken to restore intravascular volume, 26% patients require vasopressors in the postoperative period, and placement of an arterial line before surgery is recommended.[69] Increases in intra-abdominal pressure secondary to the perfusate and fluid shift both during and after the operation, decreases venous return, lowering effective preload, although placement of a central line is not mandated. Central venous pressure do not accurately predict end diastolic pressure and cannot dictate management of fluid responsiveness.[70] In addition, HIPEC patients are at an increased risk of central line infection versus the general population, thus strict adherence to sterile technique and hospital-designated central venous catheter care bundle must be maintained in patients who require central line placement.[71]

Increased intra-abdominal pressure, which is comparable to pneumoperitoneum in laparoscopy, also results in elevation of the diaphragm, reducing functional residual capacity and increasing airway pressures.[72] This change in lung physiology, in combination with diaphragmatic stripping, and resuscitation increases adverse pulmonary events including pleural effusions (4.6%–64%), respiratory distress (4.2%), and pneumonia (3.2%–5%).[62,73] An estimated 33% of patients will require more than 48 hours of mechanical ventilation following HIPEC and CRS.[74] Time dependent on mechanical ventilation is associated with increased PCI, duration of surgery, estimated blood loss, intraoperative fluid requirements, and blood product requirement.[75] Epidural analgesia decreases both perioperative opiate requirements and time of mechanical ventilation as well as assists with early mobilization and has been incorporated into many recently published ERAS protocols.[76,77]

HIPEC/CRS effects on hemodynamics and respiration have influenced some institutions to incorporate mandatory intensive care unit (ICU) admission. Recent evidence has demonstrated this may not be required in select patients. Age, ECOG status greater than 2, the number of organs resected, and intraoperative blood loss are predictive preoperative and intraoperative variables for ICU admission and can be used to triage these patients.[78,79]

Approximately one-fourth of patients discharged from the ICU will return. Readmission is significantly associated with PCI and need for diaphragmatic resection.[80] Despite readmission to the ICU, which is most often related to septic or hemorrhagic shock, long-term prognosis does not decrease in comparison with their counterparts who remain on the surgical floor. Thus, there should be a low threshold to screen patients back into the ICU.

Intensivists, stepdown teams, and surgery teams managing floor patients may all encounter challenges related to coagulopathy, ileus, renal insufficiency, and metabolic disturbances.

Following the procedure, nearly one-third of patients will experience prolonged ileus secondary to newly created anastomoses, fluid shifts associated with resuscitation, and HIPEC itself. As a result, some institutions have recommended immediate initiation of total parenteral nutrition on postoperative 0, whereas European Society for Clinical Nutrition and Metabolism (ESPEN) and American Society of Parenteral and Enteral Nutrition guidelines recommend enteral feeds as soon as a patient is able to tolerate them.[81,82] At this time, the potential role of alvimopan for prevention of postoperative ileus in the setting of HIPEC and CRS is being investigated in a Phase 2 clinical trial. Patients routinely have nasogastric tubes placed intraoperatively and patients should be educated on the therapeutic purpose before surgery. Nasogastric decompression is another aspect of ERAS protocol, which has received recent attention for fast-track management, but no consensus related to removal timing exists as of today.

With delayed initiation of nutrition, special attention must be paid to the diabetic population. In addition to the perfusate carrier, which can be a dextrose solution altering blood glucose levels, diabetic patients are more likely to have infectious and thrombotic complications, respiratory failure, arrhythmias, and renal insufficiency, which have led to increased ICU stays, and 30-day and 90-day mortality.[83]

CRS involving the genitourinary tract occurs in 8% of all cases but does not significantly alter morbidity.[84] A retrospective analysis investigating the utility of prophylactic ureteral stenting found no increased risk of stent complications, although to date no randomized controlled trial exists.[85] In contrast, the incidence of acute kidney injury (AKI) ranges from 18.5% to 48.0% of all cases.[85,86] In addition to intravascular depletion and increased intra-abdominal pressure resulting in decreased venous return and ultimately decreased perfusion of the kidney, the use of cisplatin, drop-in pH, inotrope use, blood loss, and PCI are all intraoperative risk factors for AKI.[75,87] Although randomized controlled trials on resuscitation have been performed, AKI was not investigated outcome. Close monitoring of urinary output maintaining 1 mL/kg per hour for the first 70 hours postoperatively has been recommended. Dopamine infusion and furosemide as measures of increasing renal perfusion are not currently recommended.

Coagulopathy is common following HIPEC and CRS, affecting 40% to 55% of all patients. International normalized ratio peaks during the first 24 hours and returns to normal after 72 hours. Platelet count also drops during these first 3 days, reaching its lowest point at 72 hours.[67,88,89] A combination of the dilutional effects of resuscitation with fluid and blood product in addition to the suppressive effects of chemotherapy and surgery lead to these changes. In contrast, postoperative thromboembolic events more commonly occur following discharge from the hospital and range from 5.6% to 13.5%. The advent of postoperative anticoagulation has significantly lowered these rates, leading some institutions to incorporate this practice into their standard of care.[41,42,90,91]

Infectious complications are estimated to occur in between 47% and 49% of patients, with surgical site infection being the most common. Infection at multiple sites can take place synchronously, and thorough investigation must take place to preclude sites other than the wound and other visible potential sources. Urinary tract infections (17%), central line infection (17%), pneumonia (6%), and intra-abdominal infections, including anastomotic leaks (8.7%), intestinal fistula (9%), and abscess, which can lead to intra-abdominal sepsis (4%) all can cause fever, leukocytosis, or alteration in hemodynamics.[43–45,51,92,93] Recent investigation has found infectious complications are independently associated 30-day morbidity, readmission rates, and survival. Preventive measures combined with early recognition and treatment are imminent.[13,75,94]

PALLIATIVE MANAGEMENT OF MALIGNANT BOWEL OBSTRUCTION AND MALIGNANT ASCITES

Peritoneal carcinomatosis implants can spread to both the parietal and visceral peritoneum. The effects of this mechanical implantation are multifactorial, leading to abnormal physiology of bowel motility, and altered resorption of peritoneal fluid. Increased vascular hyperpermeability and neovascularization within the peritoneum also lead to an overproduction of peritoneal fluid. The end results of these 2 processes lead to malignant bowel obstructions and malignant ascites: 2 problems commonly encountered in late-stage disease of peritoneal carcinomatosis.

Malignant small bowel obstruction is diagnosed both clinically and radiographically with evidence of a mechanical obstruction distal to the ligament of Treitz with peritoneal carcinomatosis, intraperitoneal metastasis, or ascites.[95] Extrinsic occlusion of the bowel lumen by recurrence of the primary tumor or metastatic lesions can lead to obstruction. Mechanical blockage can occur with invasion of disease into the mesentery or omentum and yield adhesions, promoting the development of an obstruction.

Intraluminal recurrence of the primary tumor can occlude the bowel lumen, or lead to a functional obstruction, by invading the bowel wall muscular layer, nerves, or celiac plexus.[96]

Simply having an intra-abdominal cancer history and new-onset obstruction does not mean that a recurrence or metastatic lesion is necessarily the source. Both benign and malignant etiologies must be considered in the differential diagnosis. Benign lesions resulting in bowel obstruction include adhesions, internal hernias, ventral hernias, fibrosis secondary to radiation, and desmoplastic reaction on the small bowel following HIPEC[97] Bowel obstructions, with either benign or malignant causes, are estimated to occur in between 5% and 43% of patients with a history of primary or metastatic intra-abdominal cancer. The 2 most common causes are ovarian (5.5% to 51%) and colorectal (10% to 28%) cancers, with extra-abdominal cancer etiologies including lung, breast, and melanoma.[94,98] In patients with known cancer history who presented with intestinal obstruction, 25% to 83% are secondary to benign causes of obstruction[99–102] This estimation for a benign cause drops to 10% to 30% when known recurrence has taken place.[101,102] In contrast to small bowel obstruction secondary to benign etiology, malignant bowel obstructions typically present as a partial bowel obstruction with intermittent and slowly progressing symptoms, whereas benign bowel obstructions can present with complete obstruction. These findings have led some investigators to avoid delaying surgical intervention if there is no known recurrence history. Two distinct sources of malignant bowel obstructions (MBOs) include local recurrence and peritoneal carcinomatosis. Although local recurrence is the major cause of MBO, peritoneal carcinomatosis still represents a significant source of MBO and management obstacle for the patients and providers.[103] Every evaluation of small bowel obstruction presenting in patients with peritoneal carcinomatosis must include both benign and malignant causes on the diagnostic differential.

Management of patients with MBO secondary to peritoneal carcinomatosis represents one of the most challenging aspects of surgical oncology. The NCCN recommends evaluating expected survival time when an MBO consult is encountered, and separating patients by months to years, weeks to months, and days to weeks. From there, patients with months to years of expected survival should be considered for intervention, and reversible and benign causes must be investigated. The Southwest Oncology Group is currently recruiting patients into a partially randomized clinical trial with a surgical intervention arm, and nonsurgical management arm.

On presentation, fluid resuscitation should begin, in addition to decompression with a nasogastric tube. Although an upright, KUB (kidney, ureter, and bladder), and lateral radiograph may rule in an obstructive process, CT or MRI cross-sectional imaging is typically needed to locate the exact cause. CT has a specificity of 100% and a sensitivity of 94% for localization of the site of obstruction. Cross-sectional imaging will ultimately help determine the next step, whether it be surgery, endoscopic intervention, or palliative management.[104]

While evaluating a patient with peritoneal carcinomatosis as a potential candidate for intervention, multiple factors must be taken into consideration: overall clinical status, presence of ascites, location and number of obstruction, and the presence of a palpable mass. An individualized approach is necessary, setting clear goals of care and expected survival.[97]

Differences in pathophysiology between small and large bowel obstruction highlight the discrepancies that exist in terms of the duration of postoperative symptom relief. Aabo and colleagues[105] found the origin of small bowel obstruction was most often secondary to serosal carcinomatosis in contrast to a single tumor site associated with large bowel obstruction. Relief from obstructive symptoms was achieved in only 44% of small bowel patients, and lasted only 2 months, compared with 6 months of palliation for large bowel obstruction. Not all cancers are equal for overall survival following presentation with MBO. Colorectal and neuroendocrine tumors are associated with increased survival. Inferior survival is also associated with synchronous site of MBO, noncolorectal primary, and presence of ascites.[106] Although conflicting evidence exists regarding overall survival between MBO patients with peritoneal metastasis versus peritoneal metastasis with systemic metastasis, local recurrence does have improved overall survival when compared with peritoneal carcinomatosis.[105,107]

Various outcomes have been studied quantifying postoperative outcomes, including clearance to discharge the patient home, symptom relief, and tolerance of an oral (PO) diet. The ability to tolerate PO during the postoperative period ranges from 30% to 100% as reported by Cousins and colleagues.[108] This was also supported by Olson and colleagues[97] Symptom improvement ranges from 42% to 80%. However, recurrent obstructions after surgical intervention occur in between 10% and 47% of patients. Improvement was significantly better for local recurrence versus peritoneal carcinomatosis: 75% versus 61%.[107–109]

Median survival after diagnosis of MBO ranges from 26 to 273 days, and can be differentiated for 2 distinct patient populations, labeled as high or low risk.[109] Overall median survival after the surgical intervention was 64 to 112 days for all patients with MBO.[105,107,110] Patients with no associated ascites or palpable mass who had return of bowel function in the postoperative period survived between 154 and 192 days versus 26 to 36 days in patients with ascites, palpable mass, and slow return of bowel function.[109] The presence of ascites alone reduces both symptom-free survival and recurrence-free survival with as little as 100 mL present in the abdomen. Higashi and colleagues found that malignant bowel obstruction recurred in as few as 9 days for this group, versus 61 days in the nonascites group.[111]

Complications following surgical intervention for MBO range from 7% to 44%, whereas postoperative mortality ranged from 6% to 32%. Given the high risk for morbidity and mortality combined, and relatively short overall survival, 34% to 87% of these patients are discharged home following their surgery whereas 22% to 31% of patients will spend their remaining life in the hospital. Unfortunately, successful operation and discharge from the hospital does not preclude patients from recurrent MBO or symptoms. From 26.7% to 100% had relief of obstructive symptoms for the remainder of their lives. Reobstruction occurs from 0% to 63% of the time[100,104,105,107–110,112]

Patients with large-volume ascites, multiple points of obstruction, poor performance status, or those who prefer less invasive measures, can opt for endoscopic procedures, such as stenting or percutaneous enterogastric tube placement depending on lesion location. Lesions proximal to the ligament of Treitz, either in the small bowel or with local mass effect leading to gastric outlet obstruction, are candidates for stenting, as are those with distal colorectal lesions. These procedures can serve as palliation or bridge therapy with "technical success rates" ranging from 88% to 100%, allowing earlier ability to tolerate when compared with surgical patients and no difference in overall survival while offering a shorter length of stay.[97,113] Some investigators have recommended patients with an intermediate life expectancy of at least 30 days be considered for endoscopic procedure, whereas those with more than 60 days who satisfy previously mentioned conditions, be considered for bypass or resection. Stent placement for gastric outlet syndrome can be limited by reobstruction, which warrants additional intervention when compared with surgical bypass. This further supports endoscopic intervention as a treatment for patients who fall into the intermediate overall survival prognostic time period category.[114]

In additional to mechanical obstruction, the nausea and vomiting that arise from distension can be treated with venting percutaneous endoscopic gastrostomy (PEG) for patients with diffuse peritoneal disease. Technical success ranges from 94% to 98% despite stomach encasement and diffuse ascites: 2 factors that were traditionally seen as contraindications to a percutaneous procedure. This may also preclude a patient from being a surgical candidate.[115,116]

The use of HIPEC for palliation of symptomatic ascites was first introduced by Ma and colleagues[95] for primary peritoneal mesothelioma with maximally invasive laparotomy and surgical debulking, and was later targeted for nonbulky disease with laparoscopy. This expanded the treatment of malignant ascites associated with colorectal, gastric adenocarcinoma, and ovarian cancer in addition to the already established primary peritoneal mesothelioma.[117–119] Measurement of successful palliation among these studies has had multiple definitions ranging from need-for-repeat paracentesis, radiologic (CT vs ultrasound) evidence of ascites, and clinical recurrence that presents with abdominal distension, decreased tolerance for PO, and nausea and vomiting. Success rates range from 83% to 100% resolution with minimal complications. Reported complications associated with the procedure were 6% to 27% and include deep vein thrombosis, surgical site infection, and gastroparesis. Median overall survival was 66 to 203 days. This success rate of overall survival and minimal complications justifies the utility of palliative HIPEC for management of malignant ascites.

SUMMARY

Treatment of peritoneal mesothelioma, or peritoneal metastasis from colorectal, appendiceal, ovarian, and pseudomyxoma peritonei can be accomplished with CRS and HIPEC with curative intent. Patient selection and overall survival are dependent on PCI, which reflects overall tumor burden within the abdomen, and influences the completeness of cytoreduction. Compressive forces from metastatic growth can yield symptoms including pain, decreased appetite, and increased abdominal girth. Bowel obstruction and abdominal ascites are ominous signs suggesting unresectability. Patients should be evaluated by a multidisciplinary tumor board and workup includes laboratory tests and CT of chest, abdomen, and pelvis to evaluate PCI, rule in resectability, and rule out metastatic disease. Diagnosis laparoscopy is useful both in the preoperative setting for diagnosis but also in the operative setting before laparotomy. Operative goals include complete cytoreduction with no microscopic disease, which is supplemented with hyperthermic chemotherapy to target all remaining disease smaller than 2.5 mm. Pulmonary and infectious complications are common during the postoperative setting and patients may have an extended length of stay in the hospital. ICU admission is not mandatory, but age, ECOG status greater than 2, the number of organs resected, and intraoperative blood loss should all be considered when triaging a patient postoperatively. Patients presenting with late-stage disease may experience partial or complete bowel obstruction and distension associated with malignant ascites. Although obstruction typically can be treated conservatively, decompressive PEG tubes, bypasses, or resection are sometimes needed. Last, patients who are refractory to diuresis or paracentesis who present with decreased quality of life secondary to malignant ascites may benefit from palliative HIPEC.

DISCLOSURE

No financial conflicts of interest to disclose.

REFERENCES

1. Miller JA, Wynn WH. Malignant tumor arising from endothelium of peritoneum, and producing mucoid ascitic fluid. J Pathol Bacteriol 1908;12:267–78.
2. Fernandez RN, Daly JM. Pseudomyxoma peritonei. Arch Surg 1980;115(4): 409–14.
3. Antman KH, Blum RH, Greenberger JS, et al. Multimodality therapy for malignant mesothelioma based on a study of natural history. Am J Med 1980;68: 356–62.
4. Dedrick RL. Theoretical and experimental bases of intraperitoneal chemotherapy. Semin Oncol 1985;12:1–6.
5. Sugarbaker PH. Peritonectomy procedures. Ann Surg 1995;221:29–42.
6. Moolgavkar SH, Meza R, Turim J. Pleural and peritoneal mesotheliomas in SEER: age effects and temporal trends, 1973-2005. Cancer Causes Control 2009;20:935–44.
7. Henley SJ, Larson TC, Wu M, et al. Mesothelioma incidence in 50 states and the District of Columbia, United States, 2003-2008. Int J Occup Environ Health 2013;19:1–10.
8. Eltabbakh GH, Piver MS, Hempling RE, et al. Clinical picture, response to therapy, and survival of women with diffuse malignant peritoneal mesothelioma. J Surg Oncol 1999;70:6–12.
9. Alexander HR Jr, Bartlett DL, Pingpank JF, et al. Treatment factors associated with long-term survival after cytoreductive surgery and regional chemotherapy for patients with malignant peritoneal mesothelioma. Surgery 2013;153(6): 779–86.
10. National Toxicology Program. Report on carcinogens. Research Triangle Park (NC): US Department of Health and Human Services, Public Health Service, National Toxicology Program; 2011.
11. Carr NJ, Cecil TD, Mohamed F, et al. A consensus for classification and pathologic reporting of pseudomyxoma peritonei and associated appendiceal neoplasia: the results of the peritoneal surface oncology group international (PSOGI) modified delphi process. Am J Surg Pathol 2016;40:14.
12. Chua TC, Moran BJ, Sugarbaker PH, et al. Early- and long-term outcome data of patients with pseudomyxoma peritonei from appendiceal origin treated by a strategy of cytoreductive surgery and hyperthermic intraperitoneal chemotherapy. J Clin Oncol 2012;30(20):2449–56.
13. Elias D, Gilly F, Boutitie F, et al. Peritoneal colorectal carcinomatosis treated with surgery and perioperative intraperitoneal chemotherapy: retrospective analysis of 523 patients from a multicentric French study. J Clin Oncol 2010;28:63–8.
14. Verwaal VJ, van Ruth S, de Bree E, et al. Randomized trial of cytoreduction and hyperthermic intraperitoneal chemotherapy versus systemic chemotherapy and palliative surgery in patients with peritoneal carcinomatosis of colorectal cancer. J Clin Oncol 2003;21(20):3737.
15. Elias D, Delperro JR, Sideris L, et al. Treatment of peritoneal carcinomatosis from colorectal cancer: impact of complete cytoreductive surgery and difficulties in conducting randomized trials. Ann Surg Oncol 2004;11(5):518.
16. Quenet F, Elias D, Roca L, et al. A UNICANCER phase III trial of hyperthermic intraperitoneal chemotherapy (HIPEC) for colorectal peritoneal carcinomatosis (PC): PRODIGE 7 (abstract). J Clin Oncol 2018;36 (suppl; abstr LBA3503). Abstract Available at: https://meetinglibrary.asco.org/record/158740/abstract. Accessed on July 16, 2018.

17. Prat J, Belhadj H, Berek J, et al. Staging classification for cancer of the ovary, fallopian tube, and peritoneum. Int J Gynaecol Obstet 2014;124(1):1–5.

18. van Driel WJ, Koole SN, Sonke GS. Hyperthermic intraperitoneal chemotherapy in ovarian cancer. N Engl J Med 2018;378:1363–4.

19. Townsend CM, Beauchamp RD, Evers BM, et al. Sabiston textbook of surgery: the biological basis of modern surgical practice. 20th edition. Philadelphia: Elsevier Saunders; 2017.

20. Bhatt A. Management of peritoneal metastases- cytoreductive surgery, HIPEC and beyond. Singapore: Springer Singapore; 2018.

21. DiZerega GS, Rodgers KE. The Peritoneum. New York: Springer Science & Business Media; 2012.

22. Terzi C, Arslan NC, Canda AE. Peritoneal carcinomatosis of gastrointestinal tumors: where are we now? World J Gastroenterol 2014;20(39):14371–80.

23. Ceelen WP. Peritoneal Carcinomatosis: A Multidisciplinary Approach. New York: Springer Science & Business Media; 2007.

24. Sadeghi B, Arvieux C, Glehen O, et al. Peritoneal carcinomatosis from non-gynecologic malignancies: results of the EVOCAPE 1 multicentric prospective study. Cancer 2000;88(2):358–63.

25. Klaver YL, Lemmens VE, Nienhuijs SW, et al. Peritoneal carcinomatosis of colorectal origin: Incidence, prognosis and treatment options. World J Gastroenterol 2012;18(39):5489–94.

26. Esquivel J, Sugarbaker PH. Clinical presentation of the pseudomyxoma peritonei syndrome. Br J Surg 2000;87(10):1414–8.

27. Magge D, Zenati MS, Austin F, et al. Malignant peritoneal mesothelioma: prognostic factors and oncologic outcome analysis. Ann Surg Oncol 2014;21: 1159–65.

28. Yano H, Moran BJ, Cecil TD, et al. Cytoreductive surgery and intraperitoneal chemotherapy for peritoneal mesothelioma. Eur J Surg Oncol 2009;35:980–5.

29. Cao S, Jin S, Cao J, et al. Advances in malignant peritoneal mesothelioma. Int J Colorectal Dis 2015;30:1–10.

30. Acherman YI, Welch LS, Bromley CM, et al. Clinical presentation of peritoneal mesothelioma. Tumori 2003;89:269–73.

31. Manzini Vde P, Recchia L, Cafferata M, et al. Malignant peritoneal mesothelioma: a multicenter study on 81 cases. Ann Oncol 2010;21:348–53.

32. Bushati M, Rovers KP, Sommariva A, et al. The current practice of cytoreductive surgery and HIPEC for colorectal peritoneal metastases: results of a worldwide web-based survey of the Peritoneal Surface Oncology Group International (PSOGI). Eur J Surg Oncol 2018;44. https://doi.org/10.1016/j.ejso.2018.07.003.

33. Chua TC, Al-Zahrani A, Saxena A, et al. Determining the association between preoperative computed tomography findings and post-operative outcomes after cytoreductive surgery and perioperative intraperitoneal chemotherapy for pseudomyxoma peritonei. Ann Surg Oncol 2011;18:1582–9.

34. de Bree E, Koops W, Kroger R, et al. Peritoneal carcinomatosis from colorectal or appendiceal origin: correlation of preoperative CT with intraoperative findings and evaluation of interobserver agreement. J Surg Oncol 2004;86:64–73.

35. Koh JL, Yan TD, Glenn D, et al. Evaluation of preoperative computed tomography in estimating peritoneal cancer index in colorectal peritoneal carcinomatosis. Ann Surg Oncol 2009;16:327–33.

36. Jacquet P, Jelinek JS, Chang D, et al. Abdominal computed tomographic scan in the selection of patients with mucinous peritoneal carcinomatosis for cytoreductive surgery. J Am Coll Surg 1995;181:530–8.

37. Esquivel J, Chua TC, Stojadinovic A, et al. Accuracy and clinical relevance of computed tomography scan interpretation of peritoneal cancer index in colorectal cancer peritoneal carcinomatosis: a multi-institutional study. J Surg Oncol 2010;102:565–70.
38. Bartlett DJ, Thacker PG, Grotz TE, et al. Mucinous appendiceal neoplasms: classification, imaging, and HIPEC. Abdom Radiol (N Y) 2019;44:1686–702.
39. Low RN, Barone RM, Lucero J. Comparison of MRI and CT for predicting the peritoneal cancer index (PCI) preoperatively in patients being considered for cytoreductive surgical procedures. Ann Surg Oncol 2015;22(5):1708–15.
40. Dohan A, Hoeffel C, Soyer P, et al. Evaluation of peritoneal carcinomatosis index with CT and MRI. Br J Surg 2017;104(9):1244–9.
41. Wang W, Tan GHC, Chia CS, et al. Are positron emission tomography-computed tomography (PET-CT) scans useful in preoperative assessment of patients with peritoneal disease before cytoreductive surgery (CRS) and hyperthermic intraperitoneal chemotherapy (HIPEC)? Int J Hyperthermia 2018;34(5):524–31.
42. Tabrizian P, Jayakrishnan TT, Zacharias A, et al. Incorporation of diagnostic laparoscopy in the management algorithm for patients with peritoneal metastases: A multi-institutional analysis. J Surg Oncol 2015;111(8):1035–40.
43. Laterza B, Kusamura S, Baratti D, et al. Role of explorative laparoscopy to evaluate optimal candidates for cytoreductive surgery and hyperthermic intraperitoneal chemotherapy (HIPEC) in patients with peritoneal mesothelioma. In Vivo 2009;23:187–90.
44. Iversen LH, Rasmussen PC, Laurberg S. Value of laparoscopy before cytoreductive surgery and hyperthermic intraperitoneal chemotherapy for peritoneal carcinomatosis. Br J Surg 2013;100:285–92.
45. Bastiaenen VP, Klaver CEL, Kok NFM, et al. Second and third look laparoscopy in pT4 colon cancer patients for early detection of peritoneal metastases; the COLOPEC 2 randomized multicentre trial. BMC Cancer 2019;19(1):254.
46. Husain A, Chi DS, Prasad M, et al. The role of laparoscopy in second-look evaluations for ovarian cancer. Gynecol Oncol 2001;80:44.
47. Inoue K1, Nakane Y, Michiura T, et al. Mucocele of the appendix. World J Surg 2007;31:542–8.
48. Low RN, Sebrechts CP, Barone RM, et al. Diffusion-weighted MRI of peritoneal tumors: comparison with conventional MRI and surgical and histopathologic findings—a feasibility study. Am J Roentgenol 2009;193(2):461–70.
49. Peters MG, Bartlett EK, Roses RE, et al. Age-related morbidity and mortality with cytoreductive surgery. Ann Surg Oncol 2015;22:898–904. Available at: https://doi-org.eresources.mssm.edu/10.1245/s10434-015-4624-y.
50. Votanopoulos KI, Newman NA, Russell G, et al. Outcomes of Cytoreductive Surgery (CRS) with hyperthermic intraperitoneal chemotherapy (HIPEC) in patients older than 70 years; survival benefit at considerable morbidity and mortality. Ann Surg Oncol 2013;20:3497–503.
51. Chouliaras K, Levine EA, Fino N, et al. Prognostic factors and significance of gastrointestinal leak after Cytoreductive Surgery (CRS) with Heated Intraperitoneal Chemotherapy (HIPEC). Ann Surg Oncol 2017;24:890–7. Available at: https://doi-org.eresources.mssm.edu/10.1245/s10434-016-5738-6.
52. Randle RW, Doud AN, Levine EA, et al. Peritoneal surface disease with synchronous hepatic involvement treated with cytoreductive surgery (CRS) and hyperthermic intraperitoneal chemotherapy (HIPEC). Ann Surg Oncol 2015;22:1634–8.

53. Chua TC, Yan TD, Zhao J, et al. Peritoneal carcinomatosis and liver metastases from colorectal cancer treated with cytoreductive surgery perioperative intraperitoneal chemotherapy and liver resection. Eur J Surg Oncol 2009;35:1299–305.

54. Carmignani CP, Ortega-Perez G, Sugarbaker PH. The management of synchronous peritoneal carcinomatosis and hematogenous metastasis from colorectal cancer. Eur J Surg Oncol 2004;30:391–8.

55. Leigh NL, Solomon D, Feingold D, et al. Improved survival with experience: a 10-year learning curve in hyperthermic intraperitoneal chemotherapy and cytoreductive surgery. Ann Surg Oncol 2020;27(1):222–31.

56. Verwaal VJ, Bruin S, Boot H, et al. 8-year follow-up of randomized trial: cytoreduction and hyperthermic intraperitoneal chemotherapy versus systemic chemotherapy in patients with peritoneal carcinomatosis of colorectal cancer. Ann Surg Oncol 2008;15:2426–32.

57. Reece L, Dragicevich H, Lewis C, et al. Preoperative nutrition status and postoperative outcomes in patients undergoing cytoreductive surgery and hyperthermic intraperitoneal chemotherapy. Ann Surg Oncol 2019;26(8):2622–30.

58. Vashi PG, Gupta D, Lammersfeld CA, et al. The relationship between baseline nutritional status with subsequent parenteral nutrition and clinical outcomes in cancer patients undergoing hyperthermic intraperitoneal chemotherapy. Nutr J 2013;12:118.

59. Weimann A, Braga M, Carli F, et al. ESPEN guideline: clinical nutrition in surgery. Clin Nutr 2017;36:623–50.

60. Webb C, Day R, Velazco CS, et al. Implementation of an Enhanced Recovery After Surgery (ERAS) Program is associated with improved outcomes in patients undergoing cytoreductive surgery and hyperthermic intraperitoneal chemotherapy. Ann Surg Oncol 2020;27:303–12.

61. Schmidt C, Moritz S, Rath S, et al. Perioperative management of patients with cytoreductive surgery for peritoneal carcinomatosis. J Surg Oncol 2009;100: 297–301.

62. Kapoor S, Bassily-Marcus A, Alba Yunen R, et al. Critical care management and intensive care unit outcomes following cytoreductive surgery with hyperthermic intraperitoneal chemotherapy. World J Crit Care Med 2017;6(2):116–23.

63. Eng OS, Dumitra S, O'Leary M, et al. Association of fluid administration with morbidity in cytoreductive surgery with hyperthermic intraperitoneal chemotherapy. JAMA Surg 2017;152(12):1156–60.

64. Hendrix RJ, Lambert LA. ASO author reflections: intraoperative fluid restriction during CRS-HIPEC—less is more. Ann Surg Oncol 2019;26(Suppl 3):575–6.

65. Colantonio L, Claroni C, Fabrizi L, et al. A randomized trial of goal directed vs standard fluid therapy in cytoreductive surgery with hyperthermic intraperitoneal chemotherapy. J Gastrointest Surg 2015;19:722–9.

66. de Witte P, de Witt CA, van de Minkelis JL, et al. Inflammatory response and optimalisation of perioperative fluid administration during hyperthermic intraoperative intraperitoneal chemotherapy surgery. J Gastrointest Oncol 2019;10(2): 244–53.

67. Schmidt C, Creutzenberg M, Piso P, et al. Perioperative anaesthetic management of cytoreductive surgery with hyperthermic intraperitoneal chemotherapy. Anaesthesia 2008;63:389–95.

68. Marik PE, Monnet X, Teboul JL. Hemodynamic parameters to guide fluid therapy. Ann Intensive Care 2011;1:1.

69. Waters PS, Smith AW, Fitzgerald E, et al. Increased incidence of central venous catheter-related infection in patients undergoing cytoreductive surgery and

hyperthermic intra-peritoneal chemotherapy. Surg Infect (Larchmt) 2019;20(6): 465–71.

70. Schluermann C, Hoeppner J, Benk C, et al. Intra-abdominal pressure, cardiac index and vascular resistance during hyperthermic intraperitoneal chemotherapy: a prospective observational study. Minerva Anestesiol 2016;82(2): 160–9.

71. Chen MYM, Chiles C, Loggie BW. Thoracic complications in patients undergoing intraperitoneal heated chemotherapy with mitomycin following cytoreductive surgery. J Surg Oncol 1997;66(1):19–23.

72. Preti V1, Chang D, Sugarbaker PH. Pulmonary complications following cytoreductive surgery and perioperative chemotherapy in 147 consecutive patients. Gastroenterol Res Pract 2012;2012:635314.

73. Balakrishnan KP, Survesan S. Anaesthetic management and perioperative outcomes of cytoreductive surgery with hyperthermic intraperitoneal chemotherapy: a retrospective analysis. Indian J Anaesth 2018;62(3):188–96.

74. Schmidt C, Steinke T, Mortiz S, et al. Thoracic epidural anesthesia in patients with cytoreductive surgery and HIPEC. J Surg Oncol 2010;102:545–6.

75. Cooksley TJ, Haji-Michael P. Post-operative critical care management of patients undergoing cytoreductive surgery and heated intraperitoneal chemotherapy (HIPEC). World J Surg Oncol 2011;9:169.

76. Mogal HD, Levine EA, Fino NF, et al. Routine admission to intensive care unit after cytoreductive surgery and heated intraperitoneal chemotherapy: not always a requirement. Ann Surg Oncol 2016;23(5):1486–95.

77. López-Basave HN, Morales-Vasquez F, Mendez-Herrera C, et al. Intensive care unit admission after cytoreductive surgery and hyperthermic intraperitoneal chemotherapy. Is it necessary? J Oncol 2014;2014:307317.

78. Wallet F, Maucort Boulch D, Malfroy S, et al. No impact on long-term survival of prolonged ICU stay and re-admission for patients undergoing cytoreductive surgery with HIPEC. Eur J Surg Oncol 2016;42(6):855–60.

79. Weimann A, Braga M, Harsanyi L, et al. ESPEN guidelines on enteral nutrition: surgery including organ transplantation. Clin Nutr 2006;25(2):224–44.

80. Simkens GA, Verwaal VJ, Lemmens VE, et al. Short-term outcome in patients treated with cytoreduction and HIPEC compared to conventional colon cancer surgery. Medicine (Baltimore) 2016;95(41):e5111.

81. The ILEUS Study: a phase 2 randomized controlled trial investigating alvimopan for enhanced gastrointestinal recovery after cytoreductive surgery and hyperthermic intraperitoneal chemotherapy. Available at: https://clinicaltrials.gov/ct2/show/NCT03352414. Accessed October 31, 2019.

82. Honoré C, Souadka A, Goéré D, et al. HIPEC for peritoneal carcinomatosis: does an associated urologic procedure increase morbidity? Ann Surg Oncol 2012;19:104–9.

83. Coccolini F1, Lotti M, Manfredi R, et al. Ureteral stenting in cytoreductive surgery plus hyperthermic intraperitoneal chemotherapy as a routine procedure: evidence and necessity. Urol Int 2012;89(3):307–10.

84. Angeles MA, Quenet F, Vieille P, et al. Predictive risk factors of acute kidney injury after cytoreductive surgery and cisplatin-based hyperthermic intraperitoneal chemotherapy for ovarian peritoneal carcinomatosis. Int J Gynecol Cancer 2019;29:382–9.

85. Cata JP, Zavala AM, Van Meter A, et al. Identification of risk factors associated with postoperative acute kidney injury after cytoreductive surgery with

hyperthermic intraperitoneal chemotherapy: a retrospective study. Int J Hyperthermia 2018;34:538–44.

86. Arjona-Sánchez A, Cadenas-Febres A, Cabrera-Bermon J, et al. Assessment of RIFLE and AKIN criteria to define acute renal dysfunction for HIPEC procedures for ovarian and non ovarian peritoneal malignancies. Eur J Surg Oncol 2016; 42(6):869–76.

87. Raspé C, Flöther L, Schneider R, et al. Best practice for perioperative management of patients with cytoreductive surgery and HIPEC. Eur J Surg Oncol 2017; 43:1013–27.

88. Hurdle H, Bishop G, Walker A, et al. Coagulation after cytoreductive surgery and hyperthermic intraperitoneal chemotherapy: a retrospective cohort analysis. Can J Anaesth 2017;64:1144–52.

89. Rottenstreich A, Kalish Y, Kleinstern G2, et al. Factors associated with thromboembolic events following cytoreductive surgery and hyperthermic intraperitoneal chemotherapy. J Surg Oncol 2017;116(7):914–20.

90. Baumgartner JM, Khan S. ASO author reflections: venous thromboembolism after CRS/HIPEC. Ann Surg Oncol 2019;26:758–9.

91. Arslan NC, Sokmen S, Avkan-Oguz V, et al. Infectious complications after cytoreductive surgery and hyperthermic intra-peritoneal chemotherapy. Surg Infect (Larchmt) 2017;18(2):157–63.

92. Sugarbaker PH, Alderman R, Edwards G, et al. Prospective morbidity and mortality assessment of cytoreductive surgery plus perioperative intraperitoneal chemotherapy to treat peritoneal dissemination of appendiceal mucinous malignancy. Ann Surg Oncol 2006;13:635–44.

93. Choudry MHA, Shuai Y, Jones HL, et al. Postoperative complications independently predict cancer-related survival in peritoneal malignancies. Ann Surg Oncol 2018;25(13):3950–9.

94. Soriano A, Davis MP. Malignant bowel obstruction: individualized treatment near the end of life. Cleve Clin J Med 2011;78(3):197–206.

95. Ma GY, Bartlett DL, Reed E, et al. Continuous hyperthermic peritoneal perfusion with cisplatin for the treatment of peritoneal mesothelioma. Cancer J Sci Am 1997;3:174–9.

96. Anthony T, Baron T, Mercadante S, et al. Report of the clinical protocol committee: development of randomized trials for malignant bowel obstruction. J Pain Symptom Manage 2007;34(Suppl 1):S49–59.

97. Ripamonti C, Bruera E. Palliative management of malignant bowel obstruction. Int J Gynecol Cancer 2002;12(2):135–43.

98. Davis MP, Nouneh C. Modern management of cancer-related intestinal obstruction. Curr Pain Headache Rep 2001;5:257–64.

99. Baines M, Oliver DJ, Carter RL. Medical management of intestinal obstruction in patients with advanced malignant disease. Lancet 1985;2:990–3.

100. Osteen RT, Guyton S, Steele G Jr, et al. Malignant intestinal obstruction. Surgery 1980;87(6):611–5.

101. Ketcham AS, Hoye RC, Pilch YH, et al. Delayed intestinal obstruction following treatment for cancer. Cancer 1970;25:406–10.

102. Denise JP, Douard R, Malamut G, et al. Small bowel obstruction in patients with a prior history of cancer: predictive findings of malignant origins. World J Surg 2013;38:363–9.

103. Edna TH, Bjerkeset T. Small bowel obstruction in patients previously operated on for colorectal cancer. Eur J Surg 1998;164:587–92.

104. Ellis CN, Boggs HW, Slagle GW, et al. Small bowel obstruction after colon resection for benign and malignant diseases. Dis Colon Rectum 1991;34:367–71.
105. Aabo K, Pedersen H, Bach F, et al. Surgical management of intestinal obstruction in the late course of malignant disease. Acta Chir Scand 1984;150(2): 173–6.
106. Ripamonti CI, Easson AM, Gerdes H. Management of malignant bowel obstruction. Eur J Cancer 2008;44(8):1105–15.
107. de Boer NL, Hagemans JAW, Schultze BTA, et al. Acute malignant obstruction in patients with peritoneal carcinomatosis: The role of palliative surgery. Eur J Surg Oncol 2019;45(3):389–93.
108. Cousins SE, Tempest E, Feuer DJ. Surgery for the resolution of symptoms in malignant bowel obstruction in advanced gynaecological and gastrointestinal cancer. Cochrane Database Syst Rev 2016;(1):CD002764.
109. Paul Olson TJ, Pinkerton C, Brasel KJ, et al. Palliative surgery for malignant bowel obstruction from carcinomatosis: a systematic review. JAMA Surg 2014; 149(4):383–92.
110. Legendre H, Vanhuyse F, Caroli-Bosc FX, et al. Survival and quality of life after palliative surgery for neoplastic gastrointestinal obstruction. Eur J Surg Oncol 2001;27:364–7.
111. Higashi H. Factors affecting successful palliative surgery for malignant bowel obstruction due to peritoneal dissemination from colorectal cancer. Japanese Journal of Clinical Oncology 2003;33(7):357–9.
112. Turnbull AD, Guerra J, Starnes HF. Results of surgery for obstructing carcinomatosis of gastrointestinal, pancreatic, or biliary origin. J Clin Oncol 1989;7:381–6.
113. Sebastian S, Johnston S, Geoghegan T, et al. Buckley MPooled analysis of the efficacy and safety of self-expanding metal stenting in malignant colorectal obstruction. Am J Gastroenterol 2004;99(10):2051–7.
114. Jeurnink SM1, Siersema PD, Steyerberg EW, et al. Predictors of complications after endoscopic retrograde cholangiopancreatography: a prognostic model for early discharge. Surg Endosc 2011;25(9):2892–900.
115. Campagnutta E1, Cannizzaro R, Gallo A, et al. Palliative treatment of upper intestinal obstruction by gynecological malignancy: the usefulness of percutaneous endoscopic gastrostomy. Gynecol Oncol 1996;62(1):103–5.
116. Meyer L, Pothuri B. Decompressive percutaneous gastrostomy tube use in gynecologic malignancies. Curr Treat Options Oncol 2006;7:111–20.
117. Chang E, Alexander HR, Libutti SK, et al. Laparoscopic continuous hyperthermic peritoneal perfusion. J Am Coll Surg 2001;193(2):225–9.
118. Garofalo A, Valle M, Garcia J, et al. Laparoscopic intraperitoneal hyperthermic chemotherapy for palliation of debilitating malignant ascites. Eur J Surg Oncol 2006;32(6):682–5.
119. Facchiano E, Scaringi S, Kianmanesh R, et al. Laparoscopic hyperthermic intraperitoneal chemotherapy (HIPEC) for the treatment of malignant ascites secondary to unresectable peritoneal carcinomatosis from advanced gastric cancer. Eur J Surg Oncol 2008;34(2):154–8.

Management of Rectal Cancer

Neal Wilkinson, MD

KEYWORDS

- Rectal cancer • Staging • Surgical techniques • Multimodality treatment

KEY POINTS

- The surgeon treating the patient with newly diagnosed rectal cancer must assess tumor stage (early or advanced) and tumor location (high or low) before recommending treatment. Treatment pathways exist that ensure appropriate surgical treatment while maximizing use of multimodality chemoradiation therapy.
- Surgical treatment requires a minimum of 1 cm distal margin, careful clearance of the mesorectum and radial margin using the total mesorectal excision (TME) technique, and 12 or more regional lymph nodes harvested and analyzed.
- Up front surgery cannot control locally advanced disease and multimodality treatments are highly effective. Taken together, careful preoperative planning and multidisciplinary treatment options should be favored over expedited surgical treatments.

INTRODUCTION

Rectal cancer is often presented with a dizzying array of treatment recommendations. This article clarifies and simplifies this common clinical problem from the surgical perspective. There is no discussion of open verses robotic or TaTME verses TAMIS, because I view these as tools in the armamentarium of the surgeon. Tool selection is secondary to sound oncologic technique and execution.

Because of the anatomic challenges and local recurrence potential, a more complex algorithm must be used when treating rectal cancer as opposed to colon cancer. Key to simplifying management is a clear understanding of the presenting stage (early or advance) and location (high or low). Once a rectal cancer is understood with regard to these two items (stage and location), the treatment algorithms follow a logical straightforward pathway based on solid evidence.

Patient anxiety is a major confounding factor in the treatment of rectal cancer, but must not contribute to the deviation of standard treatment norms. The patient-specific clinical dimension, although clearly important, is commonly cited as a rational for incomplete staging or expedited surgery. Patients never state that they "want an ostomy either temporary or permanent" or "want the cancer out later." Clearly explaining

1333 Surgical Services Drive, Kalispell, MT 59901, USA
E-mail address: nwilkinson@krmc.org

Surg Clin N Am 100 (2020) 615–628
https://doi.org/10.1016/j.suc.2020.02.014
0039-6109/20/© 2020 Elsevier Inc. All rights reserved.

surgical.theclinics.com

the best treatment options with time for follow-up questions and second opinions may be better than initiating ill-advised treatment based on inaccurate tumor staging or patient-perceived biases. Patient's fears should never result in falling into foreseeable avoidable traps. It is critically important that the patient understand that ill-advised treatment often results in an early recurrence often followed by palliative colostomy and ultimately severe and difficult-to-control pain. Treatment decisions need to be based on complete understanding of the cancer, stage and location, to avoid poor results.

HISTORICAL PERSPECTIVE
Surgery First

Historically upfront surgical resection was the principle means of treating advanced rectal cancer and provides an excellent historical perspective for what to expect with a surgery-first approach. Rectal cancer treatments before the Miles procedure had no resemblance to current treatment and are not discussed further but can be reviewed in an excellent paper by Galler and colleagues.[1] The Miles procedure, first described in 1908, was the first to report on the need for radical resection of upward, downward, and lateral zones to control rectal cancer. Surgical management of the downward spread of disease required perineal resection often well beyond modern required distal margins. Miles procedure mortality was excessive; initially reported to be 31% and improving with experience to 10% over many decades.[2] Radical surgery applied to locally advanced disease committed the patient to a permanent colostomy, a perineal wound, and offered limited long-term survival. Radical surgery when applied to early stage disease may have achieved better survival but with the previously mentioned undesirable collateral damage.

Examining the pathologic specimens and clinical outcome of rectal cancers treated by radical surgery, a better understanding of "downward" tumor spread evolved. A more limited definition of the adequate distal margin changed from perineal skin to the more limited "5 cm rule." By limiting distal resections to 5 cm, the Hartmann procedure spared the morbidity and added mortality from the perineal portion of the procedure. Subsequent studies further decreased the distal rectal margin (DRM) from 5 cm to 1 cm based on sound pathologic data. In 1983, Williams and coworkers[3] reported on 50 abdominoperineal (APR) resections with curative intent, all predating neoadjuvant therapy. They demonstrated that 76% of cases had no distal pathologic intramural spread and 14% had distal spread of less than 1 cm. The remaining 10% of patients with distal spread greater than 1 cm was associated with poorly differentiated, node-positive tumors. They concluded that 90% of rectal cancers had no distal intramural spread (beyond 1 cm) and strict use of the 5 cm rule results in unnecessary sphincter loss. When greater margins were required for distant intramural spread, the outcome would not be altered by more radical surgery. This adaptation provided equivalent oncologic margins in the downward direction but offered nothing with regard to lateral margin status.

In 1998, Heald and coworkers[4] reported on a 20-year experience with meticulous surgical technique in the treatment of rectal cancer and demonstrated that removing the entire embryologic mesorectum was critically important. This technique, total mesorectal excision (TME), was associated with a dramatic improvement of local recurrence rate: 2% at 5 and 10 years in patients carefully selected for surgery.[4] It is important to recall that Heald's excellent results were comprised of selected "curative" surgical cases. When Heald included the remaining 25% of patients with less than curative surgery recurrence rate rose to 32%. Local recurrence was associated with extramural vascular invasion, a positive circumferential radial margin (CRM), and the need for a perineal resection despite a technically sound TME procedure. Heald's key contributions to the surgical effort are two-fold: surgical techniques are critical to ensure a complete resection achieving a low recurrence rate; and adverse tumor features cannot be overcome by technique alone especially when perineal resection is required.

Modern radical surgery using appropriate distal margins and sound TME technique can control rectal cancers confined to the mesorectum with limited distal spread. One can argue that performing a wide lateral dissection or TME while limiting the distal margins could be considered the "optimal" surgery for a patient with newly diagnosed rectal cancer. Radical surgery (TME and appropriate distal margin) should be the minimum standard for any surgery-first approach but this tactic omits critical nuances with regard to location, radial margin, and stage. Preoperative knowledge of stage and location of the tumor are required to know when it is appropriate to perform surgery first. Surgery-first approach should primarily be reserved for selected patients with early stage rectal cancers preferably in a high location when sphincter preservation is contemplated. Surgery first approach in early stage (T2N0) low rectal cancers is reasonable if low pelvic anastomosis is safe or not desired, such as in the setting of incontinence. Up-front surgery for advanced stage disease cannot be advocated if any adverse features are present, such as anticipated positive margin (lateral or distal) or node-positive disease where induction therapy has been proven to be more effective.

PRESENTATION AND CLINICAL EXAMINATION

The presentation of rectal cancer can vary widely from a completely asymptomatic patient undergoing screening examination to the symptomatic mass with bleeding or impending obstruction. Many referrals are accompanied by endoscopic and histologic diagnosis. Most surgeons who are comfortable treating rectal cancer should also be comfortable repeating the clinical and endoscopic examination. Much is written about the optimal examination technique with regards to physical and endoscopic assessment. Regardless of preference and level of comfort with differing techniques, several important features (**Table 1**) need to be assessed by the operating surgeon. My preferred work-up includes obtaining a pertinent clinical history and performing a detailed rectal examination followed by limited endoscopy (flexible sigmoidoscopy) at the initial clinic visit.

- *Patient features:* sphincter strength and function, frailty with regard to multimodality tolerance, and risk of pelvic anastomosis leak and protective measures to include temporary or permanent ostomy.
- *Rectal examination:* distance of tumor to sphincter, tumor mobile or fixed, if fixed to sphincter or lateral pelvis sidewall, radial location of tumor (anterior, posterior), and transanal options if early stage.
- *Endoscopic examination:* measurement of proximal and distal tumor extent, rectal wall involvement limited or circumferential; tattoo marking if considering induction therapy; potential for obstruction; risk of bleeding; repeat biopsy may be indicated to prove invasive malignancy or differentiate squamous or adenocarcinoma histology.

ANATOMY OF THE RECTUM

There is still an active and ongoing debate regarding the definition of the rectum. At the simplest level, the rectum begins where the sigmoid colon ends but how to define this

Table 1
Initial treatment by stage, early verses advanced

	Early Stage T1 or T2 and N0	Advanced Stage T3 or T4 or N+ or + CRM
Low <10 cm	Surgery: TME and 1-cm DRM transanal resection (only T1)	Long-course XRT Total neoadjuvant therapy No role for surgery first
High >10 cm	Surgery: TME and 1-cm DRM sphincter preservation	Short or long course XRT Total neoadjuvant therapy Surgery followed by adjuvant chemo[a]

[a] Stage II only in European centers of excellence where surgical technique is optimized and institutionally reproducible.[10] XRT, radiation therapy.

anatomic location clinically is controversial. With high rectal cancer, clear differentiation between the sigmoid colon and the rectum is difficult. Body habitus (obesity, height), sex (male, female), and measurement tool (ridged or flexible endoscopy, MRI) may influence the assessment of this anatomic boundary and a simplistic 12- or 15-cm delineation may be inaccurate. For example, a thin short female may have a sigmoid cancer at less than 12 cm, whereas a morbidly obese tall male may have a rectal cancer greater than 15 cm. Most nationally recognized guidelines select either 12 or 15 cm to mark the clear difference between colon and rectum without regard to overlapping lesions or patient variability. National Surgical Adjuvant Breast and Bowel Project defined rectal cancer inclusion in R-04 as "tumor located less than 12 cm from the anal verge."[5] The National Comprehensive Cancer Network guidelines provide the following definitions: "rectum is the last part of the large intestine and is about 5 inches long" and "portion of bowel located below the pelvic inlet (an imaginary line drawn from the sacral promontory to the top of the pubic symphysis)."[6] In a recent consensus paper, more than 11 different definitions were used to define the rectum using differing anatomic landmarks and/or modalities including endoscopy, computed tomography (CT), and MRI.[7] Based on expert review, this group defined the rectum as "below the sigmoid take off," where this boundary is defined by the junction of the mesocolon and mesorectum. MRI is the preferred modality to define this division point over alternative common criteria, such as 12 cm or 15 cm from anal verge, anterior peritoneal reflection, or sacral promontory. This definition requires cross-sectional imaging, preferably MRI to determine and accurately assess (**Fig. 1**). Previously cited definitions may be easier to use but are more likely to include sigmoid cancers in a rectal definition than would be defined using the sigmoid take off by MRI. The importance of clearly defining a sigmoid lesion from a rectal lesion is to avoid including a sigmoid cancer in the complexities of rectal cancer treatment. Overlapping tumors straddling the junction of the sigmoid and rectum would require judgment where a conservative clinical recommendation would be to treat as high rectal cancer that many benefit from multimodality therapy.

The rectum is subdivided into three zones often referred to as low (0–5 cm), mid (5–10 cm), and high (10–15 cm) when measured from the anal verge.[8] A bimodal description defines low rectal cancers between 0 and 7 cm (up to 10 cm) and high rectal cancers greater than this level until the sigmoid is reached. It is critically important to determine the anal verge or 0 cm location on external clinical examination. The rectal sphincters always reside within the low rectal zone but may vary in the thin patient from 0 to 2 cm compared with the obese patient 2 to 4 cm, where the anal verge is

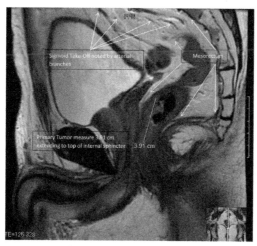

Fig. 1. Sigmoid mesorectum and rectal mesorectum are defined by MRI to identify the boundaries of the rectum. This is most important to avoid including sigmoid cancers into the complexities of rectal cancer treatment.

often difficult to visualize and measure because of gluteal folds. Anal sphincters are fortunately easier to appreciate and when considering sphincter-preserving surgery the most critical measurement is the distance between the superior aspect of the internal sphincter and the inferior aspect of the tumor. This distance either accommodates or cannot accommodate the pelvic anastomosis with regard to adequate margins and sphincter function. Low tumors often require APR because of sphincter involvement; midtumors may require downstaging and accepting minimal margins to accommodate the low pelvic anastomosis. In general any palpable tumor (assuming the average surgeon's index finger is 8–10 cm) should be defined as either low/midrectal cancer where there is risk of sphincter loss either anatomic or functional. However, any tumor above digit reach should technically have adequate margin for sphincter preservation with or without downstaging. Unfortunately, patient variability with regard to obesity, sex, and stature can greatly impact surgical options.

RADIOLOGIC STAGING: COMPUTED TOMOGRAPHY, MRI, AND ENDOSCOPIC RECTAL ULTRASOUND

Radiologic staging of a newly diagnosed rectal cancer is sound basic practice. The "symptomatic cancer" cannot be rationalized as a reason for omitting preoperative staging. A good quality CT of the chest/abdomen and pelvis with contrast should be the initial test to rule out metastatic disease and/or identify locally advanced disease. Tumor location can often be identified but tumor staging (T and N stage) is notoriously inaccurate with CT alone (**Fig. 2**). PET imaging is not recommended or indicated unless CT scan identifies equivocal findings that may impact on decisions regarding treatment.

Any tumor that falls within rectal boundaries (discussed previously) should be staged with either endoscopic rectal ultrasound (ERUS) or rectal MRI (preferred). Complete tumor staging includes defining three distinct items: (1) T stage, (2) N stage, and (3) the circumferential margin status (clear or involved). Exact tumor location is measured well in relation to anal verge and sphincter complex. When staging

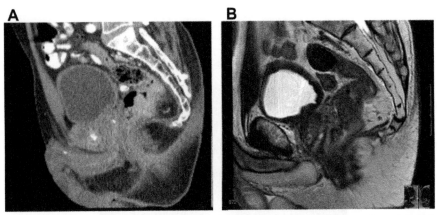

Fig. 2. (*A*) Comparison between staging CT and MRI. CT demonstrates circumferential thickening for rectum consistent with known rectal malignancy. No anatomy is seen with regard to prostate, bladder, or seminal vesicle involvement. (*B*) MRI demonstrates distance from tumor to sphincter is 2.7 cm with mesorectal fat involvement (T3); enlarges abnormal superior rectal lymph nodes (N1) with clear circumferential margin.

demonstrates locally advanced disease then upfront chemoradiotherapy should be considered. Differing modalities have differing sensitivities and specificities that favor one modality over another. Overall MRI was favored as the best modality to locally stage rectal cancer in a recent consensus expert panel; 91% of experts favored MRI over ERUS or CT alone for local staging.[9] MRI plus ERUS was recommended in early stage disease to better define the invasion of muscularis mucosa when local resection is contemplated. ERUS is superior at distinguishing T1 from T2 tumors with a specificity approaching 86% as compared with MRI at 69%.[10] ERUS primary utility is to confirm suspected T1 lesion when transanal resection is contemplated. Where MRI is far superior to all other modalities is assessing the circumferential margin, which can predict a positive surgical margin despite TME (**Fig. 3**). ERUS and CT are not able to identify the mesorectal fascia and in locally advanced disease fail to identify CRM involvement. Rectal MRI has supplanted ERUS for staging of most rectal cancers being enrolled in clinical trials. MRI for rectal cancer requires an experienced radiologist to protocol the study and interpret the results. Regardless of the modality selected, proper quality control is critical to meet and attain the specificities and sensitivities reported in published series. A well done MRI provides excellent local staging (T stage and CRM involvement) and clearly documented anatomic location with regard to sphincter complex. With regard to lymph node metastasis, all modalities are equally insensitive in the range of 55% to 69%.[9] Lymph node size alone cannot be used to distinguish between benign reactive or malignant. ERUS and MRI can distinguish specific morphologic criteria (irregular borders or mixed signal intensity) within the lymph node and have better specificity as compared with CT scanning. Small lymph nodes can still harbor malignant cells and an unremarkable lymph node pattern on imaging cannot be used to justify limiting full nodal clearance with TME techniques.

In summary, MRI is favored by expert panels and is mandatory in clinical trials; MRI provides accurate T stage and CRM involvement in advanced disease. MRI can determine sphincter involvement and or clearance. ERUS is a useful adjunct in early stage disease where local treatment is contemplated. Nodal staging is frequently inaccurate and may lead to understaging/overstaging with all modalities.

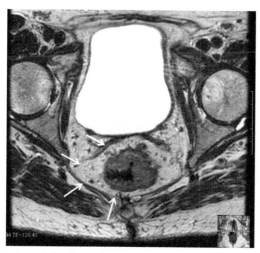

Fig. 3. Clear visualization of the circumferential radial margin (*arrows*) is identified in a patient with low rectal cancer T3N1. CT and ERUS fail to clearly identify this margin and when involved with tumor result in positive radial margin despite sound TME.

TREATMENT

Rectal cancer is organized into four distinct groups based on specific identifiable features that include stage early or advanced and location high or low. Using this framework, four discrete treatment pathways are followed that ensures appropriate surgical treatment that maximizes effective use of multimodality chemoradiation therapy. Disease stage is dichotomized into early and advanced with main diverting element being the utility of adjuvant therapy be it in the preoperative or postoperative setting. In general, stage I (T1 or T2 and N0) is the only stage that requires no additional therapy and surgery alone is indicated. Advanced stages in rectal cancer includes all stages higher than stage I to include stage II (T3 or T4 N0), stage III (any N+), and stage IV (any M+) where surgery alone is almost universally inferior. Location simply refers to the proximity to the anal sphincters, as discussed previously. In general, when a lesion is palpable (less than 8–10 cm) it should be considered low and carries a higher risk of local recurrence and sphincter loss or poor function. Sphincter preservation or sphincter loss needs to be addressed in terms of surgical planning and patient consent. In all advanced stages, multimodality therapy is indicated and selecting the sequence is critically important. However, the high rectal lesion should be more amenable to surgical resection with lower risk of recurrence and lower risk of sphincter loss especially in early stage disease. Timing of multimodality therapy is more forgiving the higher the lesion in question as detailed in **Table 1**.

Early Stage Low Rectal Cancer

Surgery alone should be considered the standard therapy for early stage cancer determined by ERUS or MRI to be T1 or T2 N0 lesion where primary low anastomosis is technically possible. The CRM should be clear of tumor for any early stage disease confined to the rectal wall. Functional outcomes vary directly with status of baseline sphincter function, which needs to be assessed carefully. Stage I (T1N0 and T2N0) rectal cancers treated with complete TME and low anterior resection with primary anastomosis plus or minus temporary diversion provides excellent oncologic outcome. There is strong evidence that distal margin of 1 cm is sufficient in preventing local recurrence (**Fig. 4**). There is no role for adjuvant chemotherapy or radiation therapies if surgery is technically sound; no perforation, intact mesorectum, and adequate lymph node harvest. Surgery alone demonstrates excellent long-term oncologic results and should act as a baseline to compare lesser treatments discussed next.

Radical surgery is the clear option for the healthy young patient where sphincter preservation is possible (eg, the 45-year-old thin woman with a T2 lesion at 8 cm where a standard low anterior resection with low anastomosis is associated with excellent functional and oncologic outcomes). Unfortunately, the low rectal cancer at the sphincter level poses a particular problem where complete resection requires perineal resection with permanent end colostomy to achieve a negative margin. Even with aggressive surgery, the low tumor anatomy is associated with higher local recurrence.[11] Worse outcome is postulated to be related to technical factors related to difficultly clearing the lateral margins or coning down and/or inadvertent rectal wall perforations at tumor site (see discussion regarding extralevator planes). Early stage disease at the sphincter complex level suffers from undesirable local recurrence and morbidity of perineal wound and permanent stoma.

Alternatives have evolved to address these issues but careful selection and execution are required to avoid local recurrence in an otherwise curable disease. Local full-thickness excision has been extensively studied. For ERUS staged Tis or T1 lesions, full-thickness negative margin resection has excellent long-term oncologic and functional outcome. There are clear indications for transanal resection but more importantly clear contraindications. Lesions must have favorable criteria: no unfavorable histology to include poorly differentiated histology, lymphovascular, or perineural invasion; less than 30% wall involvement; and favorable location and size.[12] Until recently, only the low rectal lesion was accessible via the transanal approach. Today higher

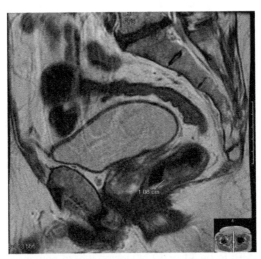

Fig. 4. Low rectal cancer 1.08 cm from superior aspect of internal sphincter T2N0. Limited sphincter margins for sphincter-preserving anterior resection and poor candidate for transanal resection (T2N0). Patient received chemoradiation therapy that resulted in a complete response and is undergoing active surveillance without resection. Based on recent meta-analysis the risk of local recurrence is 22.1% with 96% of recurrences occurring within the first 3 years.

lesions are amendable to full-thickness minimally invasive approach. Of special note, for higher lesions where full-thickness resection is planned, the lesion in question should still be below the peritoneal reflection to avoid entering the peritoneal cavity. With full-thickness margin negative resection the local recurrence rates are predictably favorable in properly selected patients and technically successful surgery.[13]

When an endoscopic lesion cannot be proved to harbor malignancy yet is not amendable to endoscopic resection, a transanal resection can furnish and confirm final pathology. If the transanal resection meets favorable criteria (T1 full thickness and margin negative) then treatment is complete. If a poorly differentiated lymphovascular invasion other high-risk feature T1 or any T2 lesion is found, then local recurrence is unacceptably high using transanal resection alone; recurrence rate between 20% and 30% for otherwise curable disease.[14] The full-thickness transanal resection may also complicate subsequent surgery and anastomosis; it is best to avoid falling into these clinical situations than trying to rectify them. To avoid falling into this trap, consider limited resection of the low rectal lesion for histologic assessment followed by ERUS and staged transanal resection of only confirmed early stage (less than T2) well-differentiated rectal adenocarcinomas. This is also one way to avoid performing a full-thickness resection of an unanticipated squamous anal cancer, which unfortunately only complicates and delays the necessary and more effective treatment.

One of the most vexing clinical situations is the early stage unfavorable histology or T2 rectal cancer low within the sphincter zone. Transanal resection is associated with unacceptable recurrence rates for what should be curable disease. Use of chemoradiation therapy for stage I disease is not clearly indicated off clinical trial. The updated results of ACOSOG Z6041 conclude that organ preservation following chemoradiation therapy can be offered in selected patients who refuse or are not candidates for transabdominal resection.[15] Preoperative downstaging treatment followed by full-thickness resection may be discussed on an individual basis at multidisciplinary format. How to manage the complete response to treatment adds further winkle to this particular scenario. Long-term survival in patients demonstrating a complete response to induction therapy is maturing. A recent meta-analysis examining the oncologic and survival outcomes of the watch and wait approach demonstrated that 22.4% of patients achieve an early clinical complete response and of those only 22.1% fail locally. Salvage surgery was possible in 88% and the 3-year overall survival was 93.5%.[16] This analysis was not limited to early stage disease but provides an excellent reference when debating surgery for curable early stage disease. Until that time, patient counseling regarding radical resection with colostomy needs to be balanced uncertainty of lesser surgery or even observation for a highly curable disease.

Early Stage High Rectal Cancer

Early stage high rectal cancers should be treated in manner similar to distal colon cancers. Based on preoperative staging and height assessment (distance from anal verge) the surgical and functional outcomes should be excellent. A significant difference between surgical treatments of the high rectal cancer verses sigmoid colon cancer is obtaining reasonable distal margin and adequate mesorectal clearance. In colonic tumors, the recommended margin of 5 cm remains primarily to ensure adequate lymph node clearance in a location where 5-cm margins should not compromise the anastomosis. Adequate mesorectal clearance remains critically important even when margins are limited to obtain adequate representative nodal stations. In the high rectal cancer resection, 1-cm margin length plus mesorectal clearance are equally important. CRM should be clear in all early stage rectal cancers if complete and technically sound TME is undertaken. Unfortunately, despite TME being established and taught in surgical residency for decades the completeness of the mesorectal envelope remains incomplete or violated at an alarming rate. Variability in training, level of experience, and technical expertise are important when approaching the high early rectal cancer. Measuring and documenting your institution and individual rate of complete mesorectal envelope provides an excellent quality measure and should be actively monitored and improved on. A safe and adequate resection of a high rectal cancer should not compromise adequate lymph node clearance, sphincter preservation, and pelvic anastomosis. Low pelvic anastomosis with inherent risk of leaks and functional issues unfortunately remains.

Final pathology may confirm or in some cases alter clinical staging, in which case further therapy is necessary. For example, should final pathology identify T3 or N1 disease, proper adherence to surgical standards is paramount. The surgeon must ensure that the CRM and DRM margins are clear and adequate lymph nodes are harvested (by convention 12 or more). In summary, for early stage high rectal cancer optimal surgery should cure most patients. When final pathology identifies more advanced disease, the initial surgery must be of adequate quality to ensure that local recurrence is minimized and to be followed by effective adjuvant therapy.

Late-Stage Low Rectal Cancer

Late-stage low rectal cancer benefits most from early induction chemoradiotherapy followed by radical resection. Local and distant recurrences remain problematic and one of the most important surgical roles is to execute required surgical procedures with minimal morbidity to enable ongoing and timely treatment. Complete staging and careful assessment of local symptoms (bleeding or obstruction) are paramount. In a symptomatic case, laparoscopic diverting colostomy is more appropriate than surgical resection when facing positive CRM, extensive nodal disease, or sphincter involvement.

Rectal MRI is extremely helpful at assessing tumor involvement of the circumferential margin, adjacent organs, and sphincters. Surgical margins and en bloc multiorgan resections are used to achieve a negative margin but only in an optimized situation and following completed induction therapy, most commonly long-course chemoradiotherapy. It is important to recognize that in the advanced setting disease distal margins do not conform to standard 1 cm required for early stage disease. Before induction therapy numerous authors demonstrated that between 5% and 10% of advanced rectal cancers extend beyond 1 cm.[3,17,18] The benefits of induction therapy are to obtain distal margin clearance where sphincter loss or positive margin is anticipated. When the DRM or sphincters are involved, then long-course radiation therapy and or systemic therapy may provide vital downstaging of the margin before surgery. In advanced but resectable low rectal cancer, technical factors play an important role in controlling recurrence. Bowel perforation during resection must be avoided by staying lateral to the sphincter complex during the perineal portion. In recent national audit 20.9% of perineal resections suffered from positive circumferential margin.[19] Technical factors to include anorectal perforation and thinning of rectal wall because of coning in on sphincters are postulated to be causative and may be equally important as tumor biology. Extralevator dissection with en bloc resection of exterior sphincters and levators can decrease positive circumferential margins.[20] Unfortunately, this technique alone has not improved disease-free survival or overall survival when comparing standard APR resection with extralevator APR.[21,22] Optimization of induction therapy plus adequate technically sound radical resection is the best means of controlling local disease to counter for adverse tumor biology.

There is active debate regarding the management of complete clinical response to induction therapy where the experience with wait and watch is maturing. The survival data and salvage therapy are promising in highly selected cases. Selecting a safe subgroup to monitor without performing surgical resection requires compliant patients, frequent follow-up, and critical decision making on recurrence.

Late-Stage High Rectal Cancer

Late-stage high rectal cancer with positive CRM or DRM involvement (beyond 1 cm) are clear indication for delaying surgical treatment in favor of induction therapy, either chemoradiation therapy or chemotherapy. Any positive margin is associated with early recurrence and cancer-related death.[23] Nodal involvement, although inaccurate in clinical staging (discussed previously), should also favor preoperative therapy to avoid requiring postoperative pelvic radiation and inherent delays in treatment related to anastomotic complications. Preoperative radiation ensures that rectal primary is radiated and thus derives a benefit from downstaging while protecting the small bowel that resides in the pelvis following surgery. Short- or long-course radiation therapy is used if the CRM is clear. When the CRM is involved, then long-course radiation therapy and/or systemic therapy may provide vital downstaging of this margin before surgery. North American surgical oncology and colorectal communities favor induction therapy before surgery for almost all locally advanced rectal cancers. In cases with clear CRM and adequate distal margin, short-course radiation therapy is a reasonable option because downstaging is not required to achieve an R0 resection. European centers of excellence often recommend up front surgery followed by adjuvant chemotherapy in instances where MRI staging is favorable and technical factors are institutionally controlled.[9] The results of up front chemotherapy and selective use of radiation have been examined in a recent clinical trial.[24] The result and conclusions will be forthcoming in the near future. Total neoadjuvant therapy followed by surgery is an active area of clinical study.[25]

The utility of long- or short-course radiation therapy or preoperative systemic therapy should be discussed in a multidisciplinary fashion because each has merits and risks. Clinical trials presently cannot clearly advocate for one modality of induction therapy over another: combined chemoradiation, chemotherapy and selective radiation, or long- or short-course radiation. In the near future, clinical trial results may further define the optimal modality. The surgeon must first decide if adjuvant therapy is required, then consider the merits and risk of the differing modalities. Items to consider in multidisciplinary discussion include: radiation therapy should be delivered in a preoperative setting if deemed necessary, postoperative radiation should be avoided whenever possible, short-course radiation treatment does not provide downstaging but likely provides equivalent oncologic results, and duration of systemic chemotherapy (3 months vs 6 months) is proving equivalent in the adjuvant setting. Taken together, we have recently seen promising results in treating high rectal cancers (T3N0M0) with short-course radiation therapy followed by surgery and 3 months of systemic chemotherapy with excellent oncologic and functional outcome (**Fig. 5**). The benefits of this regimen are that it uses all effective modalities, minimizes long-term neuropathy, decreases radiation duration and time to surgery significantly, and decreases total treatment time from 10 to 12 months to 4 to 6 months.

Metastatic Rectal Cancer

In the metastatic setting the surgeon must balance symptom control with treatment delays that result from complications related to either the symptomatic tumor or surgical complications. Obstruction warrants diverting colostomy rather than radical

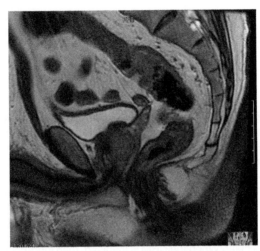

Fig. 5. High advanced rectal cancer overlapping rectosigmoid distribution. Superior aspect of tumor falls within distribution of sigmoid mesentery, and the inferior aspect within mesorectal distribution. Patient received short-course radiation therapy followed by surgery and 3 months of adjuvant therapy bringing the duration of treatment to 4 to 6 months.

resection in all advanced low tumors. Obstruction and bleeding in a high lesion may be the only clinical presentation where surgical resection should be contemplated and risk of surgery must be balanced with inherent risk of delays in treatment. It is critically important to acknowledge that multimodality treatment of advanced rectal cancers is excellent and may provide years of effective disease control. Surgical resection of rectal primary may have a clear role once disease control is established, most commonly through effective multiagent chemotherapy. Proper timing and use of radiation therapy is helpful, and active surgical participation is required. Controlling metastatic disease may ultimately enable curative options and when this is not possible, palliative management of pelvic disease still plays a role in controlling often disabling pain and poor quality end of life.

FINAL RECOMMENDATIONS

All patients with a newly diagnosed rectal cancer should be carefully assessed for tumor stage and location before surgical treatment. Most effective staging modality requires CT chest/abdomen/pelvis with intravenous contrast and rectal MRI and selective use of ERUS in early stage disease. Up front surgery cannot control locally advanced disease and multimodality treatments are highly effective. Taken together, careful preoperative planning and multidisciplinary treatment options should be favored over expedited surgical treatments. Up front surgery is indicated in select clinical scenarios with carefully assessed patient presentations. When sphincter preservation is not at stake (high rectal cancer or medical necessity for colostomy) margins between 1 and 2 cm provide greater than 95% local control. TME dissection should extend beyond the distal margin for safe mesorectal control. Wider margins may benefit patients with more advanced-stage disease. At lower levels where sphincter preservation becomes dependent on margin status, lesser margins provide near equivalent local control at 1 cm and even closer. Negative margin is essential because a prohibitively high rate of local failure occurs with a positive radial or distal margin. The surgeon's role is to execute a technically sound radical resection, wide lateral dissection, and limiting the distal margins, using preoperative adjuvant therapy when indicated to ensure optimal local control.

DISCLOSURE

The author has nothing to disclose.

REFERENCES

1. Galler AS, Petrelli NJ, Shakamuri SP. Rectal cancer surgery: a brief history. Surg Oncol 2011;20(4):223–30.
2. Lange MM, Rutten HJ, van de Velde CJ. One hundred years of curative surgery for rectal cancer: 1908-2008. Eur J Surg Oncol 2009;35(5):456–63.
3. Williams NS, Dixon MF, Johnston D. Reappraisal of the 5 centimetre rule of distal excision for carcinoma of the rectum: a study of distal intramural spread and of patients' survival. Br J Surg 1983;70(3):150–4.
4. Heald RJ, Moran BJ, Ryall RD, et al. Rectal cancer: the Basingstoke experience of total mesorectal excision, 1978-1997. Arch Surg 1998;133(8):894–9.
5. NSABP clinical trials overview: protocol R-04. Available at: http://www.nsabp.pitt.edu/R-04.asp. Accessed January 27, 2020.
6. NCCN guidelines version 1.2020 rectal cancer. Available at: https://www.nccn.org/professionals/physician_gls/default.aspx#rectal. Accessed January 27, 2020.
7. D'Souza N, de Neree Tot Babberich MPM, d'Hoore A, et al. Definition of the rectum: an international, expert-based Delphi consensus. Ann Surg 2019; 270(6):955–9.
8. Costa-Silva L, Brown G. Magnetic resonance imaging of rectal cancer. Magn Reson Imaging Clin N Am 2013;21(2):385–408.
9. Lutz MP, Zalcberg JR, Glynne-Jones R, et al. Second St. Gallen European Organisation for Research and Treatment of Cancer Gastrointestinal Cancer Conference: consensus recommendations on controversial issues in the primary treatment of rectal cancer. Eur J Cancer 2016;63:11–24 [published correction appears in Eur J Cancer. 2016 Nov;68:208-209].
10. Bipat S, Glas AS, Slors FJ, et al. Rectal cancer: local staging and assessment of lymph node involvement with endoluminal US, CT, and MR imaging–a meta-analysis. Radiology 2004;232(3):773–83.
11. Prytz M, Angenete E, Ekelund J, et al. Extralevator abdominoperineal excision (ELAPE) for rectal cancer: short-term results from the Swedish Colorectal Cancer Registry. Selective use of ELAPE warranted. Int J Colorectal Dis 2014;29(8): 981–7.
12. São Julião GP, Celentano JP, Alexandre FA, et al. Local excision and endoscopic resections for early rectal cancer. Clin Colon Rectal Surg 2017;30(5):313–23.
13. Monson JR, Weiser MR, Buie WD, et al, Standards Practice Task Force of the American Society of Colon and Rectal Surgeons. Practice parameters for the management of rectal cancer (revised). Dis Colon Rectum 2013;56(5):535–50.
14. Steele GD Jr, Herndon JE, Bleday R, et al. Sphincter-sparing treatment for distal rectal adenocarcinoma. Ann Surg Oncol 1999;6(5):433–41.
15. Garcia-Aguilar J, Renfro LA, Chow OS, et al. Organ preservation for clinical T2N0 distal rectal cancer using neoadjuvant chemoradiotherapy and local excision (ACOSOG Z6041): results of an open-label, single-arm, multi-institutional, phase 2 trial. Lancet Oncol 2015;16(15):1537–46.

16. Dattani M, Heald RJ, Goussous G, et al. Oncological and survival outcomes in watch and wait patients with a clinical complete response after neoadjuvant chemoradiotherapy for rectal cancer: a systematic review and pooled analysis. Ann Surg 2018;268(6):955–67.

17. Kwok SP, Lau WY, Leung KL, et al. Prospective analysis of the distal margin of clearance in anterior resection for rectal carcinoma. Br J Surg 1996;83(7):969–72.

18. Shirouzu K, Isomoto H, Kakegawa T. Distal spread of rectal cancer and optimal distal margin of resection for sphincter-preserving surgery. Cancer 1995;76(3): 388–92.

19. Rickles AS, Dietz DW, Chang GJ, et al. High rate of positive circumferential resection margins following rectal cancer surgery: a call to action. Ann Surg 2015; 262(6):891–8.

20. West NP, Anderin C, Smith KJ, et al, European Extralevator Abdominoperineal Excision Study Group. Multicentre experience with extralevator abdominoperineal excision for low rectal cancer. Br J Surg 2010;97(4):588–99.

21. Klein M, Colov E, Gögenur I. Similar long-term overall and disease-free survival after conventional and extralevator abdominoperineal excision-a nationwide study. Int J Colorectal Dis 2016;31(7):1341–7.

22. Lehtonen T, Räsänen M, Carpelan-Holmström M, et al. Oncological outcomes before and after the extralevator abdominoperineal excision era in rectal cancer patients treated with abdominoperineal excision in a single centre, high volume unit. Colorectal Dis 2019;21(2):183–90.

23. Nelson H, Petrelli N, Carlin A, et al. Guidelines 2000 for colon and rectal cancer surgery. J Natl Cancer Inst 2001;93(8):583–96.

24. Prospect: chemotherapy alone or chemotherapy plus radiation therapy in treating patients with locally advanced rectal cancer undergoing surgery. Available at: https://clinicaltrials.gov/ct2/show/NCT01515787. Accessed Jaunary 27, 2020.

25. Veliparib, pembrolizumab, and combination chemotherapy in treating patient with locally advanced rectal cancer. Available at: https://clinicaltrials.gov/ct2/show/NCT02921256. Accessed Jaunary 27, 2020.

Anal Cancer

Anne N. Young, MD, MSCR*, Elizabeth Jacob, MD, Patrick Willauer, MD,
Levi Smucker, MD, Raul Monzon, MD, Luis Oceguera, MD

KEYWORDS

- Anal cancer • Squamous cell carcinoma • Anal canal • Adenocarcinoma

KEY POINTS

- Define the anatomy of the anal canal.
- Discuss the main types of anal canal carcinomas and their treatment.
- Discuss evaluation and management of a patient with suspected anal cancer.

INTRODUCTION

As of 2019, anal cancer has approximately 8300 new cases diagnosed annually and causes approximately 1200 deaths a year. It is a rare cancer that comprises approximately 3% of all gastrointestinal malignancies.[1] The anatomy of the anal canal and histology of the cells within it play a role in guiding diagnosis and determining therapy. Unfortunately, in the United States, women and patients of lower socioeconomic status present with more advanced stages of anal cancer, hence are more likely to die from it than men and patients with a higher socioeconomic status.[2]

Patients with anal cancer present with a variety of symptoms that frequently are confused with benign anorectal disease, usually hemorrhoids. Rectal bleeding, pain, and pruritus are the most common presenting symptoms. A high index of suspicion is needed in those at high risk for anal cancer, who include patients with untreated human immunodeficiency virus, those who are immunocompromised, men who have sex with men, women with cervical cancer, patients with a history of radiation to the pelvis and rectal region, and people with history of human papillomavirus (HPV). HPV has been associated with up to 93% of anal squamous cell carcinomas (SCCs).[3]

The anatomy of the anal canal gives insight into the tumor origin and treatment. The anal canal is 3.5 cm to 4 cm in total length and can be divided in 2: the anatomic canal and the surgical canal. The anatomic canal is 2 cm from the dentate or pectineal line and extends distally to the anal verge. The surgical canal is defined as the region from the dentate line, extending 2 cm proximal to the anorectal ring. The superior extent of the surgical canal can be palpated on digital rectal examination as a tight muscular

General Surgery Department, Bassett Medical Center, 1 Atwell Road, Cooperstown, NY 13326, USA
* Corresponding author.
E-mail address: anne.young@bassett.org

Surg Clin N Am 100 (2020) 629–634
https://doi.org/10.1016/j.suc.2020.02.007
0039-6109/20/© 2020 Elsevier Inc. All rights reserved.

surgical.theclinics.com

junction, and it represents where the rectum enters the puborectalis sling. The distinction between the anatomic and surgical canal is the dentate line, and this is clinically important because it marks the transition in mucosa, and, therefore, the types of tumors that arise from the different cell types. The cell types from the proximal region of the canal to the distal area are glandular, transitional, and squamous. Subsequently, these cell types give rise to adenocarcinoma, basaloid or nonkeratinizing SCC, and keratinizing SCC.

The dentate line also is important because it distinguishes the lymphatic drainage of tumors that occur proximal or distal to this landmark. If a tumor originates above the dentate line, it tends to drain into the internal iliac nodes. If a tumor originates below the dentate line, lymphatic drainage tends to be into the inguinal nodes. This distinction is relevant for adequate treatment.

The anal margin extends from the anal verge distally toward the perineum and is defined as skin tissue within 5 cm to 6 cm of the anal verge (**Fig. 1**). The cell type here is keratinizing squamous cells containing hair follicles. Cancers arising from this area are perianal skin cancers and are treated as skin cancers like anywhere else in the body. Their treatment is not included in this review.

This article discusses the most commonly encountered anal canal tumors, the evaluation of these tumor, and their management. In general, the initial evaluation of a patient with a suspected anal canal cancer includes a thorough history and physical examination, including palpation of the inguinal node basins, inspection of the anal verge, digital rectal examination, and anoscopy. Diagnostic biopsies usually are obtained during a rectal examination under anesthesia, and endoscopic evaluation of

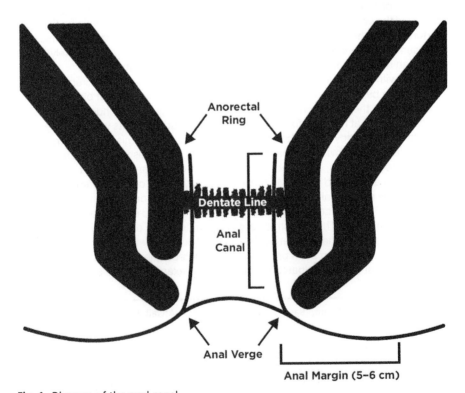

Fig. 1. Diagram of the anal canal.

the colon as indicated. Once a pathology diagnosis is made, imaging studies to define clinical staging include computed tomography scans of the chest, abdomen, and pelvis. A magnetic resonance image of the pelvis also is obtained to evaluate local invasion of the tumor and pelvic/inguinal lymph nodes. A positron emission tomography/computed tomography scan can be added for better evaluation of nodal status and evaluation of distant metastases. Staging is based on the size of the primary tumor, extent of lymph nodes involved, and presence of distant metastasis.

SQUAMOUS CELL CARCINOMA

SCC represents the most commonly found invasive cancer in the anal canal, making up 80% of all anal canal cancers.[4] There are 4 histologic subtypes—squamous, transition zone, basaloid or cloacagenic, and mucoepidermoid—all of which are evaluated and treated in the same way. Once pathologic diagnosis and the clinical staging have been completed, the treatment is based on the stage of the patient.

Treatment of SCC has dramatically changed over the past 40 years. Historically, treatment was based mostly on surgery, either local or radical excision with an abdominal perineal resection (APR). After the landmark work of Dr Nigro in the 1970s, however, treatment of SCC dramatically shifted to chemoradiation therapy, with improved outcomes.[5] Specifically, the Nigro protocol, as it is known, includes chemotherapy with 5-fluorouracil and mitomycin with 45 Gy to 60 Gy radiation and has resulted in 5-year overall survival rates in the range of 70% to 90%.[6] Current guidelines recommend that post-treatment evaluation begins with digital rectal examination (DRE) at 8 weeks to 12 weeks after completion of treatment. If there is a complete clinical response, then surveillance is recommended every 3 months to 6 months with DRE, palpation of inguinal lymph nodes, and anoscopy. If post-treatment evaluation suggests persistent disease, however, examination under anesthesia should be done to confirm. Patients should be followed for a maximum of 6 months after completion of the treatment, to assess for complete regression by the end of that interval. If there is persistent disease at 6 months, this indicates failure of chemoradiation alone. The patient should be re-evaluated for regional and distant metastases, and, if no metastases is identified, an APR should be considered.[7]

Local surgical excision can be offered to patients with superficially invasive SCCs, which are defined as tumors that are completely excised, with less than 3 mm of basement membrane invasion, and less than 7 mm of horizontal spread. In cases of recurrence after local excision, chemoradiation therapy should be considered. If there is failure to respond to this, then salvage therapy with an APR then is considered.

ADENOCARCINOMA

Primary anal canal adenocarcinoma is rare. It accounts for approximately 10% to 20% of anal cancers.[8] It is the second most common malignancy of the anal canal after SCC, but it is considered more aggressive. This malignancy arises histologically from glandular cells, which are found proximal to the dentate line. It is difficult to classify these cancers as either rectal or anal cancer, especially if the site of the tumor is at the anorectal junction, which is at the superior point of the surgical anal canal. It is for this reason that a majority of these types of cancers are considered to represent rectal cancers that have spread distally. To make the distinction, if the center of the tumor is 2 cm or more proximal to the anorectal ring, it is considered rectal cancer. If the center is within 2 cm or less from the dentate line, it is considered anal canal cancer.[7,8] This distinction is important because rectal adenocarcinoma follows a different TNM classification for staging. Risk factors specific to adenocarcinoma of the anal canal include a history of chronic inflammation, for example, Crohn disease, a history of anal fistulas, and a history of chronic fissures.

The treatment of a primary anal canal adenocarcinoma includes local surgical excision for T1 tumors and neoadjuvant chemoradiation therapy followed by radical surgical resection (APR) for all other tumors. Tumor stage and grade of differentiation, however, are the most significant prognostic factors for survival.

In addition to adenocarcinoma originating from the anal glands, there is a rare form of intraepithelial adenocarcinoma, known as extramammary Paget disease. This disease could originate from apocrine glands or develop as a result of underlying adenocarcinoma. Patients typically present with pruritus, anal tenderness, and bleeding. Physical examination reveals scaling and tan-colored plaques in the perineum. The treatment of Paget disease is wide local excision if it is determined there is no underlying malignancy on biopsy. If there is an underlying malignancy, this is managed with an APR.[9]

ANAL MELANOMA

Anal melanoma is another rare malignancy, representing 1% to 4% of all anal canal tumors and 0.3% of all melanomas. It is the most common location of malignant melanoma in the gastrointestinal tract. It carries a very poor prognosis, with 5-year survival typically 33%.[10]

It tends to affect whites and has a slight female predominance. It presents most commonly with anorectal bleeding, anal pain, change in bowel habits, a palpable mass, or tenesmus. Anal melanomas have varied appearances, from a small polypoid lesions to large ulcerated ones protruding into the rectal vault, most of which are pigmented. These lesions often are misdiagnosed as a thrombosed hemorrhoid and this delay in accurate diagnosis worsens their prognosis. Lymph node metastases are common at the time of presentation in the inguinal lymph nodes, internal iliac nodes, or mesorectal nodes.

Anal melanoma is staged and managed according to the current guidelines for cutaneous melanoma. Biopsy is recommended to confirm the suspected diagnosis. Histologic features, such as tumor with necrosis and perineural invasion, seems associated with increased relapse and low survival.

Anal melanoma typically is managed with excision. There is debate regarding whether to undertake wide local excision versus APR, because disease-specific survival between each does not seem to be significantly different.[11] Although APR provides better local control, overall survival does not seem to be affected by the type of operation as much as by margin status. Thus, wide local excision is recommended when technically feasible. Prognosis is based primarily on stage at time of presentation, and the 5-year survival rates for patients with local disease (defined as an invasive neoplasm confined to the organ of origin), regional spread (defined as an invasive neoplasm that extends directly into surrounding organs or tissues or to regional lymph nodes), and distant spread (defined as spread to parts of the body remote from the primary tumor) are 32%, 17%, and 0%, respectively.[12] Adjuvant chemotherapy and radiation are recommended based on patient stage.

BASAL CELL CARCINOMA

Basal cell carcinoma (BCC) of the anal canal accounts for 0.2% of all anal cancers.[13] BCC typically is found in areas of the skin with high ultraviolet light exposure. Risk factors for BCC include preexisting skin conditions, such as basal cell nevus syndrome or xeroderma pigmentosum, as well as any history of chronic inflammation, previous radiation, trauma, or burns. Similar to BCC found in other areas of the skin, these lesions typically present with a central ulceration and a raised pearly border. They commonly are misdiagnosed as hemorrhoids or anal fissures.

Biopsy is required for histology to distinguish this lesion from the basaloid variant of SCC, which has an earlier metastatic potential and a more aggressive course,[14] because BCC rarely invades or metastasizes. Per current guidelines, any anal canal BCC is considered a high-risk lesion. Although there is no defined margin for excision, wider surgical margins are recommended because a tumor may demonstrate subclinical extension. When the lesion extends into the anal canal and/or deep into the surrounding tissues, APR is recommended.

EXAMINATION AND SURGICAL TECHNIQUES

Anoscopy is the primary form of examination, usually preceded by digital rectal examination. For anoscopy, ensure that the patient is in the left lateral decubitus or jackknife position if tolerated. Also ensure that the anoscope is well lubricated, and that the obturator is fully inserted. Insert slowly after the relaxation of sphincter muscles. The obturator is taken out for examination of mucosa. The anoscope is removed completely prior to viewing a separate area of mucosa with reinsertion. This avoids rotation, which could lead to pinching and abrasions.

Wide local excision typically is performed for small tumors under the aforementioned indications during the time of rectal examination under anesthesia with the patient in the jackknife position. Electrocautery typically is used to extend incisions circumferentially and deep to the small lesion, taking care to avoid injury to sphincters. An anoscope may be used.

SUMMARY

Anal cancer, although rare, can prove to be a devastating diagnosis. It commonly is misdiagnosed as a benign lesion, resulting in delays in diagnosis and treatment. The foundation for successful therapy includes a timely diagnosis, accurate staging, and routine surveillance. Surgeons are encouraged to maintain a high degree of suspicion for malignancy and to have a low threshold to biopsy any anal canal lesions when indicated.

DISCLOSURE

The authors have nothing to disclose.

REFERENCES

1. American Cancer Society. Cancer facts & figures 2019. Atlanta (GA): American Cancer Society; 2019.
2. Celie KB, Jackson C, Agrawal S, et al. Socioeconomic and gender disparities in anal cancer diagnosis and treatment. Surg Oncol 2017;26(2):212–7.
3. Joseph DA, Miller JW, Wu X, et al. Understanding the burden of human papillomavirus-associated anal cancers in the US. Cancer 2008;113(10 Suppl): 2892.
4. Siegel RL, Miller KD, Jemal A. Cancer statistics, 2019. CA Cancer J Clin 2019; 69(1):7.
5. Leichman L, Nigro N, Vaitkevicius VK, et al. Cancer of the anal canal. Model for preoperative adjuvant combined modality therapy. Am J Med 1985;78(2):211.

6. Bartelink H, Roelofsen F, Eschwege F, et al. Concomitant radiotherapy and chemotherapy is superior to radiotherapy alone in the treatment of locally advanced anal cancer: results of a phase III randomized trial of the European Organization for Research and Treatment of Cancer Radiotherapy and Gastrointestinal Cooperative Groups. J Clin Oncol 1997;15:2040–9.

7. Edge SB, Byrd DR, Compton CC, et al, editors. American Joint Committee on cancer staging manual. 7th edition. New York: Springer; 2010. p. 165.

8. Anwar S, Welbourn H, Hill J, et al. Adenocarcinoma of the anal canal—a systematic review. Colorectal Dis 2013;15:1481–8.

9. McCarter MD, Quan SH, Busam K, et al. Long-term outcome of perianal Paget's disease. Dis Colon Rectum 2003;46:612–6.

10. Klas JV, Rothenberger DA, Wong WD, et al. Malignant tumors of the anal canal: the spectrum of disease, treatment, and outcomes. Cancer 1999;85(8):1686–93.

11. Malik A, Hull TL, Floruta C. What is the best surgical treatment for anorectal melanoma? Int J Colorectal Dis 2004;19(2):121–3.

12. Podnos YD, Tsai NC, Smith D, et al. Factors affecting survival in patients with anal melanoma. Am Surg 2006;72(10):917–20.

13. Beck DE, Roberts PL, Saclarides TJ, et al, editors. The ASCRS textbook of colon and rectal surgery. Springer Science & Business Media; 2011.

14. Graham RP, Arnold CA, Naini BV, et al. Basaloid squamous cell carcinoma of the anus revisited. Am J Surg Pathol 2016;40(3):354–60.

Neuroendocrine Tumors of the Pancreatobiliary and Gastrointestinal Tracts

Morgan Bonds, MD[a], Flavio G. Rocha, MD[a,b],*

KEYWORDS

- Neuroendocrine • Carcinoid • Small intestine • Pancreas • Appendix
- Liver metastases

KEY POINTS

- Incidence of neuroendocrine tumors is increasing.
- Somatostatin receptor PET is an ideal modality for localization and staging.
- Lymph node metastases are a significant predictor of recurrence and survival in gastro-enteropancreatic neuroendocrine tumors.
- Cytoreduction may improve overall survival in metastatic neuroendocrine tumors.

INTRODUCTION

Neuroendocrine tumors (NETs) are rare neoplasms of the gastroenteropancreatic tract. As a result, these tumors tend to be discovered incidentally, on either radiologic or pathologic review. The incidence of NETs in the gastroenteropancreatic tract has significantly increased since the 1970s, with many of these being localized at the time of diagnosis.[1,2] These factors lead to significant involvement from the general surgeon in the management of these tumors. This article focuses on recent updates in the pathophysiology, diagnosis, treatment, and prognosis of NETs of the pancreatobiliary (PB) and gastrointestinal (GI) tracts.

RELEVANT ANATOMY AND PATHOPHYSIOLOGY

Neuroendocrine cells arise from the neural crest cells of the embryonic ectoderm. They comprise 1% of the gut mucosa and 1% to 2% of the pancreatic gland volume; the extrahepatic bile duct mucosa also contains neuroendocrine cells.[3] In their normal state, different types of neuroendocrine cells produce specific hormones to aid in digestive or metabolic functions, such as gut motility, stimulation of digestive

[a] Section of General, Vascular, and Thoracic Surgery, Virginia Mason Medical Center, 1100 Ninth Avenue, CS-G6, Seattle, WA 98101, USA; [b] University of Washington, Seattle, WA, USA
* Corresponding author. 1100 Ninth Avenue, CS-G6, Seattle, WA 98101.
E-mail address: flavio.rocha@virginiamason.org

Surg Clin N Am 100 (2020) 635–648
https://doi.org/10.1016/j.suc.2020.02.010
0039-6109/20/© 2020 Elsevier Inc. All rights reserved.

enzymes, or glucose storage. Tumors can arise from any of these neuroendocrine cells, and as such, malignancies can develop throughout the gastroenteropancreatic tract (**Box 1**).

When NETs form, they can be nonfunctioning. Functioning tumors that arise in the midgut or hindgut do not result in symptoms because the liver removes the hormones from the blood, a phenomenon called first-pass effect. However, hormonal symptoms from these tumors can manifest once liver metastases have occurred and the excess hormones are able to enter the systemic circulation directly. **Table 1** lists the names of functioning NETs, the hormone produced, and possible primary tumor location.

CLINICAL PRESENTATION
Nonfunctioning

Nonfunctioning NETs typically have few associated symptoms in early stages. The most common presentation for these tumors is nonspecific abdominal pain that leads to cross-sectional imaging. Intestinal NETs may present with GI bleed and anemia. Occasionally, the NETs will grow large enough to obstruct the extrahepatic bile duct or the GI tract, causing jaundice or bowel obstruction, respectively. Many appendiceal NETs cause appendicitis-like symptoms (right lower quadrant pain and nausea). Rarely, an intraabdominal mass is palpated on physical examination, leading to further diagnostic workup.

Functioning

Patients with functioning NETs present symptoms of the excess hormones they produce. These symptoms are typically severe enough to initiate diagnostic workup; however, they may present with abdominal pain or obstructive symptoms as described above.

- Serotonin-producing (carcinoid): Presenting symptoms are diarrhea, sudden skin flushing, asthmalike wheezing/shortness of breath, and edema. This syndrome can also lead to right-sided heart valvular disease, resulting in these patients presenting with right-sided heart failure. It should be noted that these symptoms typically only present once distant metastases have developed.[4]
- Insulinoma: Patients with insulinomas present with symptoms of hypoglycemia due to excess insulin production. These symptoms include fatigue, anxiety, sweating, unsteadiness, pale skin, and new onset cardiac arrhythmias. Whipple triad is the classically described presentation of hyperinsulinemia: symptoms

---

Box 1
Anatomic locations pancreatobiliary and gastrointestinal of neuroendocrine tumors

Small intestine

Appendix

Colon

Rectum

Stomach

Pancreas

Extrahepatic bile ducts

Ampulla of Vater

Table 1
Functioning neuroendocrine tumors and primary location

Tumor Name	Hormone Produced	Primary Tumor Locations
Carcinoid[a]	Serotonin	Small intestine Appendix Colon Rectum Stomach Pancreas Ampulla of Vater Extrahepatic bile duct
Insulinoma	Insulin	Pancreas
Glucagonoma	Glucagon	Pancreas
Gastrinoma	Gastrin	Stomach Small intestine Pancreas Ampulla of Vater
Somatostatinoma	Somatostatin	Small intestine Pancreas Ampulla of Vater
VIPoma	Vasoactive intestinal peptide	Pancreas

[a] Symptoms only occur once distant metastases occur.

consistent with hypoglycemia, documented hypoglycemia (<55 mg/dL) when those symptoms are present, and resolution of symptoms with documented increase in blood glucose levels.[5] Excess insulin administration must be excluded by measuring c-peptide, a component of endogenous proinsulin molecules.

- Glucagonoma: The classic presentation for glucagonoma is necrolytic migratory erythema, stomatitis, weight loss, and diabetes.[6]
- Gastrinoma: This NET produces Zollinger-Ellison syndrome, which consists of abdominal pain from gastric ulcer, gastroesophageal reflux, and watery diarrhea.[7] Recalcitrant peptic ulcer disease should raise concern for the presence of a gastrinoma. This is the most common pancreatic NET in multiple endocrine neoplasia type 1.
- Somatostatinoma: Somatostatinoma is a rare NET that presents with hypochlorhydria, steatorrhea, and diabetes.[8]
- Vasoactive intestinal polypeptide (VIP)oma: These tumors secrete excess levels of vasoactive intestinal peptide that results in hypersecretory diarrhea similar to cholera. This results in weight loss and acute kidney injury.[9]

DIAGNOSTIC PROCEDURES

The diagnostic algorithm for gastroenteropancreatic NETs can be seen in **Fig. 1**. With the increased utilization of computed tomography (CT) imaging, nonfunctioning NETs tend to be found incidentally during the workup for vague symptoms. The use of intravenous contrast timed in both the arterial and the portal venous phase is instrumental in identifying these lesions because they tend to be hyperenhancing on arterial phase and isoenhancing in later phases. This characteristic holds true for NETs in all locations, as can be seen in **Fig. 2**. Benefits of CT include its wide availability, rapidity of the examination, and relative convenience for the patient. However, this modality

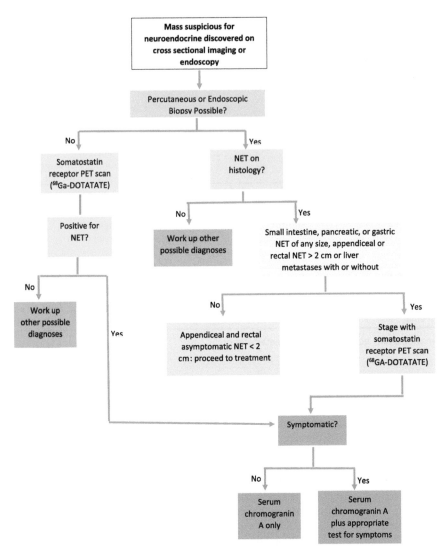

Fig. 1. Diagnostic procedures for suspected NET.

has a tendency to miss small liver metastases as well as primary tumors, especially in the small bowel.

MRI is an additional tool in the diagnosis of NETs. It is a particularly useful examination for investigating lesions in the liver. The use of hepatocyte-phase contrast has been shown to improve the contrast-to-noise ratio as well as increase interobserver agreement regarding the number and size of NET metastases in the liver when compared with intravenous contrast imaging alone.[10] The drawbacks of MRI are the prolonged test time and patient limitations (metallic implants, claustrophobia, or inability to hold breath).

Biopsy of suspected NETs is recommended when found on imaging or endoscopy. Biopsy allows for a definitive diagnosis to be established as well as evaluation of tumor

A   B

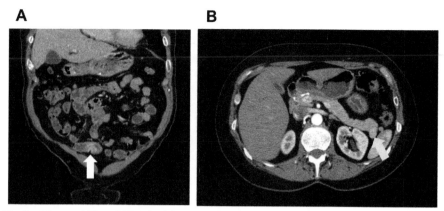

Fig. 2. CT scan of PB and GI NETs. (A) NET in the terminal ileum (*white arrow*). (B) PNET in the pancreatic tail (*yellow arrow*).

characteristics, such as grade, that can alter testing and treatment decisions. NETs of the colon, rectum, stomach, and duodenum can be biopsied via endoscopy, and this generally occurs at the time of discovery. Endoscopic ultrasound can provide access tumors in the pancreas. Liver metastases are best sampled percutaneously, although endoscopic ultrasound is a secondary option.

Tumor staging is not indicated for all NETs. Colorectal and appendiceal NETs that are smaller than 2 cm have very low potential for metastases; thus, these tumors do not require a complete staging workup. However, if a biopsy of these smaller tumors have high-risk features (high Ki67, poorly differentiated), staging should be considered. Tumors in the small bowel are typically diagnosed at a later stage because they are difficult to visualize on cross-sectional imaging and rarely cause symptoms until after they have metastasized (typically to lymph nodes). For this reason, small bowel NETs, large NETs in the aforementioned locations, and metastatic NETs should be staged before initiating treatment. Somatostatin receptor (SSRT)-PET is the imaging modality of choice to stage NETs. This test uses ^{68}Ga-DOTATATE, which binds to SSRTs, allowing localization of NETs. An intersociety consensus statement deemed SSRT-PET imaging the most appropriate imaging modality for staging NETs because of its superiority over octreotide scintigraphy and cross-sectional imaging. Use of intravenous contrast in conjunction with this nuclear medicine study improves sensitivity.[11] Often, liver metastases are the initial presentation of gastroenteropancreatic NETs. Locating the primary tumor can be done with SSRT-PET. A prospective study compared blinded reports of SSRT-PET with the same patient's pentetreotide scintigraphy and anatomic imaging (CT or MRI). SSRT-PET was the only modality to identify a primary lesion that was previously unknown and detected a total of 95.1% of all lesions compared with 45.3% and 30.9% by anatomic imaging and pentetreotide scintigraphy, respectively.[12] Because of its improved sensitivity, SSRT-PET has replaced octreotide scintigraphy as the modality of choice for localizing and staging NETs. **Fig. 3** demonstrates how SSRT-PET can localize the primary tumor in a patient diagnosed with NET liver metastases.

The most common serum test for NETs is chromogranin A. Chromogranins are a class of secreted proteins produced by neuroendocrine cells, and they are produced by a variety of organs.[13] As such, elevated chromogranin levels raise suspicion for the presence of NET but provide no indication of where the tumor is located. This

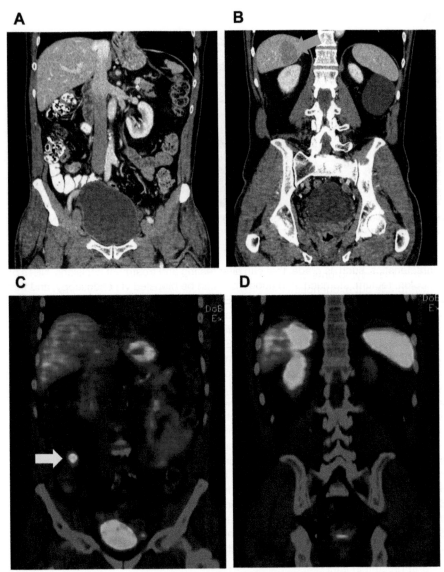

Fig. 3. SSRT PET. (*A, B*) CT scan of patient with biopsy-proven NET liver metastasis (*blue arrow*) and unknown primary. (*C, D*) SSRT-PET imaging demonstrating the primary tumor in the terminal ileum (*yellow arrow*) and again demonstrating the liver metastasis.

biomarker can be positive in functional and nonfunctional NETs. Even small residual NET will result in persistent elevation of chromogranin levels.[14] The only commercially available test is for chromogranin A, which is not elevated in all patients with NETs. When chromogranin A is elevated, it is generally used to monitor for recurrence or treatment response of NETs. Clinicians should be aware that use of proton pump inhibitors can falsely elevate these levels. However, there is evidence to suggest that elevated chromogranin A levels can be useful in prognosis. A recently published paper looking to develop a recurrence risk score for pancreatic NETs found that a pretreatment chromogranin A level greater than 5 times the upper limit of normal was associated with worse overall survival and recurrence-free survival.[15] This extreme elevation in chromogranin A often presents without other high-risk features, and the investigators included it in their suggested recurrence risk scoring system for counseling patients.[15]

Carcinoid syndrome occurs rarely (10%) in the setting of NETs. As described above, patients with carcinoid syndrome experience flushing and diarrhea because of an overproduction of serotonin by the neoplastic cells. The liver typically metabolizes excess serotonin secreted by gastroenteropancreatic NETs before it reaches systemic circulation to cause symptoms. A metabolite of this process is 5-hydroxyindoleacetic acid (5-HIAA), which is excreted in the urine. A 24-hour urine 5-HIAA level can be elevated in patients with or without carcinoid syndrome and can aid in diagnosis of NET. It can also be used as a monitoring test. However, be aware that certain foods and medications can cause false elevation of urine 5-HIAA level. This test is rarely used because functional imaging has improved.

Other functional NETs, typically pancreatic NETs, have individual biomarkers that are used for their diagnosis. Insulinomas will produce excess insulin, resulting in Whipple triad symptoms described above. A serum c-peptide should always be drawn to rule out exogenous insulin as the culprit. Gastrinomas create gastric ulcers because copious amounts of hydrochloric acid are produced in response to excess gastrin stimulation. It is recommended that gastrin levels be measured off proton pump inhibitors because it can falsely elevate serum gastrin levels. Equivocal gastrin serum levels (<2000 pg/mL fasting) require a gastrin stimulation test be performed, whereby secretin is administered followed by serum gastrin examination. An increase greater than 110 pg/mL is diagnostic of a gastrinoma. Serum levels of glucagon, somatostatin, and VIP can be measured to confirm clinical diagnoses of functional pancreatic NETs.

TREATMENT AND CLINICAL OUTCOMES

The ideal treatment of NETs is resection of all macroscopic disease seen at presentation. However, this is not always an option depending on the anatomic distribution of metastatic disease in the lymph nodes and liver. Because gastroenteropancreatic NETs occur in a range of locations, the surgical options also vary.

Small Intestine

Small bowel NETs are the most common NET to develop distant metastases. They tend to present in later stages because they rarely have specific symptoms and are difficult to visualize on cross-sectional imaging. However, despite these unfortunate circumstances, patients who present with small bowel NET in advanced stages have a median survival of 56 months.[2] Overall survival increases to 161 months when cytoreduction is undertaken.[16] Thus, an aggressive approach should be pursued for all patients with small intestine NETs.

Oncologic resection of localized small bowel NET is the gold standard. The North American Neuroendocrine Tumor Society (NANETS) still recommends performing open resection because it allows for the palpation of the entire small bowel for synchronous bowel tumors. However, laparoscopic exploration is recognized as a valid approach in certain cases.[17] Laparoscopy allows for a thorough peritoneal search for metastases (an essential step) without requiring large incisions that can be debilitating to the patient. An alternative to the open surgical approach is to perform the small bowel resection laparoscopically and then run the small bowel through a small extraction incision before performing the anastomosis.

Small intestine oncologic resection includes resection of regional lymph nodes and is typically done by resecting the mesentery associated with the segmental arterial supply of the primary tumor. A 2019 multi-institutional study of small intestine NETs found that finding a positive lymph node was more likely if 8 or more regional lymph nodes were sampled. The same study found that patients with fewer than 8 lymph nodes examined had similar 3-year recurrence-free survival regardless of how many of the nodes were positive. However, patients with 8 or more lymph nodes resected did demonstrate a difference in 3-year recurrence-free survival between patients with 4 nodes positive for NET (79.9%) versus those with 1 to 3 nodes positive (89.6%) versus those with negative lymph nodes (92.9%).[18] This finding suggests that the surgeon should aim to harvest at least 8 lymph nodes for adequate staging in small bowel NETs. Grossly positive nodes involving the base of the mesentery should be referred to an NET specialty center for evaluation of resection, particularly if they are causing symptoms.[17]

As mentioned earlier, cytoreduction of metastatic small bowel NETs improves overall survival. Woltering and colleagues[16] reported their experience with cytoreduction of metastatic NETs originating from all sites, of which 65% were small bowel NETs. The most common intraoperative finding at the time of cytoreduction was encasement of the mesenteric vessels followed by direct mesenteric extension of the tumor without mesenteric vessel involvement. Median overall survival was 161 months with 5-, 10-, and 20-year overall survival of 84%, 67%, and 31%, respectively, after cytoreduction of small intestine NETs. In the group that could only have 70% to 89% of their NET disease resected, the median overall survival was 148 months. The NANETS guidelines agree that peritoneal and liver metastases debulking should occur when possible for small intestine NETs but do not currently support the use of hyperthermic intraperitoneal chemotherapy.[17]

Appendix

In contrast to small bowel NETs, appendiceal NETs are typically found in early stages because they can occlude the appendiceal lumen and cause appendicitis even when they are relatively small in size. Most of these tumors are diagnosed on pathologic examination after appendectomy, so generally there is limited preoperative diagnostic workup.

Lymph node metastases are a significant predictor of survival in appendiceal NETs. A study using the Surveillance, Epidemiology, and End Result database looked at 613 patients with appendiceal NETs, both pure and mixed types. When looking at the entire cohort, having a pure NET type and tumor less than 2 cm independently predicted an improved survival on multivariate analysis, whereas lymph node positivity was associated with worse overall survival (hazard ratio of 11.682). Lymph node metastases remained a significant independent factor for poor overall survival when the 2 subtypes were separated for analysis; however, it was a worse prognostic sign for mixed type NETs (hazard ratio 17.471 mixed type vs 5.295 for pure type).[19]

Because lymph nodes are important for staging appendiceal NETs, and lymph nodes are not usually harvested at the time of appendectomy, the decision of when to perform an oncologic resection can be challenging (**Box 2**). Guidelines from the National Comprehensive Cancer Network recommend that appendiceal NETs confined to the appendix measuring 2 cm or smaller can be treated by appendectomy alone, whereas tumors greater than 2 cm, positive resection margin, or grossly positive lymph nodes should undergo staging imaging of CT, MRI, or SSRT-PET followed by

---

Box 2
Indications for right hemicolectomy in appendiceal neuroendocrine tumors

Right hemicolectomy recommended for all of the following:
- Greater than 2 cm
- Located at the appendiceal base
- Positive resection margin after appendectomy
- Grossly positive lymph nodes

Mid or tip of appendix 1 to 2 cm should be considered for right hemicolectomy if the following:
- Lymphatic invasion present
- Vascular invasion present
- Grade 2

---

right hemicolectomy.[20] The European Neuroendocrine Tumor Society consensus guidelines recommend right hemicolectomy for all tumors greater than 2 cm, any size tumor that involves the appendiceal base, positive resection margins after appendectomy, or more than 3 mm of mesoappendiceal extension. For tumors between 1 and 2 cm located in the tip or mid portion of the appendix, these guidelines recommend considering right hemicolectomy if vascular or lymphatic invasion is seen on pathology and for tumors that are grade 2 (Ki67, 3%–20%).[21] Despite these guidelines, it has recently been reported that one-third of appendiceal NETs smaller than 2 cm are undergoing right hemicolectomy and one-third of tumors larger than 2 cm are being treated with appendectomy alone.[22] Lack of appropriate staging, although not affecting survival, does limit the discussion the surgeon has with the patient regarding prognosis and choosing appropriate surveillance.

Pancreas

Nonfunctioning pancreatic neuroendocrine tumors (PNET) are being diagnosed more frequently in the era of modern imaging. These tumors, compared with pancreatic adenocarcinoma, have low malignant potential. This has led to much debate about what to do with nonfunctional PNETs that are not associated with genetic syndromes because the patient may not experience any negative effects during their lifetime. A retrospective study at a single institution found on histology that 14.4% of PNETs less than 2 cm had microinvasion or nodal metastases, and zero had liver metastases. This article concluded that these lesions can be observed.[23] A case-control study comparing resection and observation of PNETs less than 3 cm supported this conclusion. During the follow-up interval, the median tumor size had not changed, and there was no evidence of metastases in the observation group. Most of the resected group (95%) had low-grade pathologic condition. No patient died of their NET whether they were observed or resected.[24] This finding supports observing smaller PNETs. However, there are studies that support resection of all PNETs, including those smaller than 2 cm. A National Cancer Data Base study of PNETs less than 2 cm found the 5-year overall survival to be significantly lower in the observed cohort compared with those who underwent resection (34.3% vs 82.2%). Observation was also independently associated with death when controlled for tumor grade, tumor size, tumor location, nodal status, age, and comorbidities.[25] The decision of whether to observe small PNETs must be individualized to the patient. They must be reliable and willing to undergo routine surveillance. The decision should be made by the patient after having an informed discussion with the surgeon and review of the case at a multidisciplinary tumor board.

Small PNETs that do not involve the main pancreatic duct can be resected by simply enucleating the tumor. Resection of larger PNETs (>2 cm) typically requires a formal pancreatectomy. Lesions in the head of the pancreas are resected via pancreaticoduodenectomy and those in the tail are resected by distal pancreatectomy. Tumors in the body of the pancreas can be approached in several ways. A subtotal pancreatectomy can be performed, but a large volume of healthy gland will be sacrificed for a lesion with low malignant potential. Another option is central pancreatectomy, which involves dividing the pancreas proximal and distal to the tumor and constructing either a pancreaticogastrostomy or pancreaticojejunostomy with the distal portion of the gland (**Fig. 4**). This procedure is a difficult one with a high risk of pancreatic fistula and must be approached cautiously.

Of the operations mentioned above, central pancreatectomy and enucleation tend to result in low nodal harvest. Positive lymph nodes have been shown to be independently associated with PNET disease-specific survival. Node positivity correlates with tumor size. Greater than 50% of PNETs greater than 2 cm have positive nodes on resection, and 25% of tumors 1 to 1.9 cm have positive nodes.[26] Because lymph nodes are required for accurate staging, they need to be considered when devising the surgical approach.

Surveillance after the resection of PNETs is an important component of caring for these patients. However, the risk of recurrence is not the same for all of these tumors because of heterogeneity of this group. A recent study proposed a novel score to predict recurrence of PNETs. It assigned different points for the following variables: lymph node positivity, tumor functionality, tumor size, and tumor Ki67. Low, intermediate, and high risk of recurrence groups were then created and validated. This international group recommended 12-month surveillance for the low-risk group, 6-month surveillance for the intermediate group, and 3-month surveillance for the high-risk group.[27]

Gastric Carcinoid

Gastric NETs (or carcinoids as they are commonly named) are rare tumors even among other NETs. These tumors arise from enterochromaffin-like cells that regulate

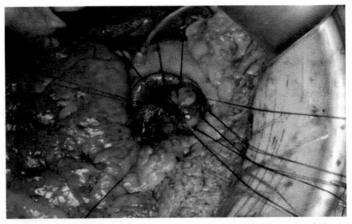

Fig. 4. Pancreaticogastrostomy in a central pancreatectomy. The tail of the pancreas is brought through the posterior wall of the stomach, and the pancreatic capsule is sutured full thickness to the posterior stomach. The anterior gastrostomy is then closed in 2 layers.

gastric acid production via histamine. As such, these neoplasms are associated with elevated gastrin levels and achlorhydria. There are 4 types of gastric NETs,[28] as follows:

- Type I: This type is the most common type of gastric carcinoid comprising 70% to 80% of these tumors. They arise from autoimmune chronic atrophic gastritis, which can lead to intrinsic factor deficiency. Women are more likely to be diagnosed with this type than men. They are often multifocal.
- Type II: Type II lesions are associated with Zollinger-Ellison syndrome and multiple endocrine neoplasm type 1 disorders as discussed above. It is estimated that 30% of this type of gastric carcinoid will metastasize.
- Type III: This type is the most aggressive with 50% to 100% estimated to metastasize. They are more common in men than women. These sporadic lesions arise from normal gastric mucosa and have no associated elevation in gastrin.
- Type IV: These are poorly differentiated NETs that are typically not amenable to surgical resection and are best treated with systemic chemotherapy.

A recent retrospective study of 79 patients investigated the impact of surgical approach on the outcomes of patients with gastric carcinoids. The group found that patients with type II and IV tumors almost universally had a formal gastrectomy, whereas those with type I and type III tumors had equal rate of formal gastrectomy versus local resection. Interestingly, overall survival was worse in those undergoing formal gastrectomy than in those who had a local resection even when types II and IV were excluded. It was concluded that tumor biology contributes more to survival than resection strategy when treating gastric NETs.[29]

Liver Metastases

The management of metastases of NETs to the liver is a complex topic. Extensive progress has been made in this area in recent years, especially in the nonsurgical management. In this section, the authors discuss the role surgery has in this disease and briefly describes the available medical therapy.

Complete resection of liver NET metastases is indicated if feasible. Patients with hormonal symptoms, such as carcinoid syndrome, show a reduction in symptoms with resection of liver metastases.[30] However, often the disease within the liver is so diffuse that complete resection and preservation of enough liver to retain function is not possible. Debulking of NET liver metastases has been shown to improve median survival of patients with nonhormonal symptoms when compared with those undergoing resection for palliation in retrospective studies (89.2 months vs 50.0 months); patients with complete resection of liver metastases have a median survival of 112.5 months.[31] The question of how much tumor needs to be removed to provide a survival benefit is constantly being readdressed as nonsurgical therapy improves. It has been shown that achieving greater than 70% cytoreduction of PNET liver metastases improves progression-free and overall survival and improves the progression-free survival in small bowel NET metastases. Progression-free survival is improved when 90% cytoreduction of liver metastases can be achieved, but not overall survival.[32] Combination of resection and ablation can be used in attempt to preserve liver volume.

Historically, octreotide has been the first line of treatment for patients with metastatic and symptomatic gastroenteropancreatic NETs. Octreotide long-acting release treatment has been shown to stabilize two-thirds of disease in metastatic midgut NETs. The effect was more prominent in patients with low-volume liver disease and those who had undergone resection of their primary tumor.[33] Everolimus has had similar results in delaying progression of metastatic PB and GI tract NETs as well as trend to longer overall survival.[34] Peptide receptor radionuclide therapy (PRRT) with lutetium-177–labeled somatostatin analogues can extend overall survival of metastatic PNETs to 71 months and metastatic midgut NETs to 60 months.[35] PRRT response can be predicted by the maximum standardized uptake value (maxSUV) on SSRT-PET imaging and is likely not beneficial for tumors with maxSUV less than 16.4.[36] The evaluation and treatment of metastatic PB and GI NETs are complicated and multimodal. A multidisciplinary approach at an experienced center is recommended.

SUMMARY

The diagnosis and treatment of gastroenteropancreatic NETs have evolved significantly. Currently, with proper surgical and medical management, the outcomes of these tumors can be improved even in the setting of metastatic disease. The use of SSRT-PET has improved the ability to detect small tumors, which allows for appropriate surveillance or therapy based on the evidence stated above. General surgeons need to be aware of what is available when managing patients with NETs as the incidence of this disease continues to increase.

DISCLOSURE

The authors have nothing to disclose.

REFERENCES

1. Dasari A, Shen C, Halperin D, et al. Trends in the incidence, prevalence, and survival outcomes in patients with neuroendocrine tumors in the United States. JAMA Oncol 2017;3(10):1335–42.
2. Yao JC, Hassan M, Phan A, et al. One hundred years after "carcinoid": epidemiology of and prognostic factors for neuroendocrine tumors in 35,825 cases in the United States. J Clin Oncol 2008;26(18):3063–72.
3. Kim JY, Hong SM. Recent updates on neuroendocrine tumors from the gastrointestinal and pancreatobiliary tracts. Arch Pathol Lab Med 2016;140:437–48.
4. Thorson A, Biorck G, Bjorkman G, et al. Malignant carcinoid of the small intestine with metastases to the liver, valvular disease of the right side of the heart (pulmonary stenosis and tricuspid regurgitation without septal defects), peripheral vasomotor symptoms, bronchoconstriction, and an unusual type of cyanosis: a clinical and pathologic syndrome. Am Heart J 1954;47(6):795–817.
5. Whipple AO, Frantz VK. Adenoma of islet cells with hyperinsulinism: a review. Ann Surg 1935;101(6):1299–335.
6. Mallinson CN, Bloom SR, Warin AP, et al. A glucagonoma syndrome. Lancet 1974;304:1–5.
7. Ellison EH, Wilson SD. The Zollinger-Ellison syndrome: re-appraisal and evaluation of 260 registered cases. Ann Surg 1964;160(3):512–28.
8. Larsson LI, Holst JJ, Kuhl C, et al. Pancreatic somatostatinoma. Clinical features and physiological implications. Lancet 1977;309:666–8.
9. Long RG, Bryant MG, Mitchell SJ, et al. Clinicopathological study of pancreatic and ganglioneuroblastoma tumors secreting vasoactive intestinal polypeptide (VIPomas). Br Med J 1981;282:1767–71.
10. Morse B, Jeong D, Thomas K, et al. Magnetic resonance imaging of neuroendocrine tumor hepatic metastases: does hepatobiliary phase imaging improve

lesion conspicuity and interobserver agreement of lesion measurements? Pancreas 2017;46(9):1219–24.

11. Hope TA, Bergsland E, Bozkurt MF, et al. Appropriate use criteria for somatostatin receptor PET imaging in neuroendocrine tumors. J Nucl Med 2018;59(1):66–74.

12. Sadowski SM, Neychev V, Millo C, et al. Prospective study of ^{68}Ga-DOTATATE positron emission tomography/computed tomography for detecting gastro-entero-pancreatic neuroendocrine tumors and unknown primary sites. J Clin Oncol 2016;34(6):588–96.

13. Wiedenmann B, Huttner WB. Synaptophysin and chromogranins/secretogranins–widespread constituents of distinct types of neuroendocrine vesicles and new tools in tumor diagnosis. Virchows Arch 1989;58:95–121.

14. Eriksson B, Oberg K. Peptide hormones as tumor markers in neuroendocrine gastrointestinal tumors. Acta Oncol 1991;30(4):477–83.

15. Fisher AV, Lopez-Aguiar AG, Rendell VR, et al. Predictive value of chromogranin A and a pre-operative risk score to predict recurrence after resection of pancreatic neuroendocrine tumors. J Gastrointest Surg 2019;23:651–8.

16. Woltering EA, Voros BA, Beyer DT, et al. Aggressive surgical approach to the management of neuroendocrine tumors: a report of 1,000 surgical cytoreductions by a single institution. J Am Coll Surg 2017;224:434–47.

17. Howe JR, Cardona K, Fraker DL, et al. The surgical management of small bowel neuroendocrine tumors: consensus guidelines of the North American Neuroendocrine Tumor Society. Pancreas 2017;46:715–31.

18. Zaidi MY, Lopez-Aguiar AG, Dillhoff M, et al. Prognostic role of lymph node positivity and number of lymph nodes needed for accurately staging small-bowel neuroendocrine tumors. JAMA Surg 2019;154(2):134–40.

19. Ciarrocchi A, Pietroletti R, Carlei F, et al. Clinical significance of metastatic lymph nodes in the gut of patients with pure and mixed primary appendiceal carcinoids. Dis Colon Rectum 2016;59(6):508–12.

20. Shah MH, Goldner WS, Benson AB, et al. NCCN clinical practice guidelines in oncology: neuroendocrine and adrenal tumors. Version 1. 2019. 2019. Available at: https://www.nccn.org/professionals/physician_gls/pdf/neuroendocrine_blocks.pdf. Accessed July 27, 2019.

21. Pape U-F, Niederle B, Costa F, et al. ENETS consensus guidelines for neuroendocrine neoplasms of the appendix (excluding goblet cell carcinomas). Neuroendocrinology 2016;103:144–52.

22. Heller DR, Jean RA, Luo JL, et al. Practice patterns and guideline non-adherence in surgical management of appendiceal carcinoid tumors. J Am Coll Surg 2019; 228:839–51.

23. Bettini R, Partelli S, Boninsegna L, et al. Tumor size correlates with malignancy in nonfunctioning pancreatic endocrine tumor. Surgery 2011;150:75–82.

24. Sadot E, Reidy-Lagunes DL, Tang LH, et al. Observation versus resection for small asymptomatic pancreatic neuroendocrine tumors: a matched case-control study. Ann Surg Oncol 2016;23(4):1361–70.

25. Sharpe SM, In H, Winchester DJ, et al. Surgical resection provides an overall survival benefit for patient with small pancreatic neuroendocrine tumors. J Gastrointest Surg 2015;19:117–23.

26. Curran T, Pockaj BA, Gray RJ, et al. Importance of lymph node involvement in pancreatic neuroendocrine tumors: impact on survival and implications. J Gastrointest Surg 2015;19:152–60.

27. Zaidi MY, Lopez-Aguiar AG, Switchenko JM, et al. A novel validated recurrence risk score to guide a pragmatic surveillance strategy after resection of pancreatic

neuroendocrine tumors: an international study of 1006 patients. Ann Surg 2019; 270(3):422–33.

28. Burkitt MD, Pritchard DM. Review article: pathogenesis and management of gastric carcinoid tumours. Aliment Pharmacol Ther 2006;24:1305–20.

29. Crown A, Kennecke H, Kozarek R, et al. Gastric carcinoids: does type of surgery or tumor affect survival? Am J Surg 2019;217:937–42.

30. Que FG, Nagorney DM, Batts KP, et al. Hepatic resection for metastatic neuroendocrine carcinomas. Am J Surg 1995;169(1):36–43.

31. Chakedis J, Beal EW, Lopez-Aguiar AG, et al. Surgery provides long-term survival in patients with metastatic neuroendocrine tumors undergoing resection for non-hormonal symptoms. J Gastrointest Surg 2019;23:122–34.

32. Maxwell JE, Sherman SK, O'Dorisio TM, et al. Liver-directed surgery of neuroendocrine metastases: what is the optimal strategy? Surgery 2016;159(1):320–35.

33. Rinke A, Muller HH, Schade-Brittinger C, et al. Randomized study on the effect of octreotide LAR in the control of tumor growth in patients with metastatic neuroendocrine midgut tumors: a report from the PROMID study group. J Clin Oncol 2009;27:4656–63.

34. Yao JC, Fazio N, Singh S, et al. Everolimus for the treatment of advanced, nonfunctional neuroendocrine tumours of the lung or gastrointestinal tract (RADIANT-4): a randomised, placebo-controlled, phase 3 study. Lancet 2016; 387:968–77.

35. Brabander T, van der Zwan WA, Teunissen JJM, et al. Long-term efficacy, survival, and safety of [177Lu-DOTA^0, Tyr^3] octreotate in patients with gastroenteropancreatic and bronchial neuroendocrine tumors. Clin Cancer Res 2017;23(16): 4617–24.

36. Kratochwil C, Stefanova M, Mavriopoulou E, et al. SUV of [^{68}Ga]DOTATOC-PET/CT predicts response probability of PRRT in neuroendocrine tumors. Mol Imaging Biol 2014. https://doi.org/10.1007/s11307-014.0795-3.

Soft Tissue Tumors of the Abdomen and Retroperitoneum

Michael K. Turgeon, MD[a], Kenneth Cardona, MD[b],*

KEYWORDS

- Retroperitoneal sarcoma • Desmoid tumors • Surgery • Multimodality therapy
- Active surveillance

KEY POINTS

- Retroperitoneal sarcomas are composed of numerous histiotypes, each with its unique tumor biology that impacts presentation, recurrence, survival, and management.
- The cornerstone of primary retroperitoneal sarcoma management is curative-intent resection, although its extent remains debatable.
- Multidisciplinary management at high-volume centers is crucial for evidence-based, patient-tailored treatment strategies that span multimodality therapy.
- Recent efforts to standardize the management of desmoid tumors support the preference for active surveillance (ie, wait and watch) over medical or surgical intervention.

INTRODUCTION

Soft tissue tumors of the abdomen and retroperitoneum encompass a broad range of rare neoplasms with varying degrees of clinical behavior ranging from benign intra-abdominal tumors, which have no significant clinical impact to the patient, to locally aggressive tumors and/or malignant tumors such as retroperitoneal sarcomas (RPS), which can be associated with considerable morbidity and mortality.

Benign intra-abdominal and retroperitoneal tumors are uncommon and have diverse etiologies, including but not limited to duplication and mesenteric cysts, lymphoceles, lymphangiomas, lipomas, and peripheral nerve sheath tumors, with mesenteric fibromatosis and sclerosing mesenteritis comprising the prevailing diagnoses.[1] Both mesenteric fibromatosis and sclerosing mesenteritis are inflammatory, fibrotic diseases that affect and involve the mesentery. Notably, mesenteric

a Division of Surgical Oncology, Department of Surgery, Winship Cancer Institute, Emory University, 1365 Clifton Road, Northeast, Building B, Suite 4100, Office 4201, Atlanta, GA 30322, USA; b Division of Surgical Oncology, Department of Surgery, Winship Cancer Institute, Emory University, 550 Peachtree Street, Northeast, 9th Floor, Suite 900, Atlanta, GA 30308, USA
* Corresponding author.
E-mail address: ken.cardona@emory.edu

Surg Clin N Am 100 (2020) 649–667
https://doi.org/10.1016/j.suc.2020.02.011
0039-6109/20/© 2020 Elsevier Inc. All rights reserved.

fibromatosis (or abdominal desmoid) is a benign, locally aggressive subtype, which constitutes 8% of all cases of fibromatosis, and can be associated with considerable morbidity, and in certain instances, mortality owing to the local involvement of the mesenteric vasculature or intestinal tract.[2] It is critical to differentiate benign tumors from their malignant counterparts because histology-guided management impacts therapeutic protocols that span the spectrum of observation (ie, active surveillance), medical therapy with cytotoxic or biologic agents, radiation therapy, and surgical resection.[3,4]

The most common malignant soft tissue tumors encountered within the abdomen and retroperitoneum are sarcomas. In the abdomen, gastrointestinal stromal tumors make up the majority of malignant visceral sarcomas encountered.[5,6] In the retroperitoneum, the most prevalent sarcoma histiotypes identified are (i) liposarcomas, (ii) leiomyosarcomas, and (iii) solitary fibrous tumors.[6,7]

Historically, treatment strategies for RPS extended broadly across all histiotypes. More recently, increasing recognition of the impact of sarcoma histiotype on oncologic outcomes has led to a growing trend in histiotype-specific management of RPS.[8] Furthermore, the site of origin influences the natural history of sarcomas with RPS having a much higher risk of recurrence, nearly 2-fold when compared with their trunk and extremity counterparts.[9] Thus, as the management of abdominal and RPS continues to evolve, it is critical for a multidisciplinary team of clinicians with expertise in the management and treatment of sarcomas to be involved to guide management strategies.[10,11]

This review focuses on the diagnostic evaluation, surgical management, and multimodality therapy of soft tissue tumors of the abdomen and retroperitoneal tumors, with a particular focus on RPS and desmoid tumors.

RETROPERITONEAL SARCOMAS

In 2019, there will be an estimated 13,000 new cases of soft tissue sarcomas, which accounts for less than 1% of all adult cancers within the United States, with RPS accounting for 16% of these cases.[12,13] Although the majority of sarcomas arise de novo, a variety of risk factors have been identified that predispose individuals to the development of a sarcoma, for instance, previous exposure to radiation and certain genetic syndromes (eg, Gardner syndrome and Li-Fraumeni syndrome).[14] With more than 75 histologic subtypes of soft tissue sarcomas identified to date, the natural history, recurrence risk, and treatment approach can be highly variable, complex, and depend on not only the specific sarcoma histiotype, but also on the anatomic location. In other words, a specific sarcoma histiotype may be treated in a certain way if located in the extremity and treated in a completely different way if located within the retroperitoneum.

Therefore, appropriate histiotype diagnosis is critical to the management of patients with RPS and tissue sampling should be strongly considered in every case. A tissue sample is obtained via an image-guided core needle biopsy to allow for in-depth histopathologic analysis and for molecular testing when indicated. It is paramount that a core of tissue and not a simple aspiration of cells (ie, fine needle aspiration) be performed to allow for complex immunohistochemical and fluorescence in situ hybridization studies to be performed on a representative sample of the tumor.[15,16] With the complexity of the histomorphologic and cytomorphologic features of RPS, it is our recommendation to engage the expertise of a dedicated sarcoma pathologist.

With regard to sarcomas of the retroperitoneum, the 3 most common histiotypes encountered in clinical practice are (i) liposarcoma (53%–63%), leiomyosarcoma

(15%–23%), and solitary fibrous tumors (5%–7%) (**Table 1**).[17–19] We focus our discussion on these 3 subtypes. However, it is important to note that many other sarcoma histiotypes can develop in the retroperitoneum.

- Liposarcomas are the most common RPS histiotype.[12] These lipomatous neoplasms arise from adipocytic cells and are further categorized into 3 subtypes: (i) well-differentiated and dedifferentiated liposarcomas, (ii) myxoid and round cell liposarcomas, (iii) and pleomorphic liposarcomas.[20] Well-differentiated and dedifferentiated liposarcomas have a predilection for the retroperitoneum, whereas myxoid, round cell, and pleomorphic liposarcomas more frequently develop within the trunk and/or extremities.[21] However, when myxoid and round cell liposarcomas are found in the retroperitoneum, they likely represent metastatic foci from a primary truncal/extremity tumor.
- Well-differentiated liposarcomas are low-grade tumors with a propensity for local recurrences and very rarely, if ever, metastasize. In contrast, dedifferentiated liposarcomas are considered intermediate or high-grade tumors that have a more aggressive clinical course with a predisposition for both local and distant metastasis. More specifically, for well-differentiated liposarcomas, the 5-year local recurrence rate is reported to be 18% to 41%, with a 5-year distant recurrence rate of less than 1%, and a 5-year overall survival of 66% to 92%.[18,19,22] Patients with well-differentiated liposarcomas commonly succumb to local recurrences of disease and not widespread metastasis, although approximately 10% of patients with well-differentiated tumors will dedifferentiate (ie, become high grade or more aggressive) at some point in their disease course.[23] Thus, it is crucial to optimize the likelihood of success of the index operation with the consultation of surgeons with an expertise in the management of RPS.
- In contrast, high-grade, dedifferentiated liposarcomas have increased rates of both local (45%–58%) and distant recurrences (25%–44%) at 5 years.[18,19,22] For dedifferentiated liposarcomas, not only is surgery essential for local control, but also multimodality therapy should be considered and discussed in a multidisciplinary setting to address the higher potential for the development of distant disease. Unsurprisingly, 5-year overall survival is 42% to 53%.[18,19,22]
- Leiomyosarcomas are the second most common type of sarcoma seen in the retroperitoneum, accounting for 15% of all RPS.[6,18] These tumors arise from smooth muscle cells primarily found within blood vessels, specifically the large veins of the retroperitoneum (eg, inferior vena cava, renal veins, iliac veins, and gonadal veins), although they can develop from small, unnamed veins as well.

Table 1				
Recurrence patterns and survival based on histiotype				
Histiotype	**Percent Makeup of RPS (%)**	**Five-Year Local Recurrence Rate (%)**	**Five-Year Distant Recurrence Rate (%)**	**Five-Year Overall Survival (%)**
Liposarcoma (well-differentiated)	28–34	18–41	<1	66–92
Liposarcoma (dedifferentiated)	23–32	45–58	25–44	42–53
Leiomyosarcoma	15–23	6–18	51–56	56–58
Solitary fibrous tumor	5–7	7–9	18–35	78–84

Data from Refs.[18,19,22]

Leiomyosarcomas have a distinct tumor biology when compared with liposarcomas such that these tumors have lower rates of local recurrences (6%–18% at 5 years) and high rates of systemic disease (distant recurrence rates of 51%–56% at 5 years), which translates to an overall survival of 56% to 58%.[18,19,22]

- Solitary fibrous tumors, previously known as hemangiopericytomas, are malignant tumors that predominantly arise from serosal membranes, including the meninges, pleura, and peritoneum. Solitary fibrous tumors have a variable natural history, although they more commonly have an indolent course with rare instances of metastasis. The 5-year local recurrence rates are 7% to 9%, with 5-year distant metastasis rates of 18% to 35%, and a 5-year overall survival of 78% to 84%.[18,19,22]

As stated elsewhere in this article, other sarcoma subtypes can develop in the retroperitoneum and these include, but are not limited to, malignant peripheral nerve sheath tumors, synovial sarcomas, and Ewing and "Ewing-like" sarcomas. Of note, these tumors are more commonly seen in young adults. Finally, it is important that the treating clinician recognize that other tumors can mimic RPS, such as lymphoma, primary germ cell tumors, adrenal tumors, renal tumors, and metastatic testicular cancer, emphasizing the importance of multidisciplinary discussion of patients with retroperitoneal tumors and the consideration of tissue sampling.

Clinical Presentation

RPS are typically asymptomatic until its growth is large enough to compress surrounding structures and, even then, the presenting symptoms can be vague and nondescript, spanning early satiety, abdominal discomfort or fullness, and in rare instances, bowel obstruction. Given the potential space of the retroperitoneum, RPS often presents as a large mass, 70% of which are larger than 10 cm, with a median tumor size of 15 cm at presentation.[24,25]

Specifically, liposarcomas present as a large, asymptomatic abdominal mass. Symptoms arise from displacement or compression of surrounding organs from mass effect (**Fig. 1**). Another not infrequent presentation of liposarcomas is an inguinal hernia containing a large "lipoma." This represents a small component of the larger retroperitoneal tumor herniating through the inguinal canal. In contrast, leiomyosarcomas present as a smaller mass and, owing to potential impairment of venous blood

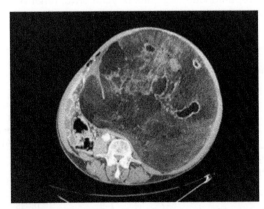

Fig. 1. Axial image of a large well-differentiated liposarcoma. (*Courtesy of* A. Gronchi, MD, Milan, Italy.)

flow, symptoms such as unilateral or bilateral leg swelling can occur, depending on the location. When localized to the retroperitoneum, solitary fibrous tumors can present with a palpable mass with associated pain, although they are more often diagnosed incidentally on imaging.

Diagnosis

For RPS, computed tomography (CT) scanning is the preferred imaging modality, which differs from the truncal and extremity sarcomas, where MRI is considered the standard imaging modality. Cross-sectional imaging of the abdomen and pelvis, typically with CT scans, is used to define the extent of the tumor burden and interface with adjacent viscera and vascular structures, which is essential for surgical planning. The liver and peritoneum should be evaluated for evidence of metastasis. Given that 14% of patients with high-grade RPS (eg, dedifferentiated liposarcomas and leiomyosarcomas) present with synchronous lung metastases, the addition of a staging CT scan of the chest is appropriate.[26] An MRI of the abdomen and pelvis is adopted in situations where there is a contraindication to intravenous contrast during CT scanning or where further delineation of vascular involvement is required. There is less of a role for PET, although there is interest in its use to better differentiate tumor grade before obtaining a tissue diagnosis.[27] There are no specific serum markers for sarcoma.

In the current era of RPS management, a tissue sample, obtained via CT-guided core needle biopsy, is part of the standard diagnostic algorithm. A biopsy is necessary for diagnosis, particularly in patients with resectable disease being considered for neoadjuvant therapies or patients with locally advanced or unresectable disease. Although concerns have been expressed regarding the risk of needle tract seeding, the benefits far outweigh the risks. Current retrospective reviews report needle tract seeding rates of less than 1%.[28] These rates are likely even lower with the use of modern coaxial sheathed biopsy needles.[29] Despite low rates of tumor seeding, the biopsy trajectory should still be carefully considered. A posterior or posterolateral approach is preferred, and an anterior or transabdominal approach should be avoided to prevent peritoneal contamination. Further, an incisional or open biopsy should not be attempted for RPS given the increased risk for tumor rupture and seeding of the abdominal cavity. This strategy is a departure from the diagnosis of truncal or extremity sarcomas, where an incisional biopsy is commonly completed by the surgeon performing the definitive resection.[28]

The recent, updated American Joint Committee on Cancer/Union for International Cancer Control eighth edition provides staging recommendations, although it is limited in its applicability because the existing criteria do not account for histologic subtype, which is a well-known prognostic indicator for RPS. In an era of personalized medicine, nomograms have been widely implemented to better predict recurrence and survival with higher specificity for an individual patient. In 2013, Gronchi and colleagues[30] established a nomogram specifically for RPS. The nomogram is based on 523 patients identified at 3 institutions and incorporates age, tumor size, grade, histologic subtype, multifocality, and extent of resection to calculate disease-free survival and overall survival. This system is now incorporated in their free application, "Sarculator," available on smart phones or other electronic devices.[31] Other accessible, clinically relevant prognostic models are available through the Memorial Sloan Kettering Cancer Center web site, including nomograms for liposarcoma survival after initial surgery, sarcoma-specific death after surgery, and sarcoma-specific death after local recurrence.[32–34]

Treatment

Surgery remains the cornerstone of treatment for RPS. Currently, the role of multimodality therapy (ie, radiation and/or chemotherapy in addition to surgery) remains a subject of debate. Although it has been extensively studied in primary truncal and extremity sarcomas, there are limited data specific to patients with RPS. Therefore, the role for multimodality therapy should be discussed within the context of a multidisciplinary setting on a case-by-case basis.

Referral to a specialized sarcoma center

With the complexity of clinicopathologic factors that impact patient outcomes, it is our recommendation that patients with RPS be referred to a center with expertise in RPS management, at least for their initial evaluation, because the best chance of cure is at presentation.[35,36] Doing so avoids the unnecessary duplication of diagnostic studies and ultimately decreases the time to carrying out definitive therapeutic plans. Further, the expertise of a multidisciplinary team can be applied to tailor individual treatment regimens with the prospect of clinical trial enrollment. To this point, a retrospective review of 35,784 patients across 26 sarcoma centers by Blay and colleagues[37] demonstrated a statistically significant reduction in risk of local relapse-free survival (hazard ratio [HR], 0.65; 95% confidence interval [CI], 0.61–0.72; $P = .0001$), disease-free survival (HR, 0.84; 95% CI, 0.79–0.88; $P<.001$), and 5-year overall survival (HR, 0.68; 95% CI, 0.61–0.74; $P<.001$) when compared with low-volume hospitals. Furthermore, Keung and colleagues[38] corroborated these findings in a large retrospective review of 6950 patients treated at high- versus low-volume centers. The study findings suggested that increased surgeon volume and more experienced treatment teams are likely contributors to these improved outcomes. Thus, our recommendation is to refer patients with RPS to a center with clinicians who have expertise in the management of patients with RPS who can offer a multidisciplinary assessment.

Surgery

Curative-intent resection with complete gross removal of the tumor remains the standard of care, particularly in patients with resectable, localized disease. Characteristics rendering RPS unresectable include extensive vascular involvement with no reconstruction options, including the aorta at the level of the celiac axis and superior mesenteric artery, multifocal peritoneal implants (sarcomatosis), distant metastasis, bilateral renal involvement, extensive disease of the liver hilum, and spinal cord involvement.[39] Often, given the tumor dimensions and extent of local invasion in the retroperitoneum as well as the abutment of nearby abdominal viscera, surgery with a wide negative margin proves challenging. The determination of resectability is crucial before intervention to optimize the index operation and to minimize the risk of recurrence.

Surgical approach

Owing to the typically large tumor size of a retroperitoneal tumor, a midline laparotomy incision from xiphoid to pubis generally allows for optimal exposure. There should be an initial assessment for sarcomatosis (peritoneal disease) to ensure surgery is not contraindicated. The retroperitoneum is then assessed and the tumor mobilized. In instances where there is invasion or involvement of the adjacent viscera, there is widespread agreement among sarcoma surgeons that an en bloc resection of such organs be performed with the goal of achieving a margin negative resection with dissection carried through normal tissue planes uncontaminated by tumor. Thus, not uncommonly, the kidney, adrenal gland, colon, pancreas, spleen, and psoas fascia/muscle are removed en bloc with the tumor (**Fig. 2**).[22] In a series of 114 patients, multivisceral resection was required in 83% of patients who received a complete resection.[39] Given the preference for hematogenous spread, it is very rare for RPS to spread to regional lymph nodes; therefore, a lymphadenectomy is not routinely necessary.[18]

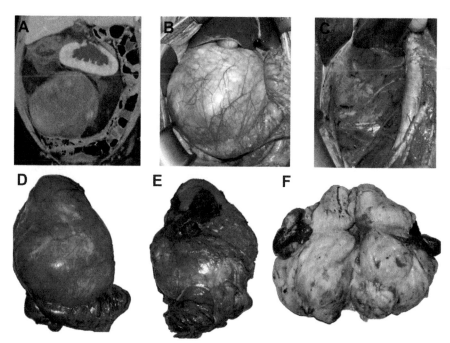

Fig. 2. (A) Coronal imaging of a dedifferentiated liposarcoma. (B) View of a RPS and displaced abdominal viscera upon entry into the abdomen. (C) View of right retroperitoneum after en bloc resection of tumor with the right colon, kidney/adrenal, and psoas musculature. (D) Anterior view of surgical specimen with tumor, right colon, kidney/adrenal, and psoas musculature. (E) Posterior view of surgical specimen with tumor, right colon, kidney/adrenal, and psoas musculature. (F) Bisected surgical specimen cleared of associated organs and structures. (Courtesy of A. Gronchi, MD, Milan, Italy.)

More recently, an extended or compartmental resection is becoming the preferred operative strategy for patients with RPS at select sarcoma centers. This procedure involves removing all adjacent viscera and associated structures on the ipsilateral side to the RPS, regardless of true tumor invasion or involvement. For instance, a right retroperitoneal liposarcoma would typically require a right colectomy, right nephrectomy and adrenalectomy, and resection of the psoas musculature en bloc with the tumor. Introduced in Europe in 2009, Bonvalot and colleagues[40] and Gronchi and colleagues[41] demonstrated the usefulness of replicating a liberal 1- to 2-cm margin seen in truncal and extremity sarcomas in grossly unaffected adjacent structures. Bonvalot and colleagues[40] highlighted a significant decrease in 5-year local recurrence (29% vs 48%; P = .007) with this approach. Gronchi and colleagues[41] demonstrated similar improved 5-year local recurrence rates (approximately 25% vs 55%; P<.0001). Notably, there was no statistical difference in the 5-year overall survival in these initial studies. Three years later, Gronchi and colleagues[42] published a follow-up study that reported a compartmental resection had lower rates of locoregional recurrence for low and intermediate grade tumors only. An extended or compartmental resection approach may be more appropriate for liposarcomas rather than leiomyosarcomas given the associated higher risk of local recurrence evident in liposarcomas. Of course, the patient's unique characteristics and potential morbidity and mortality of the operation itself should be taken into careful consideration. Despite these findings, the prevailing consensus at most centers in the United States at this time is to pursue a macroscopically negative resection with the removal of a single tumor specimen and contiguous organs, without a compartmental resection.[43] Given the ongoing debate surrounding the optimal surgical approach, treatment decisions are best discussed in a multidisciplinary tumor board setting at a sarcoma center.

Major vascular resection

Vascular resection is more commonly seen in patients with retroperitoneal leiomyosarcoma as well as other sarcoma histiotypes (eg, dedifferentiated liposarcoma) with evidence of direct invasion or involvement of associated structures. Vascular involvement is present in approximately 34% of patients with RPS and is associated with significant morbidity.[44,45] In appropriately selected candidates, there is a role for major vascular resection and reconstruction. A matched case-control study of 50 of patients diagnosed with truncal, extremity, and RPS compared patients with and without vascular reconstruction.[46] There was no significant difference in 5-year local recurrence (51% vs 54%; $P = .11$) or 5-year overall survival (59% vs 53%; $P = .67$), suggesting equivalent oncologic outcomes. In a 2019 retrospective review of 67 patients with RPS who underwent inferior vena cava or iliac vein resections, Ferraris and colleagues[47] demonstrated acceptable 5-year overall survival, 5-year local recurrence, and 5-year distant metastasis of 56.2%, 12.4%, and 51.5%, respectively. Patients who require major vascular resection and reconstruction should still be considered for surgery. It can be performed safely, particularly in the hands of experienced surgeons, and should not be considered an absolute contraindication to resection.[48,49]

Margin status

The retroperitoneum poses unique challenges for obtaining a resection margin free of disease with R0 resection (macroscopic or microscopic cancer not demonstrable at the resection margin) rates of 40% to 53%.[50,51] It is well-established that a complete resection is an independent predictor of both recurrence-free survival and overall survival.[52] Although there may be a trend that R1 resections (microscopic residual cancer at the resection margin) carry an increased risk for local recurrence, there is no clear overall survival advantage comparing an R0 and R1 resections in the retroperitoneum.[17,22,25,53–57] Thus, an R1 resection is acceptable and is not an indication for adjuvant radiation therapy in patients with RPS specifically with liposarcomas. As expected, there is a clear survival advantage comparing an R0/R1 to an R2 resection (gross residual cancer remains).[25,58] Noncurative surgery is defined as an operation that leaves gross residual disease (R2 resection).

Palliative Surgery

Palliative-intent (debulking) surgery should be selectively offered as a strategy for patients with unresectable or advanced disease with intractable symptoms of abdominal pain and/or bowel obstruction.[59] The surgeon should take into account tumor biology, patient comorbidities, the risk of the operation, and expected survival, all within the context of the patient's wishes. Our recommendation is that palliative surgery only be offered for symptom control in select patients.

Intraoperative Radiation Therapy

Intraoperative radiation therapy enables the delivery of targeted radiation to the tumor bed while minimizing toxicity to the surrounding normal tissue. Given the promising local control rates seen with extremity sarcomas, efforts have been made to apply this to RPS.[60] In 1993, Sindelar and colleagues[61] performed the only prospective, randomized study of 35 patients with RPS comparing intraoperative radiation therapy and postoperative radiation therapy with postoperative radiation therapy alone. The study suggests improved locoregional control in the combination postoperative radiation therapy and intraoperative radiation therapy cohort versus the postoperative radiation therapy alone, although there was no significant difference in overall survival noted between groups (time to locoregional recurrence, 63 months vs 38 months; $P = .40$). A retrospective review at the Memorial Sloan Kettering Cancer Center in 2000 of 32 patients and a subsequent series in 2002 of 87 patients by Petersen and colleagues[62] with RPS also evaluated the role of high-dose intraoperative radiation therapy.[63] These single-institution studies also suggest similar rates of improved local control (5-year disease-free recurrence of 74% vs 54%; $P = .04$).[63] An interim analysis of a more recent phase I/II trial by Roeder and colleagues[64] of 27 patients revealed encouraging locoregional control rates of 72% and 5-year overall survival rates of 74%. Despite possible improvement in local control, intraoperative radiation therapy has not been shown to universally provide a survival benefit; thus, its systematic use is not recommended outside the scope of a clinical trial.

Neoadjuvant Therapy

Given the high rates of recurrence, both local and distant depending on the RPS histiotype, there is significant interest in identifying multimodality approaches to improve recurrence rates and survival outcomes in patients with RPS. At this time, however, there is no definitive consensus on the optimal neoadjuvant regimen.

Neoadjuvant radiation therapy

Local recurrence rates, specifically for liposarcoma, can be considerable, and are among the main causes of death in patients with this histiotype. Therefore, adjuncts to complete surgical resection that may decrease the risk of a local recurrence have been an area of interest for sarcoma clinicians. Radiation therapy in truncal and extremity sarcomas has been shown to decrease local recurrence rates in various clinical trials. In regard to RPS, there are notable advantages to providing radiation therapy before surgery. Benefits include the displacement of radiosensitive organs from the radiation field by the tumor itself, identification of the gross tumor margin, smaller radiation field, potential for lower radiation doses, shorter course of treatment, and less toxicity.[65] For these reasons, current clinical guidelines strongly recommend that, when radiation is considered, it should be given in the neoadjuvant setting as opposed to the adjuvant setting. Data from 2 prospective trials that included patients with intermediate or high-grade RPS who received neoadjuvant radiation therapy had a 5-year local recurrence-free survival of 60%, disease-free survival of 46%, and overall survival of 61%, and, when compared with historical controls at that time, there was a trend toward decreased rates of local recurrence.[66]

In attempt to study the impact of preoperative radiation therapy in a prospective, randomized manner, ASCOG Z9031 compared upfront surgery with neoadjuvant radiation therapy, although the study closed early owing to inadequate patient accrual. Recently, the Surgery With or Without Radiation Therapy in Untreated Non-metastatic Retroperitoneal Sarcoma (STRASS or EORTC 62092) study, a prospective, randomized phase III trial that compared patients with primary, resectable RPS receiving neoadjuvant radiation therapy followed by surgery versus upfront surgery with the primary outcome of abdominal recurrence-free survival was completed in 2018 and reported at the American Society of Clinical Oncology meeting in 2019 (NCT01344018). Unfortunately, the study (n = 266) did not meet its primary endpoint of an improved abdominal recurrence-free survival (3-year abdominal recurrence-free survival was 60.4%; 95% CI, 0.71–1.44; $P = .954$). However, the authors did report that in an unplanned, unpowered subgroup analysis, there was an improvement in recurrence-free survival in patients with well-differentiated liposarcoma. Hence, the benefit of neoadjuvant radiotherapy is unknown but should be pursued selectively for patients with RPS.

Neoadjuvant chemotherapy

The role of neoadjuvant systemic therapy in RPS is limited and not well-defined. Although there is increasing interest in pursuing histology-specific chemotherapy regimens, this area requires ongoing study. Neoadjuvant chemotherapy has been used selectively for high-risk patients, particularly patients with histologic subtypes at increased risk for distant disease. Different histiotypes have been shown to have variable responses to chemotherapy, possibly explaining the lack of benefit seen in studies examining RPS of all histiotypes as a single cohort.[18,19,67] The use of neoadjuvant chemotherapy can be considered in cases of chemosensitive or high-risk RPS, such as synovial sarcoma, malignant solitary fibrous tumor, dedifferentiated liposarcoma, and leiomyosarcoma. A retrospective review by Miura and colleagues[68] in 2015 of 8653 patients with RPS demonstrated no survival advantage with the use of neoadjuvant or adjuvant chemotherapy. In fact, the administration of neoadjuvant chemotherapy was associated with worse survival compared with upfront surgery (40 months vs 52 months; $P = .002$). The upcoming STRASS-2 trial will further evaluate the role of neoadjuvant chemotherapy for patients with high-risk RPS (eg, dedifferentiated liposarcoma and high-grade leiomyosarcoma) with the primary outcome of disease-free survival (NCT04031677).

Neoadjuvant chemoradiation therapy

The usefulness of neoadjuvant chemoradiation is also not well-established. Sequential chemotherapy then radiation therapy can be applied only very selectively and with the guidance of a multidisciplinary team. There is no optimal chemoradiation regimen established and prospective, randomized trials are needed.

Adjuvant Therapy

Currently there is no consensus regarding adjuvant therapy for resectable disease. Adjuvant strategies are primarily used in select patients who have undergone surgery with curative intent who may receive a survival advantage.

Adjuvant radiation therapy

There is no conclusive survival advantage of radiation therapy in the adjuvant setting, although there are single-institution series that demonstrate improved locoregional control. For instance, a retrospective series at the Princess Margaret Hospital by Catton and colleagues[54] of 104 patients with RP soft tissue sarcoma managed by surgery and adjuvant radiation demonstrated an improvement in local recurrence-free survival compared with historical controls; local recurrence-free survival was 28% and 9% at 5 and 10 years, respectively ($P = .0001$). A more recent retrospective review in 2011 using the Surveillance, Epidemiology, and End Results database by Tseng and colleagues[69] of 2308 patients with RPS compared patients who received adjuvant radiation therapy with those who did not demonstrated no significant difference in 5-year overall survival (HR, 0.92; 95% CI, 0.78–1.09) and disease-specific survival (HR, 0.96; 95% CI, 0.78–1.17). In aggregate, these disparate results are likely an artifact of inconsistent dose regimens and mixed cohorts of histologic variants in addition to the inclusion of patients with primary and recurrent disease. Taken together, there is no conclusive treatment benefit of radiation therapy in the adjuvant setting. Furthermore, current guidelines strongly recommend against the administration of radiation therapy in patients with RPS in the adjuvant setting.[35]

Adjuvant chemotherapy and chemoradiation

Neither adjuvant chemotherapy nor chemoradiation are considered standard of care after curative-intent resection of RPS because the optimal timing, sequence, dosing, and choice of therapeutic agents have not been discerned. There may be an advantage for certain histologic subtypes with increased metastatic potential, including high-grade liposarcomas and leiomyosarcomas, to receive multimodality therapy. However, currently, it is strongly recommended that these therapies be explored in the neoadjuvant (preoperative) setting and not the postoperative setting.[70]

An in-depth discussion of the various cytotoxic and biologic therapeutic options currently available for sarcomas patients is beyond the scope of this review. However, to this date, first-line chemotherapy for sarcoma remains single-agent doxorubicin or combination therapy of doxorubicin with ifosfamide, versus gemcitabine-based chemotherapy regimens, primarily extrapolated from studies conducted in patients with unresectable or metastatic disease.[71] Novel agents such as trabectedin (for liposarcoma and leiomyosarcoma), eribulin (liposarcoma), tyrosine kinase inhibitors (pazopanib), MDM2, and CDK4 antagonists (palbociclib for liposarcoma) are also available and used in select cases, and immunotherapy agents are currently under investigation (**Table 2**).[72–78]

Treatment Summary

Surgery remains the cornerstone of treatment for RPS with the goal of surgery being the complete removal of all gross disease, though the extent of resection is still debatable. Per the National Comprehensive Cancer Network treatment guidelines, patients with resectable disease should proceed with upfront surgery.[79] Given the paucity of prospective, randomized control trial data and the fact that the role of multimodality therapy is often generalized from more well-established data seen in the treatment strategies used for truncal and extremity sarcoma, we favor the multidisciplinary management of RPS at high-volume, specialized sarcoma centers to determine the appropriateness of neoadjuvant radiation therapy or neoadjuvant chemotherapy and, more importantly, for consideration of a clinical trial on an individual case basis.

Table 2
Novel agents for the treatment of advanced sarcomas

Agent	Histiotype	Mechanism of Action
Trabectedin	Myxoid/round cell liposarcoma	Blocks DNA binding of transcription factor FUS-CHOP
Eribulin	Dedifferentiated liposarcoma	Microtubule inhibitor
Pazopanib, sunitinib	All liposarcoma types	Tyrosine kinase inhibitor
RG7112, RG7388	Well-differentiated and dedifferentiated liposarcoma	MDM2 antagonist
Palbociclib, flavopiridol	Well-differentiated and dedifferentiated liposarcoma	CDK4 antagonist
Nelfinavir	Well-differentiated and dedifferentiated liposarcoma	SREBP-1 inhibitor
Panobinostat	All liposarcoma types	Histone deacetylase inhibitor

Data from Refs.[72–78,95]

Recurrence

The 5-year recurrence for intra-abdominal and RPS in aggregate is approximately 50%, although as discussed elsewhere in this article, the natural history, recurrence patterns, and rates of recurrence differ among the various histiotypes (**Fig. 3**).[35] Tumor features, such as histiotype, grade, completeness of resection, tumor rupture, and the use of multimodality therapy, all impact disease recurrence.

Locally recurrent RPS represents a clinical management challenge given its high probability of re-recurrence, despite surgical intervention. It has been well-established that the ability to achieve a complete resection decreases with each operation with R0 resection rates of 57%, 33%, and 14% for the first, second, and third recurrences, respectively.[25] The role of re-resection in patients with recurrent disease remains controversial, although nomograms are available to help guide clinicians in decision-making in the context of histiotype-specific disease-free survival and overall survival estimates.

Surveillance

Long-term follow-up is necessary for patients with RPS, with sarcoma surgeons recommending life-long surveillance after curative-intent resection, as recurrence is often late. There are no randomized clinical trials evaluating surveillance strategies for patients with RPS. The National Comprehensive Cancer Network guidelines recommend a physical examination with cross-sectional imaging of the abdomen and pelvis with contrast every 3 to 6 months for 2 to 3 years, then every 6 months for the next 2 years, then annually for patients with R0 and R1 resections.[79] In the future, postoperative surveillance should be adapted to the specific RPS histiotype given the differences in

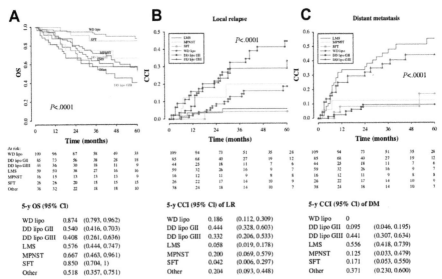

Fig. 3. (A–C) Survival, local recurrence, and distant metastasis based on RPS histiotype. DD, dedifferentiated; DM, diabetes mellitus; Lipo, liposarcoma; LMS, leiomyosarcoma; LR, local relapse; MPNST, malignant peripheral nerve sheath tumor; OS, overall survival; SFT, solitary fibrous tumor; WD, well-differentiated. (*From* Gronchi A, Miceli R, Allard MA, et al. Personalizing the approach to retroperitoneal soft tissue sarcoma: histology-specific patterns. of failure and postrelapse outcome after primary extended resection. *Ann Surg Oncol.* 2015;22(5):1447-1454; with permission.)

underlying tumor biology and disease progression. There is a concerted effort to pursue more nuanced, histology-driven approaches to surveillance, particularly for the more common subtypes, such that more indolent tumors may only require a history and physical examination and cross-sectional imaging of the abdomen and pelvis every 6 months for 3 years followed by annual clinical assessment. In contrast, more aggressive histologic subtypes may require cross-sectional imaging of the chest, abdomen, and pelvis every 3 to 4 months for 2 years, broadened to every 6 months for the next 3 years, and then annually.[80]

DESMOID TUMORS

Desmoid tumors (ie, fibromatosis) are locally aggressive soft tissue tumors without metastatic potential, comprising less than 3% of all soft tissue malignancies.[81] These rare, monoclonal fibroblasts are most often seen invading the soft tissues of the trunk, abdominal wall, and within the abdomen (mesentery). Intra-abdominal desmoids most often arise sporadically in adults 30 to 40 years of age and are with associated with mutation in the *CTNNB1* gene.[82,83] In contrast, 10% of desmoid tumors are associated with a known clinical syndrome, namely, familial adenomatous polyposis or Gardner syndrome, and carry a mutation in the *APC* gene.[84]

Desmoid tumors generally have an indolent course, although there are reported cases of rapid progression.[85] On cross-sectional imaging, desmoid tumors seem to be heterogeneous and are primarily solid. These tumors do not have specific characteristic findings that consistently distinguish them from malignant neoplasms; thus, a tissue diagnosis is necessary. Accurate diagnosis depends on morphologic, immunohistochemistry findings, and molecular genetics. This can be via a core biopsy and confirmed by a pathologist specializing in soft tissue tumors. Notably, these tumors do not need to be staged given their limited capacity for metastasis.

Efforts have been made in recent years to standardize the management of desmoid tumors with emerging data supporting the preference for initial observation (ie, active surveillance) over medical or surgical intervention for desmoid tumors at any location. With this strategy, patients receive cross-sectional imaging within 1 to 2 months of diagnosis, then every 3 to 6 months. Because desmoid tumors have high rates of recurrence ($\leq$50%) after surgical resection, which can be associated with considerable morbidity and have a spontaneous regression rate of 30%, initial observation is recommended.[86,87] For stable, asymptomatic tumors, initial observation is favored over surgery because there was no difference in disease progression for patients undergoing surgery or for patients who received conservative management.[88] Similarly, when comparing patients who were managed by initial observation to medical therapy (antihormonal therapy, nonsteroidal anti-inflammatory drugs, or chemotherapy), there was no significant difference in control of the disease.[89]

Surgery or medical therapy should be reserved for those patients who have failed active surveillance, are symptomatic (there is evidence of bowel obstruction or fistulization of tumor to bowel), or if there is concern that further growth would encroach on critical structures (eg, the root of the mesentery vasculature).[79,90] In patients where it is unlikely to obtain a margin negative resection owing to the infiltration of local structures, significant functional limitation, or an unplanned R1 resection, surveillance is preferred over re-resection or adjuvant radiation therapy. In the postoperative setting, radiation therapy is not recommended, given that there is no conclusive advantage.[91,92] Patients with disease unamenable to surgery may benefit from consultation with a sarcoma medical oncologist or radiation oncologist.[93] To determine the applicability and safety of an initial observation strategy, the initiation of medical therapy, or the consideration for resection, the international collaborative of the Desmoid Tumor Working Group recommends coordinated management with a multidisciplinary team of sarcoma clinicians at the time of diagnosis.[79,90,94]

SUMMARY

The heterogeneous nature of RPS poses unique management challenges with the cornerstone of treatment of being surgical resection. A concerted effort to improve the chances of a complete oncological resection at the time of initial diagnosis is critical in the treatment of patients with RPS and should involve a multidisciplinary team of sarcoma specialists to determine the role and sequence of surgery and multimodality therapy. Although there is a paucity of prospective, randomized controlled data, there is an increasing trend for the use of neoadjuvant radiation therapy in select histiotypes, underscoring the importance of referral to a sarcoma center. Neoadjuvant chemotherapy may have a role in select patients with chemosensitive and high-risk RPS histiotypes. With the improved understanding of tumor biology for distinct RPS histiotypes, there is an increasing role for histology-guided treatment and surveillance strategies. Continued international collaboration is crucial in determining the optimal approach for this rare and multifaceted disease process.

DISCLOSURE

The authors do not have commercial or financial conflicts of interest and no additional funding sources.

REFERENCES

1. Levy AD, Rimola J, Mehrotra AK, et al. From the archives of the AFIP: benign fibrous tumors and tumorlike lesions of the mesentery: radiologic-pathologic correlation. Radiographics 2006;26(1):245–64.
2. Mukut D, Ghalige HS, Santhosh R, et al. Mesenteric fibromatosis (desmoid tumour) - a rare case report. J Clin Diagn Res 2014;8(11):ND01–2.
3. Bala A, Coderre SP, Johnson DR, et al. Treatment of sclerosing mesenteritis with corticosteroids and azathioprine. Can J Gastroenterol 2001;15(8):533–5.
4. Tonelli F, Ficari F, Valanzano R, et al. Treatment of desmoids and mesenteric fibromatosis in familial adenomatous polyposis with raloxifene. Tumori 2003;89(4):391–6.
5. Siegel RL, Miller KD, Jemal A. Cancer statistics, 2015. CA Cancer J Clin 2015;65(1):5–29.
6. Brennan MF, Antonescu CR, Maki RG. Management of soft tissue sarcoma. New York: Springer; 2012.
7. Renne SL, Iwenofu OH. Pathology of retroperitoneal sarcomas: a brief review. J Surg Oncol 2018;117(1):12–24.
8. Olimpiadi Y, Song S, Hu JS, et al. Contemporary management of retroperitoneal soft tissue sarcomas. Curr Oncol Rep 2015;17(8):39.
9. Manoso MW, Frassica DA, Deune EG, et al. Outcomes of re-excision after unplanned excisions of soft-tissue sarcomas. J Surg Oncol 2005;91(3):153–8.
10. Birkmeyer JD, Siewers AE, Finlayson EV, et al. Hospital volume and surgical mortality in the United States. N Engl J Med 2002;346(15):1128–37.
11. Bonvalot S, Gaignard E, Stoeckle E, et al. Survival impact of surgical management in reference centers for retroperitoneal sarcoma: a nationwide study of FSG-GETO and NETSARC. J Clin Oncol 2018;36(15_suppl):11568.

12. Brennan MF, Antonescu CR, Moraco N, et al. Lessons learned from the study of 10,000 patients with soft tissue sarcoma. Ann Surg 2014;260(3):416–21 [discussion: 421–12].
13. American Cancer Society. Cancer Facts & Figures 2019. Atlanta (GA): American Cancer Society; 2019.
14. Amankwah EK, Conley AP, Reed DR. Epidemiology and therapies for metastatic sarcoma. Clin Epidemiol 2013;5:147–62.
15. Qualman SJ, Coffin CM, Newton WA, et al. Intergroup Rhabdomyosarcoma Study: update for pathologists. Pediatr Dev Pathol 1998;1(6):550–61.
16. Italiano A, Di Mauro I, Rapp J, et al. Clinical effect of molecular methods in sarcoma diagnosis (GENSARC): a prospective, multicentre, observational study. Lancet Oncol 2016;17(4):532–8.
17. Gronchi A, Casali PG, Fiore M, et al. Retroperitoneal soft tissue sarcomas: patterns of recurrence in 167 patients treated at a single institution. Cancer 2004; 100(11):2448–55.
18. Gronchi A, Miceli R, Allard MA, et al. Personalizing the approach to retroperitoneal soft tissue sarcoma: histology-specific patterns of failure and postrelapse outcome after primary extended resection. Ann Surg Oncol 2015;22(5):1447–54.
19. Tan MC, Brennan MF, Kuk D, et al. Histology-based Classification Predicts Pattern of Recurrence and Improves Risk Stratification in Primary Retroperitoneal Sarcoma. Ann Surg 2016;263(3):593–600.
20. Conyers R, Young S, Thomas DM. Liposarcoma: molecular genetics and therapeutics. Sarcoma 2011;2011:483154.
21. Linehan DC, Lewis JJ, Leung D, et al. Influence of biologic factors and anatomic site in completely resected liposarcoma. J Clin Oncol 2000;18(8):1637–43.
22. Gronchi A, Strauss DC, Miceli R, et al. Variability in patterns of recurrence after resection of primary retroperitoneal sarcoma (RPS): a report on 1007 patients from the Multi-institutional Collaborative RPS Working Group. Ann Surg 2016; 263(5):1002–9.
23. Thway K. Well-differentiated liposarcoma and dedifferentiated liposarcoma: an updated review. Semin Diagn Pathol 2019;36(2):112–21.
24. Stoeckle E, Coindre JM, Bonvalot S, et al. Prognostic factors in retroperitoneal sarcoma: a multivariate analysis of a series of 165 patients of the French Cancer Center Federation Sarcoma Group. Cancer 2001;92(2):359–68.
25. Lewis JJ, Leung D, Woodruff JM, et al. Retroperitoneal soft-tissue sarcoma: analysis of 500 patients treated and followed at a single institution. Ann Surg 1998; 228(3):355–65.
26. Billingsley KG, Burt ME, Jara E, et al. Pulmonary metastases from soft tissue sarcoma: analysis of patterns of diseases and postmetastasis survival. Ann Surg 1999;229(5):602–10 [discussion: 610–2].
27. Fu J, Song F, Cheng A. PET/CT imaging manifestations of different pathological subtypes of liposarcoma. Zhejiang Da Xue Xue Bao Yi Xue Ban 2019;48(2): 193–9 [in Chinese].
28. Berger-Richardson D, Swallow CJ. Needle tract seeding after percutaneous biopsy of sarcoma: risk/benefit considerations. Cancer 2017;123(4):560–7.
29. Singer E, Yau S, Reitz L, et al. Tumor seeding from a percutaneous renal mass biopsy. Urol Case Rep 2019;23:32–3.
30. Gronchi A, Miceli R, Shurell E, et al. Outcome prediction in primary resected retroperitoneal soft tissue sarcoma: histology-specific overall survival and disease-free survival nomograms built on major sarcoma center data sets. J Clin Oncol 2013;31(13):1649–55.

31. Forest D. Sarculator. Mobile Application.
32. Dalal KM, Kattan MW, Antonescu CR, et al. Subtype specific prognostic nomogram for patients with primary liposarcoma of the retroperitoneum, extremity, or trunk. Ann Surg 2006;244(3):381–91.
33. Kattan MW, Leung DH, Brennan MF. Postoperative nomogram for 12-year sarcoma-specific death. J Clin Oncol 2002;20(3):791–6.
34. Kattan MW, Heller G, Brennan MF. A competing-risks nomogram for sarcoma-specific death following local recurrence. Stat Med 2003;22(22):3515–25.
35. Management of recurrent retroperitoneal sarcoma (RPS) in the adult: a consensus approach from the Trans-Atlantic RPS Working Group. Ann Surg Oncol 2016;23(11):3531–40.
36. Raut CP, Callegaro D, Miceli R, et al. Predicting survival in patients undergoing resection for locally recurrent retroperitoneal sarcoma: a study and novel Nomogram from TARPSWG. Clin Cancer Res 2019;25(8):2664–71.
37. Blay JY, Honore C, Stoeckle E, et al. Surgery in reference centers improves survival of sarcoma patients: a nationwide study. Ann Oncol 2019;30(7):1143–53.
38. Keung EZ, Chiang YJ, Cormier JN, et al. Treatment at low-volume hospitals is associated with reduced short-term and long-term outcomes for patients with retroperitoneal sarcoma. Cancer 2018;124(23):4495–503.
39. Jaques DP, Coit DG, Hajdu SI, et al. Management of primary and recurrent soft-tissue sarcoma of the retroperitoneum. Ann Surg 1990;212(1):51–9.
40. Bonvalot S, Rivoire M, Castaing M, et al. Primary retroperitoneal sarcomas: a multivariate analysis of surgical factors associated with local control. J Clin Oncol 2009;27(1):31–7.
41. Gronchi A, Lo Vullo S, Fiore M, et al. Aggressive surgical policies in a retrospectively reviewed single-institution case series of retroperitoneal soft tissue sarcoma patients. J Clin Oncol 2009;27(1):24–30.
42. Gronchi A, Miceli R, Colombo C, et al. Frontline extended surgery is associated with improved survival in retroperitoneal low- to intermediate-grade soft tissue sarcomas. Ann Oncol 2012;23(4):1067–73.
43. Raut CP, Swallow CJ. Are radical compartmental resections for retroperitoneal sarcomas justified? Ann Surg Oncol 2010;17(6):1481–4.
44. Kilkenny JW 3rd, Bland KI, Copeland EM 3rd. Retroperitoneal sarcoma: the University of Florida experience. J Am Coll Surg 1996;182(4):329–39.
45. Schwarzbach MH, Hormann Y, Hinz U, et al. Clinical results of surgery for retroperitoneal sarcoma with major blood vessel involvement. J Vasc Surg 2006;44(1):46–55.
46. Poultsides GA, Tran TB, Zambrano E, et al. Sarcoma resection with and without vascular reconstruction: a matched case-control study. Ann Surg 2015;262(4):632–40.
47. Ferraris M, Callegaro D, Barretta F, et al. Outcome of iliocaval resection and reconstruction for retroperitoneal sarcoma. J Vasc Surg Venous Lymphat Disord 2019;7(4):547–56.
48. Bonvalot S, Miceli R, Berselli M, et al. Aggressive surgery in retroperitoneal soft tissue sarcoma carried out at high-volume centers is safe and is associated with improved local control. Ann Surg Oncol 2010;17(6):1507–14.
49. Tzanis D, Bouhadiba T, Gaignard E, et al. Major vascular resections in retroperitoneal sarcoma. J Surg Oncol 2018;117(1):42–7.
50. Stojadinovic A, Leung DH, Hoos A, et al. Analysis of the prognostic significance of microscopic margins in 2,084 localized primary adult soft tissue sarcomas. Ann Surg 2002;235(3):424–34.

51. Nathenson MJ, Barysauskas CM, Nathenson RA, et al. Surgical resection for recurrent retroperitoneal leiomyosarcoma and liposarcoma. World J Surg Oncol 2018;16(1):203.
52. Gyorki DE, Brennan MF. Management of recurrent retroperitoneal sarcoma. J Surg Oncol 2014;109(1):53–9.
53. Bonvalot S, Levy A, Terrier P, et al. Primary extremity soft tissue sarcomas: does local control impact survival? Ann Surg Oncol 2017;24(1):194–201.
54. Catton CN, O'Sullivan B, Kotwall C, et al. Outcome and prognosis in retroperitoneal soft tissue sarcoma. Int J Radiat Oncol Biol Phys 1994;29(5):1005–10.
55. Karakousis CP, Gerstenbluth R, Kontzoglou K, et al. Retroperitoneal sarcomas and their management. Arch Surg 1995;130(10):1104–9.
56. Singer S, Corson JM, Demetri GD, et al. Prognostic factors predictive of survival for truncal and retroperitoneal soft-tissue sarcoma. Ann Surg 1995;221(2):185–95.
57. Bremjit PJ, Jones RL, Chai X, et al. A contemporary large single-institution evaluation of resected retroperitoneal sarcoma. Ann Surg Oncol 2014;21(7):2150–8.
58. Chiappa A, Zbar AP, Biffi R, et al. Primary and recurrent retroperitoneal sarcoma: factors affecting survival and long-term outcome. Hepatogastroenterology 2004;51(59):1304–9.
59. Yeh JJ, Singer S, Brennan MF, et al. Effectiveness of palliative procedures for intra-abdominal sarcomas. Ann Surg Oncol 2005;12(12):1084–9.
60. Roeder F, Krempien R. Intraoperative radiation therapy (IORT) in soft-tissue sarcoma. Radiat Oncol 2017;12(1):20.
61. Sindelar WF, Kinsella TJ, Chen PW, et al. Intraoperative radiotherapy in retroperitoneal sarcomas. Final results of a prospective, randomized, clinical trial. Arch Surg 1993;128(4):402–10.
62. Petersen IA, Haddock MG, Donohue JH, et al. Use of intraoperative electron beam radiotherapy in the management of retroperitoneal soft tissue sarcomas. Int J Radiat Oncol Biol Phys 2002;52(2):469–75.
63. Alektiar KM, Hu K, Anderson L, et al. High-dose-rate intraoperative radiation therapy (HDR-IORT) for retroperitoneal sarcomas. Int J Radiat Oncol Biol Phys 2000;47(1):157–63.
64. Roeder F, Ulrich A, Habl G, et al. Clinical phase I/II trial to investigate preoperative dose-escalated intensity-modulated radiation therapy (IMRT) and intraoperative radiation therapy (IORT) in patients with retroperitoneal soft tissue sarcoma: interim analysis. BMC Cancer 2014;14:617.
65. Raut CP, Pisters PW. Retroperitoneal sarcomas: combined-modality treatment approaches. J Surg Oncol 2006;94(1):81–7.
66. Pawlik TM, Pisters PW, Mikula L, et al. Long-term results of two prospective trials of preoperative external beam radiotherapy for localized intermediate- or high-grade retroperitoneal soft tissue sarcoma. Ann Surg Oncol 2006;13(4):508–17.
67. Jones RL, Fisher C, Al-Muderis O, et al. Differential sensitivity of liposarcoma subtypes to chemotherapy. Eur J Cancer 2005;41(18):2853–60.
68. Miura JT, Charlson J, Gamblin TC, et al. Impact of chemotherapy on survival in surgically resected retroperitoneal sarcoma. Eur J Surg Oncol 2015;41(10):1386–92.
69. Tseng WH, Martinez SR, Do L, et al. Lack of survival benefit following adjuvant radiation in patients with retroperitoneal sarcoma: a SEER analysis. J Surg Res 2011;168(2):e173–80.
70. Almond LM, Gronchi A, Strauss D, et al. Neoadjuvant and adjuvant strategies in retroperitoneal sarcoma. Eur J Surg Oncol 2018;44(5):571–9.

71. Gronchi A, De Paoli A, Dani C, et al. Preoperative chemo-radiation therapy for localised retroperitoneal sarcoma: a phase I-II study from the Italian Sarcoma Group. Eur J Cancer 2014;50(4):784–92.

72. In GK, Hu JS, Tseng WW. Treatment of advanced, metastatic soft tissue sarcoma: latest evidence and clinical considerations. Ther Adv Med Oncol 2017;9(8): 533–50.

73. van der Graaf WT, Blay JY, Chawla SP, et al. Pazopanib for metastatic soft-tissue sarcoma (PALETTE): a randomised, double-blind, placebo-controlled phase 3 trial. Lancet 2012;379(9829):1879–86.

74. Demetri GD, von Mehren M, Jones RL, et al. Efficacy and safety of trabectedin or dacarbazine for metastatic liposarcoma or leiomyosarcoma after failure of conventional chemotherapy: results of a phase III randomized multicenter clinical trial. J Clin Oncol 2016;34(8):786–93.

75. Schoffski P, Chawla S, Maki RG, et al. Eribulin versus dacarbazine in previously treated patients with advanced liposarcoma or leiomyosarcoma: a randomised, open-label, multicentre, phase 3 trial. Lancet 2016;387(10028):1629–37.

76. Dickson MA, Schwartz GK, Keohan ML, et al. Progression-free survival among patients with well-differentiated or dedifferentiated liposarcoma treated with CDK4 inhibitor palbociclib: a phase 2 clinical trial. JAMA Oncol 2016;2(7): 937–40.

77. Tawbi HA, Burgess M, Bolejack V, et al. Pembrolizumab in advanced soft-tissue sarcoma and bone sarcoma (SARC028): a multicentre, two-cohort, single-arm, open-label, phase 2 trial. Lancet Oncol 2017;18(11):1493–501.

78. Tseng WW, Demicco EG, Lazar AJ, et al. Lymphocyte composition and distribution in inflammatory, well-differentiated retroperitoneal liposarcoma: clues to a potential adaptive immune response and therapeutic implications. Am J Surg Pathol 2012;36(6):941–4.

79. von Mehren M, Randall RL, Benjamin RS, et al. Soft tissue sarcoma, version 2.2018, NCCN Clinical Practice Guidelines in Oncology. J Natl Compr Canc Netw 2018;16(5):536–63.

80. Zaidi MY, Canter R, Cardona K. Post-operative surveillance in retroperitoneal soft tissue sarcoma: the importance of tumor histology in guiding strategy. J Surg Oncol 2018;117(1):99–104.

81. Reitamo JJ, Hayry P, Nykyri E, et al. The desmoid tumor. I. Incidence, sex-, age- and anatomical distribution in the Finnish population. Am J Clin Pathol 1982; 77(6):665–73.

82. Kasper B, Strobel P, Hohenberger P. Desmoid tumors: clinical features and treatment options for advanced disease. Oncologist 2011;16(5):682–93.

83. Giarola M, Wells D, Mondini P, et al. Mutations of adenomatous polyposis coli (APC) gene are uncommon in sporadic desmoid tumours. Br J Cancer 1998; 78(5):582–7.

84. Nieuwenhuis MH, Lefevre JH, Bulow S, et al. Family history, surgery, and APC mutation are risk factors for desmoid tumors in familial adenomatous polyposis: an international cohort study. Dis Colon Rectum 2011;54(10):1229–34.

85. Hayashi K, Takamura M, Yokoyama H, et al. A Mesenteric Desmoid Tumor with Rapid Progression. Intern Med 2017;56(5):505–8.

86. Bonvalot S, Ternes N, Fiore M, et al. Spontaneous regression of primary abdominal wall desmoid tumors: more common than previously thought. Ann Surg Oncol 2013;20(13):4096–102.

87. Gronchi A, Casali PG, Mariani L, et al. Quality of surgery and outcome in extra-abdominal aggressive fibromatosis: a series of patients surgically treated at a single institution. J Clin Oncol 2003;21(7):1390-7.

88. Penel N, Le Cesne A, Bonvalot S, et al. Surgical versus non-surgical approach in primary desmoid-type fibromatosis patients: a nationwide prospective cohort from the French Sarcoma Group. Eur J Cancer 2017;83:125-31.

89. Fiore M, Rimareix F, Mariani L, et al. Desmoid-type fibromatosis: a front-line conservative approach to select patients for surgical treatment. Ann Surg Oncol 2009;16(9):2587-93.

90. Kasper B, Baumgarten C, Garcia J, et al. An update on the management of sporadic desmoid-type fibromatosis: a European Consensus Initiative between Sarcoma PAtients EuroNet (SPAEN) and European Organization for Research and Treatment of Cancer (EORTC)/Soft Tissue and Bone Sarcoma Group (STBSG). Ann Oncol 2017;28(10):2399-408.

91. Wong SL. Diagnosis and management of desmoid tumors and fibrosarcoma. J Surg Oncol 2008;97(6):554-8.

92. Spear MA, Jennings LC, Mankin HJ, et al. Individualizing management of aggressive fibromatoses. Int J Radiat Oncol Biol Phys 1998;40(3):637-45.

93. Acker JC, Bossen EH, Halperin EC. The management of desmoid tumors. Int J Radiat Oncol Biol Phys 1993;26(5):851-8.

94. Bertagnolli MM, Morgan JA, Fletcher CD, et al. Multimodality treatment of mesenteric desmoid tumours. Eur J Cancer 2008;44(16):2404-10.

95. Matthyssens LE, Creytens D, Ceelen WP. Retroperitoneal liposarcoma: current insights in diagnosis and treatment. Front Surg 2015;2:4.

Soft Tissue Tumors of the Extremity

Christina L. Roland, MD, MS

KEYWORDS

- Soft tissue mass • Sarcoma • Lipoma • Surgery • Radiation therapy
- Chemotherapy

KEY POINTS

- Soft tissue masses that are large, fixed, or recently noticed or changing in size should prompt further investigation with preoperative imaging. MRI is the gold standard for soft tissue tumor evaluation.
- Pretreatment pathologic assessment with percutaneous core needle biopsy is critical to optimal treatment of soft tissue sarcoma.
- Multidisciplinary management of extremity and truncal soft tissue sarcoma includes a combination of margin-negative surgical resection, external beam-radiation therapy and systemic chemotherapy.
- For patients diagnosed with localized sarcoma, margin-negative surgical resection is the cornerstone of treatment. This includes resection of the biopsy site, with the goal to remove the tumor with approximately 1 to 2 cm of surrounding normal tissue.
- Current National Comprehensive Cancer Network guidelines recommend combination of wide resection + radiation therapy in patients with intermediate or high-grade sarcomas of any size (American Joint Committee on Cancer stage II, IIIA or IIIB).

INTRODUCTION

Soft tissue tumors of the extremity encompass a wide range of pathology, from benign lipomas and peripheral nerve sheath tumors to high-grade soft tissue sarcoma (STS). Although the vast majority of soft tissue extremity masses are benign, in 2019, approximately 13,000 people in the United States were diagnosed with STS, of which approximately 60% are located on the extremity and trunk.[1] Extremity STS tends to carry a better prognosis than tumors in the retroperitoneum or pelvis, which is reflected in updates to the eighth edition of the American Joint Commission on Cancer (AJCC) staging system.[2] Over the past 30 years, improvements in multimodality therapy and limb-sparing surgery have resulted in significant improvements in quality-of life and oncologic outcomes for patients with STS. However, preoperative diagnosis (usually via percutaneous biopsy) is essential as a multimodal approach with margin-negative

Department of Surgical Oncology, The University of Texas MD Anderson Cancer Center, 1400 Pressler Street, Unit 1484, Houston, TX 77030, USA
E-mail address: clroland@mdanderson.org

Surg Clin N Am 100 (2020) 669–680
https://doi.org/10.1016/j.suc.2020.02.015

surgical resection, radiation therapy, and systemic chemotherapy are critical for optimal outcomes, with local control rates exceeding 90% and 5-year survival >70% for patients with localized disease treated with multimodality therapy. Unfortunately, for those patients who develop metastatic disease, median survival is approximately 14 months,[3] highlighting the need for improved systemic therapy and optimal treatment at the time of diagnosis.

WORKUP OF SOFT TISSUE TUMORS
Imaging

Although most soft tissue tumors are benign, inaccurate preoperative assessment with unplanned resection of STS can result in poor oncologic outcomes.[4] On the contrary, routine imaging of all soft tissue masses is time-consuming and not cost-effective. Masses that are small (<2 cm), mobile, and have not changed in size over years are most likely benign, whereas masses that are large (>2 cm), fixed, or recently noticed or changing in size should prompt further investigation with imaging (**Fig. 1**).[5]

The main objective with initial imaging is to define the lesion and evaluate for concerning features, including size, location (subcutaneous or below the fascia) relation to adjacent structures, and homogeneity. To maintain normal tissue architecture, imaging should occur *before* any tumor manipulation, including biopsy or surgical excision, as complications such as hematoma or seroma make interpretation of subsequent imaging difficult.

Ultrasound is a good initial imaging modality for soft tissue tumors. Tumor size, location within the extremity/trunk (subcutaneous or subfascial), tumor heterogeneity, and ill-defined margins are features that are concerning for malignancy and require further workup.[6]

MRI is the gold standard for soft tissue tumor evaluation. Marking of the palpable lesion aids in optimizing the MRI coil and sequences. A multiphase MRI with contrast allows optimal evaluation (**Fig. 2**). T1-weighted images are useful for evaluation of lipomatous lesions, as the presence of lipid signal on a T1-weighted image that

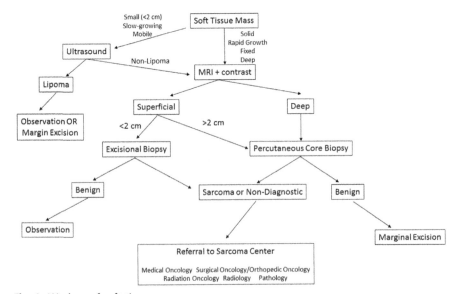

Fig. 1. Workup of soft tissue mass.

A   **B**

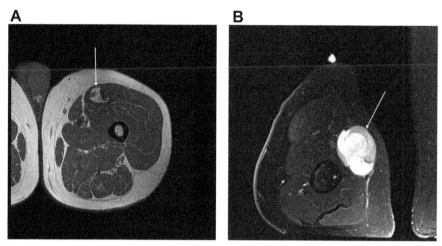

Fig. 2. MRI characteristics of benign versus malignant soft tissue tumors of the extremity. (*A*) T1 fat-suppressed image (*arrow*) of intramuscular lipoma with persistent lipid signal on fat-suppressed images. (*B*) High-grade STS (*arrow*) with characteristic hyperintense T2 signal.

suppresses with a fat-suppressed pulse is characteristic of high-grade liposarcoma.[5,7] Many soft tissue masses are hyperintense relative to skeletal muscle on T2-weighted sequences, but signal heterogeneity is suggestive of malignancy. Advanced MRI techniques, such as diffusion-weighted imaging and dynamic contrast enhancement, can aid in further characterization of concerning lesions.

Biopsy

Accurate, pretreatment pathologic assessment is critical to optimal treatment of STS. With few exceptions, nearly all extremity and trunk soft tissue masses that require surgical excision should have biopsies performed before excision (see **Fig. 1**). Image-guided percutaneous biopsy is the preferred method for tissue acquisition, as it is associated the decreased patient morbidity and low cost and has been shown to be equivalent to open biopsy in terms of diagnostic accuracy.[8,9] Once the biopsy has been planned, the goal is to minimize tumor contamination between the suspected malignancy and the surrounding, uninvolved tissues. Communication between the surgeon and the radiologist is critical for biopsy planning. Biopsy needle insertion site should be placed in the area that will be included in the future surgical specimen so that the tract can be incorporated in the definitive resection and should not traverse uninvolved muscular compartments.

Tumors either not accessible by core needle biopsy or those that have been sampled but yielded inconclusive results may require an open approach, but this should be the exception and not the rule. Incision for an open biopsy should be placed along the long axis of the extremity, to facilitate resection of the biopsy site en bloc at the time of definitive surgical treatment. Skin flaps or rotational flaps should be avoided to minimize contamination and meticulous hemostasis is crucial for preventing post biopsy hematoma.

HISTOPATHOLOGY

Once the diagnosis of STS has been made, accurate histopathologic classification is imperative to treatment planning. There are more than 70 subtypes of STS (based on the cell of origin), all of which have different local and distant recurrence risks and oncologic outcomes (**Table 1**). The diagnosis of STS using the World Health Organization classification has evolved significantly over the past 15 years, largely due to significant progress in diagnostic markers and genetic insights.[10] The most common histologic subtypes in the extremity and trunk include undifferentiated pleomorphic sarcoma (formerly malignant fibrous histiocytoma), liposarcoma, leiomyosarcoma, synovial sarcoma, and malignant nerve sheath tumors. Tumor behavior varies significantly among histologic types: for example, lymph node metastases are more common in epithelioid sarcoma, rhabdomyosarcoma, clear-cell sarcoma, angiosarcoma, and undifferentiated pleomorphic sarcoma,[11] whereas desmoid tumors are locally aggressive and nonmetastasizing.

STAGING OF SOFT TISSUE SARCOMA

For the first time since development, the AJCC staging system has separate staging systems based on tumor site (**Table 2**). Although emerging data suggests that histologic subtype is important for oncologic outcomes, the current AJCC staging system does not differentiate treatment based on subtype, only tumor grade.[2] The grading of STSs is most commonly performed according to the Fereacion Nationale des Centers de Lutte Contre le Cancer (FNCLCC) system, which uses a combination of differentiation, mitotic count, and necrosis to determine tumor grade. Under the AJCC system, extremity and trunk STS are staged using tumor size (T), lymph node involvement (N), metastasis (M), and Grade (G), although tumor grade remains the most important variable in determining outcomes (see **Table 2**).

Complete staging for an STS includes imaging of the primary tumor and evaluation for metastatic disease. Multiphase MRI is the imaging modality of choice for evaluation of extremity and trunk STS. MRI defines tumor size, muscular involvement, and relationship to neurovascular structures. For most sarcomas, the most common locations for metastases are pulmonary and computed tomography (CT) of the chest is the most common imaging modality to exclude metastatic disease. Higher risk of lung metastases are observed in tumors >5 cm and certain histologies, such as with Ewing sarcoma, malignant peripheral nerve sheath tumor, extraskeletal chondrosarcoma and pleomorphic sarcoma (see **Table 1**).

MULTIMODALITY TREATMENT

Multidisciplinary management of extremity and truncal STS includes a combination of margin-negative surgical resection, external beam radiation therapy, and systemic chemotherapy. For localized disease, this almost always includes surgical resection. Using a combined approach, local control rates are generally reported in the range of 80% to 90% (**Table 3**).[12]

Surgery

For patients diagnosed with localized sarcoma, margin-negative surgical resection is the cornerstone of treatment. This includes resection of the biopsy site, with the goal to remove the tumor with approximately 1 to 2 cm of surrounding normal tissue.[13] However, in some anatomic areas (adjacent to critical neurovascular structures), a narrower margin may be necessary to preserve function and is often safe following radiation therapy.[14] STSs are generally surrounded by a zone of compressed reactive tissue that forms a pseudocapsule, but this pseudocapsule should not be used to guide resection (enucleation). Dissection should proceed through grossly normal tissue planes not abutting the tumor. If the tumor is adjacent to or displacing major

Table 1		
Metastatic potential for most common types of extremity and trunk soft tissue sarcoma		
Low	Intermediate	High
Well-differentiated liposarcoma	Inflammatory myofibroblastic tumor	Undifferentiated pleomorphic sarcoma
Dermatofibrosarcoma pertuberans	Hemangio-endothelioma	Leiomyosarcoma
Desmoid fibromatosis	Solitary fibrous tumor	Malignant peripheral nerve sheath tumor
	Hemangio-pericytoma	Dedifferentiated liposarcoma
		Round cell liposarcoma
		Angiosarcoma
		Rhabdomyosarcoma
		Extraskeletal Ewings
		Synovial sarcoma
		Epithelioid

neurovascular structures, these do not need to be resected, but the adventitia or perineurium should be removed. Surgical clips should be placed to delineate the extent of the resection bed for patients likely to require postoperative radiation therapy.

Occasionally, vascular resection and reconstruction are necessary for en bloc resection when vessel encasement is encountered. Although postoperative complications are more common, local control rates are comparable to patients not requiring vascular resection.[15] Resection of major nerves in the extremity should be avoided unless nerve encasement by the tumor is identified. In this case, en bloc resection of the nerve is necessary and can be associated with favorable long-term functional outcomes.[16]

Bony invasion from extremity STS occurs in approximately 5% of patients and is associated with reduced overall survival. When bone invasion is identified on MRI, planned bone resection is required to obtain an adequate surgical margin. In the absence of frank cortical invasion, the periosteum is an adequate surgical margin with combined modality therapy (surgery + radiation therapy).[17]

Radiation Therapy

Historical rates of local recurrence after local excision alone for treatment of STS ranged from approximately 30% to 50%,[18] which prompted the use of radical compartmental excision and amputation as standard primary treatment for localized extremity and trunk STS. However, it was noted that although local recurrence was improved with more aggressive resection, a significant number of patients developed metastatic disease (primarily in the lungs), putting into question the role of these morbid procedures as first-line local treatment. In 1982, the National Cancer Institute (NCI) published a pivotal randomized, clinical trial evaluating amputation versus wide resection + radiation therapy (XRT) for treatment of localized extremity STS.[19] Although limb-sparing resection + radiation was associated with increased local recurrence compared with amputation, there was no difference in overall survival between the groups, which has led to limb-sparing surgery + XRT as the primary treatment modality for localized extremity and trunk sarcoma.

The evidence for combination XRT + wide resection comes from 2 randomized controlled trials (RCTs) and a number of retrospective studies. In an NCI study, patients with high-grade extremity sarcoma were randomized to limb-sparing surgery and chemotherapy ± postoperative XRT. A second cohort of patients with low-grade sarcoma were randomized to limb-sparing surgery ± XRT. In both the high-

Table 2
Eighth American Joint Commission on Cancer staging for extremity and trunk soft tissue sarcomas with associated 5-year overall survival (OS)

Stage	0	5−y OS, %
IA	T1 N0 M0 G1	85.3
IB	T2/3/4 N0 M0 G1	83.0
II	T1 N0 M0 G2/3	79.0
IIIA	T2 N0 M0 G2/3	62.4
IIIB	T3/4 N0 M0 G2/3	50.1
IV – overall	T any N0/1 M1 G any	13.9
IV – N +/M−	T any N1 M0 G any	33.1
IV – M+	T any N0/1 M1 G any	12.4

T1: $\geq$5 cm; T2: greater than 5 and $\leq$10 cm; T3: greater than 10 and $\leq$15 cm; T4: greater than 15 cm; N0: lymph node negative; N1: lymph node positive; M0: no distant metastasis; M1: distant metastasis; G1: low grade; G2: intermediate grade; G3: high grade.

From Fisher SB, Chiang YJ, Feig BW, et al: Comparative Performance of the 7th and 8th Editions of the American Joint Committee on Cancer Staging Systems for Soft Tissue Sarcoma of the Trunk and Extremities. Ann Surg Oncol 25:1126-1132, 2018; with permission.

grade and low-grade groups, treatment with the combination surgery + XRT arms was associated with reduced local recurrence by approximately 25%, which was maintained after long-term follow-up.[20,21] In a second RCT from Memorial Sloan Kettering Cancer Center, patients randomized to limb-sparing surgery + brachytherapy had improved local control compared with those treated with surgery alone.[22] The data from these 2 trials established limb-sparing surgery + XRT as standard of care for the treatment of localized STS. Neither trial demonstrated a difference in overall survival.

XRT can be delivered either in the preoperative or postoperative setting with similar oncologic outcomes but with different side-effect profiles.[23] Preoperative XRT is associated with significantly higher wound complication rates (up to 35%); however, long-term toxicity (edema, fibrosis, joint stiffness) is higher with postoperative XRT, likely due to the larger radiation field and higher XRT dose (64 Gy postoperative vs 50 Gy preoperative). The decision to include XRT in the preoperative versus postoperative setting is institution dependent, based on a variety of factors.

Based on these data, current National Comprehensive Cancer Network (NCCN) guidelines recommend combination of wide resection + XRT in patients with intermediate or high-grade sarcomas of any size (AJCC stage II, IIIA, or IIIB).[24] Surgery alone *can* be considered for patients with small, stage II STS (<5 cm, intermediate or high-grade) resected with wide margins ($\geq$2 cm). Small tumors adjacent to critical

Table 3
Randomized trials demonstrating reduction in local recurrence with adjuvant radiation therapy

	Local Control Rate	
Trial	Surgery, %	Surgery + RT, %
NCI (EBRT): 10-y	70	98.4
MSKCC (BRT): 5-y	66	89.0

Abbreviations: BRT, Brachytherapy; EBRT, external beam radiation therapy; MSKCC, Memorial Sloan Kettering Cancer Center; NCI, National Cancer Institute; RT, radiation therapy.

Data from Refs.[20–22]

structures (ie, neurovascular structures) where wide resection cannot be obtained should be considered for radiation therapy. Unfortunately, a significant number of patients do not receive NCCN guideline recommended therapy.[25] An analysis of the National Cancer Data Bank demonstrated that only 58% of patients with intermediate or high-grade STS >5 cm received NCCN guideline adherent therapy (margin-negative surgery + XRT or amputation) and those who received adherent therapy had better overall survival than those who did not (61% vs 45%, respectively), highlighting the importance of multimodality therapy in high-grade STS. Clinical trials are currently under way to evaluate for short-course preoperative therapy or reduced dose in radio-sensitive sarcomas to reduce short-term and long-term toxicity.

Systemic Therapy

Adjuvant therapy

Despite significant improvements in local control and reduced long-term morbidity with increasing limb salvage, metastasis and death remains a continued issue for patients with STS. Unfortunately, patients with large (>5 cm), high-grade tumors have a distant recurrence of at least 50% at 5 years, highlighting the need for systemic treatments. Although recognized as an unmet clinical need, data regarding the utility of systemic chemotherapy in patients with nonmetastatic STS are controversial and hotly debated. Doxorubicin, dacarbazine, and ifosfamide have consistently demonstrated response rates of approximately 20% as single-agent therapy, with higher rates reported with combination approaches. Response rates vary by histology but these agents remain the backbone for current systemic therapy regimens.[26] As an example, synovial sarcoma is considered a chemosensitive histology, with single-institution data demonstrating improvements in disease-specific survival of up to 20% with combination therapy. Early randomized trials did not differentiate based on sarcoma histology, making it difficult to evaluate the efficacy of systemic chemotherapy in individual STS subtypes. To help clarify the effectiveness of systemic chemotherapy, the Sarcoma Meta-analysis Collaboration (SMAC) in 1998 with an update in 2008, evaluated 18 studies with approximately 1900 patients in a meta-analysis.[27,28] These data demonstrated that the addition of adjuvant chemotherapy was associated with an absolute distant metastatic risk reduction of 9% and 6% improvement in overall survival, favoring systemic chemotherapy. However, the updated meta-analysis did not include 2 large randomized trials by the European Organization for Research and Treatment of Cancer (EORTC) evaluating combination doxorubicin/ifosfamide-containing regimens. Pooled analysis of these 2 trials demonstrated improved recurrence-free survival (hazard ratio 0.74, 95% confidence interval 0.6–0.92) but not overall survival.[29] Current NCCN guidelines give the option for systemic chemotherapy with a category 2B recommendation for patients with stage III disease (>5 cm, intermediate or high-grade tumors), either alone or in combination with radiation therapy as part of a multidisciplinary evaluation at a sarcoma center, given the significant risk of relapse and death.[24]

Neoadjuvant Therapy

Although traditionally administered in the postoperative or adjuvant setting, clinical practice suggests that a significant number of patients treated with systemic chemotherapy are treated in a preoperative or neoadjuvant fashion. Several possible benefits of this scenario include in vivo assessment of tumor response to evaluate efficacy, potential downstaging to facilitate margin-negative resection, and evaluation of biologic behavior of the disease, as patients with rapidly progressive tumors can potentially be spared morbid operations.[30] The only randomized trial evaluating neoadjuvant chemotherapy versus surgery alone was performed by the EORTC in the 2000s.

Unfortunately, long-term follow-up did not reveal any differences in disease-free survival.[31] However, there are several criticisms of this trial that warrant discussion. First, although most patients who developed recurrent disease did so at a distant site (63%), only approximately 50% of patients were treated with radiation therapy and a significant number of patients developed a local recurrence (12%) or a combination of local and distant recurrence (25%), which is significantly higher than expected with current multimodality therapy (local recurrence approximately 5%). In addition, there were 11 different histologies represented between the 2 groups, and current evidence suggests response to chemotherapy is histology-specific. For example, synovial sarcoma and myxoid round cell liposarcoma are associated with improvements in absolute disease-specific survival of up to 20%,[32,33] significantly higher than seen in the SMAC when all histologies are combined. Last, it is important to acknowledge that the doses of chemotherapy in this study were low, particularly for patients treated in the United States, making it difficult to make definitive conclusions from this study.

Based on the observations that response to chemotherapy is histology-specific (ie, not all histologies respond equally or to the same agents), a follow-up multicenter study from Italy, France, Spain, and Poland evaluated histology-tailored neoadjuvant chemotherapy versus standard Adriamycin/ifosfamide × 3 doses, followed by multimodality local therapy with radiation and surgical resection. Interestingly, patients in the standard chemotherapy arm had significantly better disease-free and overall survival than patients treated in the histology-specific arm, adding to the continued controversy surrounding the use of systemic chemotherapy in localized STS. It is clear, however, that patients with large, high-grade tumors remain at significant risk for the development of metastatic disease, highlighting the need for novel agents.

Novel Agents Including Immunotherapy

Recently, as the use of immunotherapy has increased substantially over the past decade, data evaluating the utility of checkpoint blockade in patients with STS have emerged. Two recent clinical trials evaluated anti-PD1 therapy and/or combination anti-PD-1/anti-CTLA-4 in patients with metastatic sarcoma.[34,35] Although a multitude of subtypes of sarcoma were enrolled, both studies demonstrated fairly consistent results. Most patients did not respond to single-agent anti-PD-1 therapy, but there were histology-specific responses, with RECIST (response evaluation in solid tumors) responses of up to 40% in patients with undifferentiated pleomorphic sarcoma up to 20% in dedifferentiated liposarcoma, leading to expansion cohorts in these 2 histologies in both studies. These results are very encouraging and have led to the development of several neoadjuvant clinical trials of checkpoint blockade in patients with surgically resectable disease, alone and in combination with radiation therapy (NCT03307616, NCT03092323, NCT03116529).

Last, in patients with metastatic or unresectable STS, recent Food and Drug Administration approvals of novel agents in specific histologies included approval of trabectedin for liposarcoma and leiomyosarcoma and eribulin for liposarcoma in patients who have failed prior systemic chemotherapy. However, these agents are currently not recommended for first-line therapy in patients with localized disease and should be considered in a multidisciplinary setting.

FOLLOW-UP

As discussed, a significant number of patients will develop recurrent disease within 5 years, highlighting the need for active surveillance. However, little data exists regarding the appropriate timing and effectiveness of surveillance strategies on outcomes. NCCN guidelines recommend history and physical examination with chest imaging and imaging of primary tumor site with MRI with and without contrast every 3 to 6 months for 2 to 3 years and then every 6 months for the next 2 years and then annually. Chest imaging is most commonly performed with a CT chest, although single-institution data would suggest that the addition of CT over chest radiograph adds little clinical benefit in patients with tumors smaller than 5 cm.[36] In addition, patients should be evaluated by occupational therapy and physical therapy for continued rehabilitation needs, as long-term morbidity such as weakness, chemotherapy-induced neuropathy, and lymphedema present after initial evaluation.

MANAGEMENT OF LOCAL RECURRENCE

Local recurrence can occur in up to 20% of patients and is associated with reduced survival.[37] However, whether the local recurrence is causative or just a marker of aggressive biopsy is unknown. An isolated local recurrence should undergo workup similar to a new primary tumor, with consideration of wide surgical resection, plus radiation therapy and consideration of systemic chemotherapy. Treatment for patients who had previous irradiation can be complicated, because reirradiation can be associated with significant long-term toxicity, including wound complications and osteonecrosis. The use of reirradiation in patients who develop a local recurrence can be performed, and early studies evaluating the use of proton reirradiation suggest favorable toxicity profile and warrant further evaluation.[38] Although wide resection with limb-sparing approach remains the mainstay of treatment, amputation should be considered to provide adequate local control if a limb-sparing option is not feasible.

MANAGEMENT OF DISTANT DISEASE

Distant metastases occur in up to 50% of patients with intermediate-grade and high-grade extremity and trunk sarcoma and represent a significant challenge. Once metastases have developed, primary treatment is systemic chemotherapy. In selected patients with low volume of metastatic disease, a long disease-free interval (>12 months), and excellent performance status, selective metastasectomy may potentially lead to improved survival in highly selected patients.[39–41] Newer, less invasive techniques, such as stereotactic body radiation, are under investigation as alternatives to metastatectomy.[42]

SUMMARY

Careful evaluation of patients with soft tissue masses is critical for optimal management of STS. Although most soft tissue masses evaluated are benign, preoperative imaging should be performed before surgical excision, especially for large, deep, fixed masses. Ultrasound is a good screening tool for low-risk lesions, with MRI follow-up for suspicious characteristics. Percutaneous biopsy of non-lipomatous masses is recommended before surgical resection and referral to a sarcoma center should be considered if STS is identified. Multimodality therapy of STS including margin-negative surgery with radiation therapy is associated with favorable local recurrence rates, although distant recurrence remains an issue in up to 50% of patients with high-grade sarcomas.

DISCLOSURE

Dr. Roland receives research funding from Bristol Myers Squibb and is supported by a research grant from The American College of Surgeons.

REFERENCES

1. American Cancer Society: sarcoma: adult soft tissue cancer. 2018. Available at: https://www.cancer.org/cancer/soft-tissue-sarcoma/about/key-statistics.html.
2. Amin MB, American Joint Committee on Cancer. AJCC cancer staging manual. 8th edition. New York: Springer; 2017.
3. Billingsley KG, Burt ME, Jara E, et al. Pulmonary metastases from soft tissue sarcoma: analysis of patterns of diseases and postmetastasis survival. Ann Surg 1999;229:602-10 [discussion: 610-2].
4. Barrientos-Ruiz I, Ortiz-Cruz EJ, Serrano-Montilla J, et al. Are biopsy tracts a concern for seeding and local recurrence in sarcomas? Clin Orthop Relat Res 2017;475:511-8.
5. Smolle MA, Andreou D, Tunn PU, et al. Diagnosis and treatment of soft-tissue sarcomas of the extremities and trunk. EFORT Open Rev 2017;2:421-31.
6. Lakkaraju A, Sinha R, Garikipati R, et al. Ultrasound for initial evaluation and triage of clinically suspicious soft-tissue masses. Clin Radiol 2009;64:615-21.
7. Ahlawat S, Fritz J, Morris CD, et al. Magnetic resonance imaging biomarkers in musculoskeletal soft tissue tumors: Review of conventional features and focus on nonmorphologic imaging. J Magn Reson Imaging 2019;50:11-27.
8. Strauss DC, Qureshi YA, Hayes AJ, et al. The role of core needle biopsy in the diagnosis of suspected soft tissue tumours. J Surg Oncol 2010;102:523-9.
9. Heslin MJ, Lewis JJ, Woodruff JM, et al. Core needle biopsy for diagnosis of extremity soft tissue sarcoma. Ann Surg Oncol 1997;4:425-31.
10. Fletcher CDM, Bridge JA, Hogendoorn PCW, et al. editors. WHO classification of tumors of soft tissue and bone. Lyon (France): IARC; 2013. p. 236-8.
11. Keung EZ, Chiang YJ, Voss RK, et al. Defining the incidence and clinical significance of lymph node metastasis in soft tissue sarcoma. Eur J Surg Oncol 2018; 44:170-7.
12. Elias AD. The clinical management of soft tissue sarcomas. Semin Oncol 1992; 19:19-25.
13. McKee MD, Liu DF, Brooks JJ, et al. The prognostic significance of margin width for extremity and trunk sarcoma. J Surg Oncol 2004;85:68-76.
14. Kim BK, Chen YLE, Kirsch DG, et al. An effective preoperative three-dimensional radiotherapy target volume for extremity soft tissue sarcoma and the effect of margin width on local control. Int J Radiat Oncol Biol Phys 2010;77:843-50.
15. Ghert MA, Davis AM, Griffin AM, et al. The surgical and functional outcome of limb-salvage surgery with vascular reconstruction for soft tissue sarcoma of the extremity. Ann Surg Oncol 2005;12:1102-10.
16. Brooks A, Gold J, Graham D, et al. Resection of the sciatic, peroneal, or tibial nerves: assessment of functional status. Ann Surg Oncol 2002;9:41-7.
17. Lin PP, Pino ED, Normand AN, et al. Periosteal margin in soft-tissue sarcoma. Cancer 2007;109:598-602.
18. Cantin J, McNeer GP, Chu FC, et al. The problem of local recurrence after treatment of soft tissue sarcoma. Ann Surg 1968;168:47-53.
19. Rosenberg SA, Tepper J, Glatstein E, et al. The treatment of soft-tissue sarcomas of the extremities: prospective randomized evaluations of (1) limb-sparing surgery plus radiation therapy compared with amputation and (2) the role of adjuvant chemotherapy. Ann Surg 1982;196:305-15.
20. Beane JD, Yang JC, White D, et al. Efficacy of adjuvant radiation therapy in the treatment of soft tissue sarcoma of the extremity: 20-year follow-up of a randomized prospective trial. Ann Surg Oncol 2014;21:2484-9.

21. Yang JC, Chang AE, Baker AR, et al. Randomized prospective study of the benefit of adjuvant radiation therapy in the treatment of soft tissue sarcomas of the extremity. J Clin Oncol 1998;16:197–203.
22. Pisters PW, Harrison LB, Leung DH, et al. Long-term results of a prospective randomized trial of adjuvant brachytherapy in soft tissue sarcoma. J Clin Oncol 1996;14:859–68.
23. O'Sullivan B, Davis AM, Turcotte R, et al. Preoperative versus postoperative radiotherapy in soft-tissue sarcoma of the limbs: a randomised trial. Lancet 2002;359:2235–41.
24. von Mehren M, Randall RL, Benjamin RS, et al. Soft tissue sarcoma, version 2.2016, NCCN clinical practice guidelines in oncology. J Natl Compr Canc Netw 2016;14:758–86.
25. Voss RK, Chiang YJ, Torres KE, et al. Adherence to National Comprehensive Cancer Network guidelines is associated with improved survival for patients with stage 2A and stages 2B and 3 extremity and superficial trunk soft tissue sarcoma. Ann Surg Oncol 2017;24(11):3271–8.
26. Canter RJ. Chemotherapy: does neoadjuvant or adjuvant therapy improve outcomes? Surg Oncol Clin 2016;25:861–72.
27. Sarcoma Meta-Analysis Collaboration. Adjuvant chemotherapy for localised resectable soft-tissue sarcoma of adults: meta-analysis of individual data. Sarcoma Meta-analysis Collaboration. Lancet 1997;350:1647–54.
28. Pervaiz N, Colterjohn N, Farrokhyar F, et al. A systematic meta-analysis of randomized controlled trials of adjuvant chemotherapy for localized resectable soft-tissue sarcoma. Cancer 2008;113:573–81.
29. Le Cesne A, Ouali M, Leahy MG, et al. Doxorubicin-based adjuvant chemotherapy in soft tissue sarcoma: pooled analysis of two STBSG-EORTC phase III clinical trials. Ann Oncol 2014;25:2425–32.
30. Wasif N, Smith CA, Tamurian RM, et al. Influence of physician specialty on treatment recommendations in the multidisciplinary management of soft tissue sarcoma of the extremities. JAMA Surg 2013;148:632–9.
31. Gortzak E, Azzarelli A, Buesa J, et al. A randomised phase II study on neoadjuvant chemotherapy for 'high-risk' adult soft-tissue sarcoma. Eur J Cancer 2001;37:1096–103.
32. Eilber FC, Eilber FR, Eckardt J, et al. The Impact of Chemotherapy on the Survival of Patients With High-grade Primary Extremity Liposarcoma. Transactions of the ... Meeting of the American Surgical Association CXXII, San Francisco, CA, April 15-17, 2004. 2004. p. 284–95.
33. Eilber FC, Brennan MF, Eilber FR, et al. Chemotherapy is associated with improved survival in adult patients with primary extremity synovial sarcoma. Ann Surg 2007;246:105–13.
34. Tawbi HA, Burgess M, Bolejack V, et al. Pembrolizumab in advanced soft-tissue sarcoma and bone sarcoma (SARC028): a multicentre, two-cohort, single-arm, open-label, phase 2 trial. Lancet Oncol 2017;18(11):1493–501.
35. D'Angelo SP, Mahoney MR, Van Tine BA, et al. Nivolumab with or without ipilimumab treatment for metastatic sarcoma (Alliance A091401): two open-label, non-comparative, randomised, phase 2 trials. Lancet Oncol 2018;19(3):416–26.
36. Fleming JB, Cantor SB, Varma DG, et al. Utility of chest computed tomography for staging in patients with T1 extremity soft tissue sarcomas. Cancer 2001;92:863–8.
37. Billingsley KG, Lewis JJ, Leung DHY, et al. Multifactorial analysis of the survival of patients with distant metastasis arising from primary extremity sarcoma. Cancer 1999;85:389–95.

38. Guttmann DM, Frick MA, Carmona R, et al. A prospective study of proton reirradiation for recurrent and secondary soft tissue sarcoma. Radiother Oncol 2017; 124:271–6.
39. Chudgar NP, Brennan MF, Tan KS, et al. Is repeat pulmonary metastasectomy indicated for soft tissue sarcoma? Ann Thorac Surg 2017;104:1837–45.
40. Ferguson PC, Deheshi BM, Chung P, et al. Soft tissue sarcoma presenting with metastatic disease: outcome with primary surgical resection. Cancer 2011;117: 372–9.
41. Okiror L, Peleki A, Moffat D, et al. Survival following pulmonary metastasectomy for sarcoma. Thorac Cardiovasc Surg 2016;64:146–9.
42. Baumann BC, Nagda SN, Kolker JD, et al. Efficacy and safety of stereotactic body radiation therapy for the treatment of pulmonary metastases from sarcoma: a potential alternative to resection. J Surg Oncol 2016;114:65–9.

Moving?

Make sure your subscription moves with you!

To notify us of your new address, find your **Clinics Account Number** (located on your mailing label above your name), and contact customer service at:

Email: journalscustomerservice-usa@elsevier.com

800-654-2452 (subscribers in the U.S. & Canada)
314-447-8871 (subscribers outside of the U.S. & Canada)

Fax number: 314-447-8029

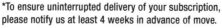

Elsevier Health Sciences Division
Subscription Customer Service
3251 Riverport Lane
Maryland Heights, MO 63043

*To ensure uninterrupted delivery of your subscription, please notify us at least 4 weeks in advance of move.

ELSEVIER

Printed and bound by CPI Group (UK) Ltd, Croydon, CR0 4YY

03/10/2024

01040481-0003